ACCREDITATION AND EVALUATION IN THE EUROPEAN HIGHER EDUCATION AREA

HIGHER EDUCATION DYNAMICS

VOLUME 5

SCOPE OF THE SERIES

Higher Education Dynamics is a bookseries intending to study adaptation processes and their outcomes in higher education at all relevant levels. In addition it wants to examine the way interactions between these levels affect adaptation processes. It aims at applying general social science concepts and theories as well as testing theories in the field of higher education research. It wants to do so in a manner that is of relevance to all those professionally involved in higher education, be it as ministers, policy-makers, politicians, institutional leaders or administrators, higher education researchers, members of the academic staff of universities and colleges, or students. It will include both mature and developing systems of higher education, covering public as well as private institutions.

The titles published in this series are listed at the end of this volume.

ACCREDITATION AND EVALUATION IN THE EUROPEAN HIGHER EDUCATION AREA

Edited by

STEFANIE SCHWARZ

*University of Kassel,
Germany*

and

DON F. WESTERHEIJDEN

*University of Twente,
Enschede, The Netherlands*

KLUWER ACADEMIC PUBLISHERS
DORDRECHT / BOSTON / LONDON

A C.I.P. Catalogue record for this book is available from the Library of Congress.

ISBN 1-4020-2796-6 (HB)
ISBN 1-4020-2797-4 (e-book)

Published by Kluwer Academic Publishers,
P.O. Box 17, 3300 AA Dordrecht, The Netherlands.

Sold and distributed in North, Central and South America
by Kluwer Academic Publishers,
101 Philip Drive, Norwell, MA 02061, U.S.A.

In all other countries, sold and distributed
by Kluwer Academic Publishers,
P.O. Box 322, 3300 AH Dordrecht, The Netherlands.

Printed on acid-free paper

Printed in the Netherlands.

Table of Contents

Preface

The massification of higher education in the second half of the 20th century and the rapid expansion of knowledge set a world-wide challenge to the higher education sector and to its relation with society, which led to a new interest in – and new forms of – quality assurance. Higher education is about teaching and learning for degrees, and about research; these processes are supported by management and administration. Quality assurance concerns the development and improvement of quality of these three areas. The subject of this book is quality assurance of the educational function in higher education in Europe. Within that still very large area we developed a perspective that concentrated on external aspects of quality assurance rather than on quality management that is internal to the institution, because that is where main driving forces for current developments are found. Policy-makers across Europe are faced with the challenge of setting the contextual demands for quality assurance of higher education institutions, balancing the demands of functions (such as economic and social development towards a knowledge society) and constituencies within their countries with demands at European and global levels. 'SOCRATES', 'Bologna' and 'GATS' are the catchwords at these levels. Due to limitations in time and resources, we could not address all of these issues, so we concentrated on accreditation and evaluation activities at the supra-institutional level, i.e. national accreditation and evaluation schemes. Our book gives a first synoptical overview for the European Higher Education Area on these issues in order to analyse commonalities and differences in policy trends.

A study of the 20 European higher education systems represented in this volume shows that the ultimate responsibility of quality assurance for degree programmes is still in the hands of the (nation-)state. This is no surprise and it makes sense, considering the ownership of higher education: All higher education systems in Europe are mainly public (with private sectors of varying but mostly small size). As the main stakeholders in the respective higher education systems, states naturally claimed ownership of both quality and its assurance. However, since the 1980s, states proved more and more willing to loosen control over higher education and especially over quality assurance. Almost all European countries have given up direct quality control. The management of evaluation and accreditation, and the handling of how to implement, watch, manage, change and monitor the quality of higher education degree programmes and institutions shifted from direct state control to (more often than not: quasi-) non-governmental institutions. This was a major change for European higher education. The newly created institutions were called evaluation committees, accreditation councils, accreditation agencies, etc. As the detailed analysis in the country reports in this volume vividly show, accreditation and evaluation institutions often overlap and have blurred boundaries. However, they are divided by one important element of definition (see Schwarz and Westerheijden in this volume): Accreditation institutions are institutions at the supra-institutional level that manage a quality assurance process of higher education institutions, degree types and/or programmes that end in a formal summary judgement that leads to formal approval regarding the respective institution, degree type and/or programme. On the other hand, evaluation procedures do not end in a formal summary judgement and do not lead directly to any type of formal approval. But the boundaries between accreditation and evaluation practices are so blurred that it is almost impossible to draw a line between the two. To put it simply: Accreditation 'borrows' so many methods from its 'older brother' evaluation, that the two sometimes seem so similar that it makes it difficult to say when 'the same is really different' or when 'different is really the same'.

Approval outside accreditation – i.e. direct state approval – was, until the 1990s, the norm for approving degree types in higher education in Europe, which functioned exclusively in a national context. But, as the 20 country reports reveal, the Bologna Process encouraged the introduction of comparable first and second cycles ('Bachelor' and 'Master') in the European Higher Education Area. For many European countries, this constituted a paradigm shift, a new mode of structuring teaching and learning. The greater the change, the more important it is that this reform process is handled with care and is accompanied by strong and stable quality assurance systems. The addition of the explicitly international Bologna perspective in many countries gave a strong impetus to the development of new quality assurance arrangements, especially accreditation schemes. In the parallel restructuring of the degree structure with Bachelor and Master and the setting up of accreditation schemes, we see a great challenge for Europe. Several countries – Germany and the Netherlands are explicit examples in this book – are struggling with the threat of an overload of work hanging over the higher education institutions as well as the accreditation and evaluation institutions. Each of the 20 European countries in this study have their own (his)stories of accreditation in the framework of evaluation activities, showing different ways of dealing with the challenge of setting up a new quality assurance scheme that demonstrates its own way of dealing with the quality of higher education institutions.

How did we go about this project that aimed to map the accreditation and evaluation activities in Europe? It started in January 2002 at the Centre for Research on Higher Education and Work, University of Kassel, in co-operation with stakeholders from higher education research and practice in Germany and throughout Europe. The goal was to investigate the current state and the dynamics of accreditation and evaluation in European countries. Stefanie Schwarz, Centre for Research on Higher Education and Work at the University of Kassel in Germany, and Don Westerheijden, Centre for Higher Education Policy Studies at the University of Twente in the Netherlands, as project coordinators, developed the project. Given the time frame and the available resources, we chose a research design that drew on a network of national and international experts of quality assurance. The design was discussed with an ad hoc working group at a one-day workshop in Frankfurt, during which we debated intensely and constructively about the outline of the country reports. After fine-tuning the outline, we sent it to all the European experts that we had selected as reporters for 21 countries (in the end, experts from 20 countries replied to our requests) in the summer of 2002. Within six months, the first drafts of the country reports were collected and commented, leading to final draft reports by March 2003. From April 10 to 13, 2003, the German Trade Union for Education and Science, together with the Education International and the Hans Böckler Foundation, convened a European Conference on 'Shaping the European Higher Education Area' where we presented our first empirical results and discussed them with the country experts and the other conference participants. After the conference, the experts were given five months to finalise their reports and again we were in close contact with the expert group. The result is the present volume which, we hope, sheds some light on the jungle of quality assurance in the European Higher Education Area.

We express our gratitude to the German Federal Ministry of Education and Research, the Hans Böckler Foundation, and the German Trade Union for Education and Science for supporting the study.

We would like to thank all the contributors for their co-operation. They provided country reports in which the reader will find many more vivid and highly useful ideas than we could use for our synopsis. Moreover, they greatly supported the project with their expertise, their enthusiasm, their patience, and also their sense of humour. They truly helped to make this work not only fruitful and interesting, but also very enjoyable.

We extend our thanks to the ad hoc working group that met in Frankfurt for constructive feedback at the beginning of the project. As their names do not appear in the book, we would like to mention them here: Thank you Karin Fischer-Bluhm (Verbund Norddeutscher Universitäten, Hamburg), Romuin Reich (Senatsverwaltung für Wissenschaft, Forschung und Kultur, Berlin), Hermann Reuke (ZEvA, Hannover), Roland Richter (Wissenschaftliches Sekretariat für die Studienreform im Land Nordrhein-Westfalen), Klaus Schnitzer (HIS, Hannover) and Ulrich Teichler (Centre for Research on Higher Education and Work, University of Kassel) for being constructive and critical with your feedback regarding the outline of this research project. Our special gratitude goes to Ulrich Teichler who gave expert advice throughout the project and guided the research design phase. We also appreciate the help and support of the staff at the Centre for Research on Higher Education and Work, University of Kassel.

Many thanks go to the 'back ground' crew, who helped to turn the draft chapters into a camera-ready manuscript. Christina Keyes, in Paris, and Meike Rehburg, in Germany (Kassel and Stuttgart), were of great help and went well beyond the actual proof-reading and formatting. Special thanks to Meike Rehburg for her valuable ideas and insights regarding the content of the final manuscript.

We would also like to thank Kluwer Academic Publishers, namely Peter Maassen and Tamara Welschot for their professional management regarding the publication.

Last but not least we would like to thank Gerd Köhler, German Trade Union for Education and Science, for his support and constructive feedback throughout the study on 'Accreditation and Evaluation in the European Higher Education Area'.

Kassel and Enschede
Stefanie Schwarz, Don Westerheijden

1 Accreditation in the Framework of Evaluation Activities: A Comparative Study in the European Higher Education Area

STEFANIE SCHWARZ & DON F. WESTERHEIJDEN

1.1 Introduction: The Study's Goals and Structure

Higher education systems in Europe are currently undergoing deep reforms. These reforms are triggered by national developments, as well as by the aim to evolve towards comparable systems and ensure the quality of the higher education systems in Europe (Bologna Process). This study was initiated by the education trade unions' goal to widen the scope of the debate on accreditation and evaluation activities in higher education in Europe from a comparative perspective. In order to provide the factual base for this discussion, we were asked to carry out a comparative study of 'accreditation in the framework of evaluation activities' in the European higher education area. Accreditation is the focus of our study, but accreditation is a policy instrument made up of two elements: evaluation and approval. Therefore, we felt it necessary to analyse these two elements in their own right. Hence, the aims of the study are to:

1. Provide an updated picture of the current situation with regard to (1) accreditation schemes, (2) other approval schemes (outside accreditation) and (3) evaluation schemes.

2. Analyse the underlying principles of the accreditation scheme(s) and how they relate to other approval and evaluation schemes ('system logic' or 'system dynamic').

3. Point out and analyse current reforms of the accreditation scheme(s) (with a view to other approval and evaluation schemes as well as supra-national developments, e.g. the Bologna process and other influences).

Our study covers all countries involved in the Bologna process. For practical reasons, we have had to limit ourselves to a sub-set consisting of all fifteen EU member states (situation as of 2003, minus Luxembourg which has a minute higher education sector), a main Western European country which is not part of the EU (Norway) and a sample of Central and Eastern European countries which entered the EU in 2004 (the Czech Republic, Hungary, Latvia, Lithuania, Poland), bringing the total to 20 countries. With regard to Central and Eastern Europe, we have reason to believe that the situation depicted below is representative of not just the countries sampled, but

S. Schwarz and D.F. Westerheijden (eds.),
Accreditation and Evaluation in the European Higher Education Area, 1–41.

also of much more of the Central and Eastern European area (Campbell & Rozsnyai, 2002).

We asked all 20 country experts of this study to provide reports on their respective system of 'accreditation in the framework of evaluation activities'. They compiled studies describing and analysing in detail how the respective accreditation and evaluation systems are institutionalised and how they are linked to other relevant developments, e.g. the Bologna Process and internationalisation trends (including GATS). From April 10 to 13, 2003, all country experts were invited to share their work and to learn about the ideas of their European colleagues in a two-day workshop at the EI/GEW Forum 'Shaping the European Area of Higher Education and Research'.

In this chapter, we will provide a synopsis of the findings of the country reports by taking the three main elements, 'accreditation', 'evaluation' and 'approval other than accreditation' as the basic structure of the sections. To maintain consistent distinctions between accreditation, evaluation and other approval schemes across all 20 country cases, we adopted the following definitions.

Accreditation schemes[1]: All institutionalised and systematically implemented evaluation schemes of higher education institutions,[2] degree types[3] and programmes[4] that end in a formal summary judgement that leads to formal approval processes regarding the respective institution, degree type and/or programme.

Approval of institutions, degree types, programmes: To grant the 'right to exist within the system' (or, respectively, to reject the 'right to exist') to an institution, degree-type, programme (e.g. charter, licence, accreditation). The approval can be carried out by several organisations or one organisation and is granted by one or more organisation(s) at the supra-institutional level.

Approval outside the accreditation scheme: All major approval schemes of higher education institutions, degree types and programmes that are not part of the accredi-

---

1   The term 'scheme' refers to the 'entire picture', the 'overall picture', the landscape of the respective three concepts of 'accreditation activities', 'approval other than accreditation activities' and 'evaluation activities'.

2   *Higher education institutions*: All organisations providing degrees at the tertiary level (ISCED 5 and 6), recognised by governmental/public agencies and/or by the general public. This definition is meant to include both public and private higher education institutions with official national recognition and 'non-official' higher education leading to degrees that may be recognised in other countries but not necessarily in the country of operation. Our intention is to keep an eye open on organisations that are active in 'transnational higher education'.

3   *Higher education degree-types:* The different degrees that are awarded by and certified through a higher education institution (e.g. Bachelor, Master, Diploma, etc.).

4   *Higher education programmes:* All education provisions within higher education institutions that lead to higher education degrees (ISCED 5 and 6).

tation scheme (e.g. approval by the state ministry that does not involve accreditation).

Evaluation schemes: All institutionalised and systematically implemented activities regarding the measurement, analysis and/or development of quality for institutions, degrees-types and/or programmes that are carried out at the *supra-institutional level*. Evaluation activities *do not* directly or indirectly lead to approval processes regarding the respective institution, degree type and programme.

Other evaluation schemes (than the just mentioned): Other types of ratings / measurements of quality that do not fulfil the criteria of the definition of *evaluation schemes*, such as institution-based evaluation.

Moreover, the term *quality assurance scheme* or *quality assurance system* will be used as an umbrella term, denoting accreditation and evaluation systems together, in contrast to approval without formal evaluative elements.

These definitions were developed with a view to the specific goals of our study and may therefore diverge somewhat from other sets of definitions. However, we are convinced that the differences with many recent or authoritative publications in the field are not substantial (cf. Sursock, 2001; Young et al., 1983). A particularly well-developed set of definitions is found in an ENQA report on 'accreditation-like practices' (Hämäläinen et al., 2001). Hämäläinen et al. also distinguish distinction between *accreditation* and *approval* '(without an explicit accreditation process)' (p. 7), but they also analyse terms that cover effects for the individual graduate, such as *recognition* of degrees and *authorisation* to practise a given profession, which are beyond the scope of this study. When discussing accreditation, they make several distinctions, i.a. official as against private accreditation. In their terms, our definition of accreditation seems targeted at 'official' accreditation, i.e. accreditation by governmental higher education authorities or their delegated agencies, leading to – as in our definition – formal approval decisions. 'Private accreditation', being voluntary and not linked to the authorities, 'may enhance a unit's reputation, but it does not alter its formal status' (Hämäläinen et al., 2001, p. 9). As will be shown below, in 'open accreditation systems' such private accreditation agencies may be given a role in the authorities' decisions, which is one of the reasons why we include them in our study. Moreover, with the current 'denationalisation' (cf. i.a. van Vught, van der Wende, & Westerheijden, 2002) of higher education we do not wish to overlook the possibility that higher education institutions attach a great deal of importance to private accreditation by narrowing our definition too much in advance.

Our study has limitations, of course. To begin with, it is limited in time: editing of the country chapters was closed in summer/fall of 2003. Hence, for newer developments the reader is referred elsewhere. Like all studies based on the voluntary co-operation of a large number of experts from very different national backgrounds, it has its limitations regarding coherent use of terms. The definitions we gave above were communicated to the authors of the country reports, and we took measures to try to ensure that they were applied in a uniform fashion. Yet some room for interpretation of the meaning of the terms remained, and more room for interpretation had to be left to the authors in linking the terms to empirical phenomena in their countries. In that sense, this study reflects some of the diversity that is often seen as both a strength and a weakness of Europe.

Another limitation lies in the aim and scope of this chapter. The wealth of information given in the 20 country chapters is more than can be analysed in any single chapter. For instance, we focused on commonalities rather than differences in order to emphasise the common ground that already exists in the area of evaluation, accreditation and approval and that can be used as a basis for further development towards a European Higher Education Area. We are aware that there are differences among the countries and that underlying principles embodied in national institutions may make the commonalities less common than they may seem at first sight. Still, we aim to show that the common approach of cross-national studies of higher education systems in Europe, in which the historical differences are often emphasised, need not be the only viable approach. Path-dependencies do not preclude convergence, especially not in a geographical area where so much interdependence has existed for so many centuries.

A final limitation that we should like to mention is the fact that time and budget could only be stretched so far. In a fast-moving area – and higher education in Europe in the wake of the Bologna Declaration certainly is a fast-moving area – perhaps it is better to have a book like this one with a relatively up-to-date picture of the evaluation and accreditation landscape, rather than a more thorough analysis that comes well after the events.

1.2   Quality in the Steering of Higher Education Before the Bologna Declaration

Quality in the sense of achieving academic excellence has always been a central value in higher education. Neave rightly stated 'quality is not "here to stay", if only for the self-evident reason that across the centuries of the university's existence in Europe, it never departed' (Neave, 1994, p. 116). Until the 1970s, quality in higher education was controlled through bureaucratic means: legal conditions for the establishment of institutions, faculties and/or programmes of study and state-provided means (funding, housing) to fulfil those conditions, centralised and formalised rules for the appointment of academic staff, similarly centralised and formalised rules for the acceptance of students, annual line-item budgets, etc.[5] And until about the 1960s or 1970s, this way of ensuring quality of higher education was fairly successful: low-quality provision of higher education was an unheard of phenomenon in the state-controlled European higher education systems. However, quality assurance as a separate instrument in university management and in government policy started in the 1970s and 1980s, when it was discovered as a new management tool in industry mimicking the successes of the Japanese economy. First, higher education in the USA was influenced, later, around 1984, the first governmental policies were implemented in Western Europe. Apart from the old isomorphism drive to copy whatever seemed successful in US higher education, and the new isomorphism drive to copy whatever seemed successful in industry,[6] there were a number of reasons why new governance tools became expedient in Western European higher education at that point in time. In sum, these were (van Vught, 1994):

- 'massification' of higher education;
- limits of central control were reached with these larger higher education systems;
- deregulation was in fashion at the time, when neo-liberalism made a forceful entry into the political arena;
- government budget limits were reached, again because of the massification of higher education but also more generally because governments under the neo-liberal influence were not willing to increase the share of public to private earnings even more to maintain the welfare state.

This put 'value for money' high on the agenda, which resulted in higher education institutions being given autonomy to do 'more with less', as one of the half-serious, half-sarcastic slogans went. As Trow observed quite sharply, evaluation policies indicated the breakdown of the traditional degree of trust in society that higher education was functioning at high quality (Trow, 1994, 1996). A danger inherent in evaluation policies is that '[i]f accountability and evaluation are reduced to a primarily technical exercise by way of rigid output measures and overly standardised evaluation exercises, then the essential debate about the values and assets which HEIs are best suited to pursue for society is clearly at risk' (Reichert & Tauch, 2003, p. 102). This rise of societal demands for accountability has been documented exten-

---

5   The United Kingdom and Ireland have been exceptions in this trend of bureaucratic centralised control on the European continent. British universities were more autonomous, but they too were subject to national rules (e.g. Acts of Parliament) for their establishment and there was national funding (although the British mechanism for distributing money, the University Grants Council, gave much more autonomy to the academic oligarchy) (Clark, 1983).

6   We stress 'seems' here, because of the mimetic character of much of this copying behaviour, witnessed by the fact that many similar 'fads' fade away without leaving many traces after a number of years (Birnbaum, 2000).

sively, not only in higher education, but also and especially in public administration (cf. Brignall & Modell, 2000; Enders, 2002; Lane, 2000; Rowley, 1996).

The implementation of quality assurance mechanisms in higher education systems first started in some Western European countries in the middle of the 1980s. In Central and Eastern Europe, they were introduced from 1990 onwards. However, the aims and goals attached to quality assurance were quite different in Western and Central/Eastern Europe at the outset.

The 'pioneer countries' in Western Europe – the United Kingdom, France and the Netherlands – introduced their first formal quality assurance policies around 1985. In 1990, Denmark was the first follower of these pioneers, and from then on, the 'quality movement' spread to the rest of Western Europe. The conditions of higher education in Western Europe were similar for some countries and quite different for others, as were the tendencies to mimic. For example, the main motor to establish accreditation in most Nordic countries was the desire to expand open access and equal opportunity for mass higher education by creating new regional colleges and new study programmes as counterparts to the large traditional universities. In other countries both North and South (Germany, Italy, the Netherlands), low efficiency of the higher education system was the major issue to be solved by quality assurance.

An important tool in spreading the external evaluation was the European Union's Pilot Project, which was launched in 1994 (Management Group, 1995). It consisted of evaluation exercises involving one or two programmes in two knowledge areas in all (then) EU countries.

In 1998, as a late consequence of the EU's pilot project, the Commission of the EU made a recommendation to establish and support a network of the EU member states' quality assurance agencies (Kern, 1998). This network, the European Network of Quality Assessment Agencies (ENQA), became operational in 2000. By 2002, it had 36 member organisations and 30 government members. With a voluntary but exclusive membership, ENQA is heterogeneous in nature. The character of its operation is professional – a body of quality assurance experts – rather than political, although its work inevitably has political consequences. ENQA is very aware of this.

That same year, just before the Sorbonne and Bologna Declarations changed the whole scene, two inventories were made of the situation of quality assurance in Western Europe (Centre for Quality Assurance and Evaluation of Higher Education, 1998; Scheele, Maassen, & Westerheijden, 1998). From both, it can be concluded that almost all Western European countries at that moment had a government policy to assess quality in higher education. (The most notable exceptions were Germany, Italy and Greece.) Spontaneous serious involvement of universities in quality assurance without governmental policies were rare exceptions, although existent (witness e.g. the dozens of universities that volunteered for the CRE's Institutional Evaluation Programme). And if universities engaged in quality assurance voluntarily, the effectiveness tended to be much more marked than when complying with government-initiated policies (Brennan & Shah, 2000).

The Central and Eastern European countries advanced rapidly regarding evaluation and accreditation activities. With the demise of the Communist regimes in Central and Eastern Europe in 1989–1990, the issue of quality assurance presented itself in a very different form in this half of the continent, quickly leading to different institutional arrangements to cope with it. Before 1989, the central control of quality in Central and Eastern Europe, like in the West until the 1980s, was based on bureaucratic means. In Šebková's words in this volume: 'Quality was not evaluated or even discussed. Indeed, the high quality of education was simply declared and announced'. In (some degree of) contrast to the West, state bureaucratic control was confounded with overt and covert control mechanisms of the governing party's *nomenklatura* system (e.g. Cerych, 1993; Hendrichová, 1998; Neacsu, 1998; Sadlak, 1995; Wnuk-Lipinska, 1998).

In short, we could say that the main purposes of introducing quality assurance policies in Central and Eastern Europe included (cf. Westerheijden & Sorensen, 1999):

- Transformation of higher education curricula to eradicate Marxist-Leninist dogma.
- Rapid expansion to accommodate tremendous excess-demand for higher education (reflecting the needs of post-industrial societies in combination with the elite character of the higher education systems).
- Much freer entry to the higher education market than previously, for national private higher education institutions as well as for foreign (public and private) higher education institutions.
- Underlying these changes was the change of the relationship between the state and higher education institutions: the state retreated from its former strict central control, which led to extremely decentralised higher education systems. .

In general, the model used for quality assurance in Central and Eastern European countries was that of state-controlled accreditation of all programmes and/or institutions in the country. Accreditation was to function as a shield to keep out 'rogue' provision of higher education and maintain some form of central control in the highly decentralised higher education systems.

In sum, this shows a great divide among the different paths of development with regard to quality assurance followed in European countries. In the next section, we will look in more detail at the situation in the 20 countries of our study. For analytical purposes, we will try to group countries as much as possible, but the groupings and categories may be different for different aspects, implying that in principle there is not a *fixed* taxonomy, as summarised in geographical notions like 'the Nordic countries', 'the Mediterranean countries' or the 'Central and Eastern European countries' – even though for some limited purposes such fixed geographical categories may be useful.

1.3   Quality in the Light of Evaluation and Accreditation Activities

The countries in this study include many of those that signed the Bologna Declaration – that is why they were chosen in the first place. It was only for reasons of time and money that we could not include all of them. At the same time, we are spanning large parts of other continua. For instance, the size of the higher education systems in the countries involved ranges from small (with some 110,000 students in Latvia) to large (e.g. France, which counts more than to 2 million students in higher education). There are also unitary systems (e.g. the United Kingdom) and systems with several types of higher education institutions (e.g. France). All are to a large degree publicly funded, although the institutional arrangements differ; e.g., in the United Kingdom all public institutions are autonomous entities, while in Germany they are in many respects (e.g. personnel policy) part of the government apparatus. The arrangements regarding private higher education also vary: from non-acceptance (as in the Czech Republic before 1998) to liberal – but quality-controlled – as in the Netherlands.

When in the following we refer to 'government', in many countries this is the nation-state government. However, a number of large European countries have devolved (part of) authority over higher education to federal states within the nation, especially Germany, Spain, the United Kingdom. Belgium has another type of federalisation. Here, higher education is completely decentralised and our data (as often in European projects) are limited to the Flemish-speaking Community.

Concerning government, there is great fluidity regarding its role, ranging from passive administrative authorisation for a private body to open a higher education institution, to actively taking the initiative to create and support a public body to run a higher education institution. In this chapter we are mainly concerned with the passive side of the spectrum, i.e. with the judgement and approval, not with the issue of whether governments also actively initiate and support higher education institutions or study programmes.

In response to the GATS negotiations, both universities and students in Europe in 2000 vehemently declared that higher education in Europe was a public good (EUA & ESIB, 2002), a statement also adopted by the ministers of education (*Prague Communiqué*, 2001). And indeed, higher education in all the countries involved in the study is mainly provided by public institutions.[7] However, private higher education institutions can be found in most countries (except Greece), even though they usually service only a small proportion of the students according to official statistics (Tsaoussis, 1999; Uvalic-Tumbic, 2002). Thus, in Germany there are 43 private higher education institutions servicing just over 1 % of all students. In other countries, private higher education is much more widespread (e.g. Poland, Portugal).

1.3.1 The Three Pillars in Relation to Each Other: Evaluation, Accreditation and Approval

Quantitative Developments of Evaluation and Accreditation Activities in Europe

As indicated in section 2 of this chapter, European countries have experienced great change regarding their institutionalisation of evaluation, accreditation and 'approval other than accreditation'. The results of our study show that in the early 1990s, less than half of the European countries had started evaluation at the supra-institutional level. By 2003, all European countries had implemented supra-institutional evaluation, except for Greece (see Tables 1 and 2). According to data in the *Trends III* report, this covers 80 % of all higher education institutions in Europe (Reichert & Tauch, 2003, p. 105).

Table 1. Focus on supra-institutional evaluation activities. Year: 1992[8]

No focus on evaluation activities	Focus on evaluation activities
NO, SE, FI, ES, PT, IT, GR, DE, AT, BE(FL)	NL, DK, FR, GB, IR, HU, PL, CZ, LT, LV

Table 2. Focus on supra-institutional evaluation activities. Year: 2003

No focus on evaluation activities	Focus on evaluation activities
–	NO, SE, FI, DK, HU, PL, CZ, LT, LV, ES, PT, IT, GR(?), GB, IR, DE, AT, FR, BE(FL), NL

In most countries, evaluation activities include teaching as well as research performance (in combined or separate schemes) and may be carried out at the programme as well as at the institutional levels (cf. also: Danish Evaluation Institute, 2003). Great

---

7   In the United Kingdom: 'state-funded private institutions'.

8   For brevity's sake, we shall use ISO two-letter codes to designate countries in the tables; Flanders will be abbreviated to BE(FL).

differences are encountered when the focus is on aims and instruments of evaluation. The 2003 ENQA survey sees three predominant modes: programme evaluation, programme accreditation and institutional audit (Danish Evaluation Institute, 2003). However, the general procedures of supra-institutional evaluation in all countries largely follow the 'general model of quality assessment' (van Vught & Westerheijden, 1994).

Granting institutions and programmes 'the right to exist' was traditionally a task that was performed by the state government. Only recently, in the wake of the introduction of 'new autonomy' for higher education institutions, has the task been transferred from the state ministries to newly established supra-institutional organisations (e.g. accreditation agencies, quality assurance agencies that incorporate accreditation activities, etc.). The country experts report that all European countries have established a framework of accreditation for (parts of) higher education. The pace of the development can be characterised as rapid. Whereas in 1998 less than half the European countries in our study had implemented accreditation schemes for (parts of) higher education, in 2003 all European countries, with the exception of Greece[9] and Denmark[10], defined their system as having implemented 'some type of accreditation scheme' (see Tables 3 and 4).

Table 3. State approval versus accreditation scheme with evaluation activities. Year: 1998

State approval	Accreditation scheme with evaluation activities
NO, SE, FI, DK, ES, PT, IT, GR, DE, AT, FR, BE(FL), NL, LT	HU, PL, CZ, LV, GB, IR

Table 4. State approval versus accreditation scheme with evaluation activities. Year: 2003

State approval	Accreditation scheme with evaluation activities
DK, GR(?)	NO, SE, FI, HU, PL, CZ, LT, LV, ES, PT, IT, GB, IR, DE, AT, FR, BE(FL), NL

Denmark is the only country in Europe that explicitly does not see any added value in shifting from its well-functioning evaluation scheme in combination with state approval to an accreditation scheme in combination with evaluation activities.

---

9   At the time of writing the reports in this volume, evaluation was proposed in Greece, but the policy process had not come to a conclusion. Accreditation was a concept beyond the Greek discussion.

10 Nevertheless, even in Denmark accreditation is part of the policy instruments, viz. for private tertiary study programmes that want to apply for government funding. However, this is an 'accreditation' performed solely by staff of the national evaluation agency (cf. the remarks on France below).

Whereas evaluation activities follow a common general approach in all European countries, accreditation is not following any type of common general approach at present in Europe. The main differences in the accreditation schemes across Europe can be defined as follows: '

(1) There are currently no patterns that demonstrate comparable structures of accreditation schemes. For example, the accreditation activities range from approval procedures of 'degree programmes at one type of higher education institution' (e.g. Austria) to 'all institutions and all programmes' (e.g. Hungary). The key players are quite different in the European countries, some countries have started agencies at the supra-institutional level (e.g. Germany, Spain), others have accreditation only for professional fields by professional bodies (e.g. Ireland, Spain before 2003), other countries regard the state ministry as the 'accreditation agency' in co-operation with the respective quality assurance agencies (e.g. Finland).

(2) At present, there are no patterns that demonstrate comparable methods for accreditation schemes. Moreover, a number of country reports suggest that there is no direct link between the different types of accreditation organisations connected to public authorities (e.g. accreditation agencies), and private sector agencies (e.g. professional bodies) (e.g. Spain, Portugal, the United Kingdom).

(3) The types of evaluation processes underlying the approval decision in accreditation schemes vary widely.

In sum, one can wonder if there is a common understanding of 'accreditation' amongst the contributors to the country reports – notwithstanding the definition given in this project – and more broadly, amongst the decision-makers in the European countries. We shall look into that issue in more detail later, but first, we shall continue our overview of the evaluation framework in the European countries.

Approval as an Indicator of Trust or of Lack of Autonomy?

The rise of quality assurance with evaluation and accreditation activities as a policy instrument has been interpreted as indicating a decrease in the trust in society that higher education 'delivers the goods' without giving special attention to it (Trow, 1996). Partly, an assurance of quality was implicit in the governmental regulation and funding of the overwhelmingly public systems of higher education in Continental Europe, as mentioned above. In that perspective, countries where traditional forms of approval without explicit evaluation are prevalent show a higher level of trust in higher education than countries where evaluation and accreditation are prevalent modes of control. However, the absence of formal evaluation or accreditation cannot really be taken as a sign of trust, for traditional bureaucracy was and is a powerful means of control in itself (cf. France, Greece). Indeed, the argument was often made that quality assurance was an alternative to the former strict bureaucratic control, giving more room for institutional autonomy,[11] self-regulation or bottom-up initiatives in the higher education system (e.g. Flanders pre-2003, Finland, Greece, the Netherlands pre-2003, Sweden).

Specifying what 'traditional' bureaucracy controls and what 'modern' evaluation or accreditation controls, can solve the paradox. In general, bureaucratic control focuses on inputs (staff appointments, student access, annual funding, curriculum plans), although the French process of approval of private higher education institutions only takes place after five years of operation, implying that there is some degree of interest in output. Yet even here, the main emphasis is on staff qualifications, facilities and similar input factors. In contrast, evaluation and accreditation can focus on input, process or output alike. In more traditionally-oriented evaluation and accreditation systems, the focus remains on input factors. The aim of quality assurance models developed during the 1980s and 1990s in industry, such as TQM and ISO-9000, was to draw attention to the process of 'producing' quality education and quality graduates – the latter was the funnel through which output quality came into the picture. The French case also shows the fluidity of terms – notwithstanding our efforts to develop strictly separated definitions. What is called into question by the report on developments in France is the meaning of 'evaluation': Is it necessary for evaluation to be built upon the four-step model (van Vught & Westerheijden, 1994) with self-evaluation and review panels performing site visits? Or is it enough for experts from the ministry of education to study documentation sent by a higher education institution?[12] How does the latter differ, if at all, from the rules-based and paper-based traditional bureaucratic preparation of a decision? The distinction between accreditation and evaluation is also fluid in France. As Chevaillier mentions, (internal) evaluation is a condition for accreditation (or approval) of a study programme. Still, he makes clear that without changing names of official procedures, the mechanisms through which these procedures *actually* operate, and the character *in operation* (in caricature: from a bureaucratic rubber stamp to an actual evaluation with no guaranteed outcome) may change considerably.

Accountability and Improvement Orientations

A main distinction in the analysis of quality assurance is the types of functions a system must fulfil. Weusthof & Frederiks made a distinction between four main functions (Weusthof & Frederiks, 1997):

---

11 Institutional autonomy is not the same as individual academic freedom, although in political discourse, they seem to be mingled where the main opposition is between government and higher education. The moment the discussion turns into questions of power within the higher education institution, the opposition between academic freedom and institutional autonomy becomes clear, the latter being easily equated with 'managerialism'.

12 Also the practice in some British professional organisations.

- Accountability,
- Quality improvement,
- Validation,
- Information.

It may be argued that the basic divide – inextricably linked like 'two sides of a coin' (Vroeijenstijn, 1989) – is between accountability and quality improvement. Accountability has to do with informing society (in particular the state) about the quality 'delivered' by higher education. Validation (the function of legitimising quality judgements, i.e. something accreditation is supposed to do) can be seen as a form of accountability. Therefore, in the countries with a heavy emphasis on accreditation, it may be argued that there is also an emphasis on the accountability side of the coin. Information as Weusthof & Frederiks used it is linked to the transparency issue which, at the international level, is one of the main reasons for the Bologna process; it is information for stakeholders to help them make reasoned choices (e.g. for pursuing studies, or for employing a graduate). The information function was stressed in Sweden. Quality assurance stressing accountability or information giving in itself is not a strong incentive to improve or enhance quality of higher education above the threshold level defined by e.g. accreditation standards or governmental requirements. This was shown amongst others in the research on the effects of the Dutch external quality assessment mechanism (Jeliazkova, 2001; Jeliazkova & Westerheijden, 2000). A strong drive for quality improvement therefore may need external mechanisms tuned to fulfilling this function. While agreeing that the situation is indeed like 'two sides of a coin', and more complex than a simple dichotomy would suggest, as a first approximation we should like to typify countries in the study on this dimension (Table 5). Other countries' landscape of evaluation and accreditation is so mixed that even a rough sketch seems too risky (the Czech Republic may be a good example, with both accountability-oriented accreditation and improvement-oriented evaluation).

Table 5. Broad emphasis of accreditation and evaluation systems per country: Year 2003

Accountability emphasis	Quality improvement emphasis
BE(FL), DE, HU, PT, LT, LV, NL	NO, SE, FI, DK

As a rule, quality assurance agencies, governments and higher education institutions tend to emphasise the quality improvement element. Most studies therefore find that quality improvement is the most common function of evaluation and accreditation schemes (Campbell & Rozsnyai, 2002; Danish Evaluation Institute, 2003; Reichert & Tauch, 2003). From our reading of the country reports in this volume, a different picture emerges if one tries to distil the primary focus of the schemes as they are actually implemented (Table 5, selected countries, as explained above).

An element of the validation function may also be the recognition of study programmes abroad for purposes of student mobility or for graduate employment abroad. Although until now this is mostly dealt with by means of individual level arrangements through degree recognition by higher education institutions on the advice of ENIC/NARIC offices, quality assurance is given prominence in this respect as well (Sweden). In some cases, better international recognition of the country's higher education degrees was an explicit argument to introduce accreditation (the Netherlands). This international or European dimension seems to be prevalent mostly in small countries.

Unanticipated consequences of introducing supra-institutional evaluation or accreditation schemes may include a tendency for rigidity, as attention in higher education institutions may focus on meeting (perceived) standards (hence the term 'compliance culture'; van Vught, 1989) rather than on accountability to society (also *Trends III* report, cited before). However, higher education institutions often value external evaluation and accreditation activities as a positive 'prodding' to pay attention to its important but not always urgent core value of quality education.

Another potential problem of the development of national frameworks for judging study programmes may be that they put pressure on harmonisation within countries at a time when it is claimed that diversity is needed more than ever:

- because of 'massification' of higher education (countries are setting ever higher participation targets, sometimes well above 50 % of the relevant age cohort), different types of students have different learning needs;
- in the 'knowledge society', the roles of higher education are multiplying, leading to the need to respond in different ways to different demands.

Pressure to uniformitise may ensue from methodical issues associated with the predefined criteria necessary in accreditation. They would lead to greater homogeneity instead of the diversity of approaches and competencies needed in the present-day 'massified' higher education systems and in the emerging knowledge economy. Besides, adaptation of published criteria is a time-consuming process, so that accreditation continuously runs the risk of falling behind the state of the art. Then again, accreditation criteria tend to be a compromise between the participants in the decision-making process of the accreditation organisation, leading to the criteria being a *communis opinio*, but not challenging for the development of the best programmes or units. Finally, as accreditation judgements are based on passing threshold criteria, they would tend to discourage innovation and quality improvement. Innovative approaches to accreditation criteria and processes can overcome such disadvantages at least partly, as seen, for example, in the current practices in

European EQUIS (www.efmd.be), in the American engineering accreditor ABET (www.abet.org/eac/eac2000.htm) and other professional accreditation organisations in the USA, as well as in the US regional accreditor WASC (www.wascweb.org).

Relations between Accreditation, Evaluation and Approval Schemes

Quite often, the picture depicted for foreign observers of steering quality in a country's higher education system seems to be that there is only one scheme. The country reports in this study clearly show that – as any student of the matter discovers upon closer contact with any single higher education system – the situation is never as simple as that. Even separating steering of quality from other instruments of higher education policy, as this study does, entails some distortion of the full picture. We try to overcome this limitation in two ways. One is to focus on the dynamics or driving forces. The other is to look at all (main) different supra-institutional schemes, focusing on their interaction.

For the mainly publicly-funded higher education systems that are the norm all over Europe, governmental recognition of study programmes or higher education institutions is the main decision that can be reached, as it comes with official recognition of degrees (often an important if not always necessary condition for degrees' *effectus civilis*) and with funding for the programme or institution as well as for students (i.e. student stipends, grants, loans, etc.). Governments almost invariably use a single scheme as the authoritative basis for (semi-)official recognition or approval of study programmes and/or higher education institutions. This is most explicit with governmental approval schemes and with 'state-sponsored' accreditation schemes (e.g. Flanders, the Czech Republic, Germany, France, Hungary, the Netherlands, Poland), but can be equally the case with evaluation schemes (Denmark, Sweden, the United Kingdom).

Other evaluation or accreditation schemes, in particular those under the control of the professions (as in Portugal and the United Kingdom), are important for students, as they influence their chances of entering the labour market, but are less clearly linked to governmental decision-making. In the United Kingdom, the influence of professional accreditation in some cases is offset by the reputation of the university: degrees from prestigious universities will be sought after by students even if they are not accredited by the competent professional organisation. In Portugal, representatives of the professional *Orden* often take part in the review teams of the national evaluation as 'linking pins'.

Ownership of evaluation schemes by the higher education institutions (as in the United Kingdom, Portugal, the Netherlands pre-2003) seemed to result in less direct links with governmental decision-making than 'state-sponsored schemes', yet more direct than the cases where schemes are owned by professions.

Moreover, in what can only be analysed as their marketing efforts, higher education institutions are increasingly engaged in collecting multiple accreditations voluntarily. The areas of business schools (EQUIS, AMBA, AACSB are familiar 'kite marks' here) and faculties of engineering (turning mostly towards ABET or FEANI) provide prime examples across all European countries. Even in the very core of French higher education with its tradition of an 'économie concertée', signs of increasingly aggressive marketing are visible in the establishment of the *Conférence des Grandes Écoles*.

When several accreditation or evaluation schemes exist in a country, one question becomes how they interact with each other. Is there a concerted system of one scheme complementing another, or is interference a better characterisation? Often, a fear exists in higher education institutions that interference may cause a bureaucratic overload leading to 'evaluation fatigue' because independent agencies involved in different schemes always seem to want information in their own particular format. Indeed, it seems that careful co-ordination is needed to achieve beneficial complementarity among schemes. Putting several schemes under a single agency may be a way to achieve this, as is seen in the Czech Republic. Yet there is a danger that one of the schemes will come to dominate the scene and attract most effort and attention, undermining the idea of complementarity.

The parallel existence of national evaluation or accreditation schemes with those of professions and voluntary schemes is one of the reasons for the 'evaluation fatigue' noted in our reports. In Portugal, conversations have been initiated to achieve more efficiency in this respect. In the United Kingdom, the perception of an excessive evaluation burden has been one of the main reasons for the higher education institutions' 'revolt' against the former QAA evaluation scheme, which led to the introduction of 'a lighter touch' after 2001. In the Netherlands, the existence of at least four (semi-) official evaluation schemes led to a consolidation of the three main research reviews into a single research review scheme in 2003, alongside the accreditation scheme for education.

There are, in addition, other issues of complementarity or interference than just the information delivery issue. For instance, in the Netherlands, the accreditation scheme introduced in 2003 is meant to maintain the quality improvement function that was such a prominent feature of the previous evaluation schemes. The accreditation scheme is sometimes portrayed as an addition on top of evaluation, i.e. as if they are complementary. It is not clear, however, if the knowledge that an evaluation process will be used for accreditation purposes will not lead to strategic behaviour (e.g. trying to hide weaknesses from accreditors instead of discussing them with peers). If that happened, accreditation would be interfering with the evaluation scheme.

Parallel evaluation schemes also lead to the question of whether the striving for more transparency actually leads to less transparency for the 'end users', i.e. for students, parents and employers, in other words, whether Europe's previous 'jungle of degrees' will be replaced by a 'jungle of accreditations' (Haug, 1999).[13] However, the fear of uncertainty is not the only way to look at the issue. The other side of the coin is the increased information given by different types of accreditation judgements in 'open accreditation systems' (van Vught et al., 2002). Study programmes or higher education institutions may distinguish themselves by choosing one or another type of accreditation, and in principle the 'end users' would then know more about the qualities of the institution than when only a single quality 'kite mark' were available. However, in the developing practice among business schools, which seem keen on accumulating as many accreditations as they can (in a different meaning of a 'multiple accreditation system') it becomes unclear what the marketing message to potential customers will be from sporting a whole set of accreditations – although these schools are best placed to know about marketing...

The International Scene: National Steering of Quality and Transnational Higher Education

Both globalisation and the Bologna process – insofar as the two can be separated – call the relevance of national borders into question to some degree. International mobility of students and graduates is one of the aims of the Bologna Declaration. In the analytical scheme of GATS, one of the 'modes of delivery' of transnational education is the 'commercial presence' of foreign higher education institutions in other countries. How do approval, accreditation and evaluation schemes accommodate the cross-border aspects of higher education?

Under the new Norwegian accreditation scheme, the co-ordinating agency NOKUT has been given the brief to develop a recognition policy, focusing on Norwegian students' obtaining degrees from foreign higher education institutions. This seems to be a case where the quality assurance agency is also given tasks of ENIC/NARIC agencies, where the recognition of foreign degrees on an individual basis is the core task. A difference with normal ENIC/NARIC agencies may be that, in Norwegian higher education regulation, stress is laid on developing general criteria rather than case-by-case decisions.[14]

A different view on international aspects is given by the Netherlands Accreditation Organisation, which resuscitates the Renaissance meaning of the 'nether lands' (low countries) in that it includes both the Netherlands and Flemish Belgium. In fact, this

---

13 The same could be said about evaluation schemes, not just about accreditation schemes, but that is what the discussion focuses on most often.

14 Possibly, the difference with ENIC/NARIC decision-making may not be great at all and it may just be a matter of emphasis in the regulatory texts.

is going to be a bi-national accreditation organisation, showing that national systems are no longer the only units to consider in the European higher education landscape. At the same time, this example shows the difficulty of working across state borders: the legal frameworks, although having the same intention, are not *quite* the same, and operationally the NAO is discovering that 'the devil is in the details'.

Virtually all accreditation and evaluation schemes apply to higher education institutions within the country. In some cases it was mentioned that foreign providers of higher education also have to be accredited in order to operate (Hungary, the Netherlands since 2003). On the other hand, the United Kingdom is the only country requiring (and evaluating!) British higher education institutions to apply quality assurance principles for their provision overseas.

Transnational aspects of higher education are addressed explicitly in cross-national initiatives such as the Joint Quality Initiative of a number of European countries (www.jointquality.org) and the *Tuning* project. But this is not our subject of study (cf. Farrington, 2001; Machado dos Santos, 2000; Middlehurst, 2001; Reichert & Tauch, 2003; Westerheijden & Leegwater, 2003). In most national quality assurance schemes, on the contrary, international aspects are not clearly visible (such as regular use of truly international reviewers, application of explicitly 'international' standards and criteria, attention for internationalisation/Europeanisation of curricula, etc.).

1.3.2   Accreditation in More Detail

Coverage

As a rule, *all* higher education institutions and *all* programmes at *all* main levels of bachelor, master and (less often) doctorate in a higher education system are subjected equally to accreditation schemes. There may be differences by institutional category, e.g. only universities that offer master's degrees can apply for accreditation to obtain the right to offer PhD degrees (or PhD programmes), as in the Czech Republic, Hungary, Poland. In Germany, accreditation is so far limited to the new two-cycle structure (Bachelor and Master), leaving aside the traditionally structured programmes (Magister, Diplom, etc.) Another exception to the rule of universal application is found in Austria, where the new sectors of colleges (*Fachhochschulen*) and private, postgraduate, higher education institutions are subject to accreditation, while the traditional public university sector until now is exempt from it. Similarly, in Ireland only the non-university higher education institutions are subject to direct external control of programme quality comparable to an accreditation scheme by HETAC.

It goes without saying that voluntary and professional accreditation schemes, such as business studies associations in several countries (e.g. the United Kingdom, Italy) or internationally (EQUIS), only cover units in their own field, and that, being voluntary, higher education institutions are free to take or not to take such an accreditation. For some regulated professions in some countries however, professional accreditation is practically obligatory in order to ensure graduates' access to the labour market (e.g. accountancy or engineering in the United Kingdom, engineering in Portugal).

In the majority of countries, the *study programme* is the 'unit of analysis' in accreditation schemes in Europe. That is to say that the main judgements resulting from accreditation schemes pertain to individual programmes of study (Table 6). However, the higher education institution as an organisational entity is the focus of accreditation if accreditation is used to confer a legal status on higher education institutions, e.g. as 'university college' or 'doctoral-granting university'.[15]

Table 6. Unit of judgement in accreditation schemes

Programme of study	Higher education institution
CZ, DE, HU, IT, NL, NO, PL, PT, GB, LT	AT, CZ, NO, SE

Apart from the unit or level decision, it is possible to choose *where in the educational process* to 'measure' quality, i.e. is the emphasis in the accreditation (or evaluation) scheme on input factors, process factors and/or output factors? While in our report we cannot go into that level in any detail, some contrasts are striking (Danish Evaluation Institute, 2003; the reader is referred to Hämäläinen et al., 2001; Vroeijenstijn, 2003). The countries taking part in the so-called 'Joint Quality Initiative' all emphasise that, for them, accreditation ought to depend first and foremost on the proven quality of the graduates, which is the main output factor. The country report on Italy, for instance, shows a contrasting position, in that data required for recognition of study programmes' regulations – note that it is an *ex ante* recognition of *regulations* – of the new two-cycle type concentrate on input: numbers of teaching staff, available facilities, curriculum plans, etc.

The *addressee of decisions* is often the higher education institution's main governance body (rector/president, senate/council), yet the decisions and rights or obligations that follow from them are usually confined to a single programme area, e.g. the right to offer a master's degree programme in chemical technology. Furthermore,

---

15 One difficulty in applying these rules (hence in categorising countries for the table) lies in cases where smaller units such as faculties coincide with programmes.

accreditation decisions almost invariably carry *consequences for the government*, such as the expectation that it will recognise the degrees awarded and, more materially, that it will fund (a number of) student places in the accredited programmes of study.

With their focus on study programmes, the main emphasis of accreditation schemes is education, or more specifically teaching. Especially in Central and Eastern European countries, the research prowess of the programme's academics as evidenced by their publications is used as an important indicator of input quality into the teaching process.

Actors and Ownership

Governments originated almost all accreditation schemes considered here.[16] Reasons for their interest in quality assurance were given above. In all cases, the academic community co-operated – willy-nilly perhaps, but co-operated. Willingness to co-operate may be surmised to have been fairly large in Central and Eastern Europe, given the widely shared opinion that after 1989 rapid transformation was highly desirable. The equally understandable desire to protect students in these countries from 'rogue' higher education provision regrettably was almost indistinguishable from 'market protection' by the established public higher education institutions. This resulted in a perverse system in which the underpaid professors of public higher education prevented rapid expansion of the higher education system, thus letting the unmet demand of students persist. It was then catered for by the same professors who made up for their low official income by starting 'rogue' private provision of higher education ('garage universities').[17] Similar problems of planning through state quota or *numerus clausus* leading to large unmet demand can be found in Portugal and Greece for example.

In Western Europe, there was less collusion between the state and the academic oligarchy. Similarly, and more specifically focusing on accreditation, the Dutch addition of accreditation on top of the previously existing external quality assessment scheme was defended explicitly as a means to re-establish trust in quality assurance, which was seen by stakeholders as not providing transparent information on quality (the background for the accreditation pilot by the HBO Council) and as a system of 'mutual backscratching' by the academics from public higher education institutions.

---

16   The exceptions are the professional accreditations in countries like the United Kingdom, Ireland and Portugal, as well as the accreditation (validation) of some (higher) education institutions by other higher education institutions in Ireland and the United Kingdom.

17   An argument made repeatedly and eloquently by the former president of the Free University of Amsterdam, Harry Brinkman.

The Dutch HBO Council in starting its pilot accreditation project reacted to signals from Dutch employers; this provides a clear example of indirect influence of stakeholders. It also provides one of the few examples of this phenomenon, as in most accreditation schemes the state and the academic oligarchy seem to be the only parties involved. Employers or students are mentioned only very rarely in the country reports. One exception is provided by the German *Akkreditierungsrat*, which counts representatives of stakeholders in its governing board (five representatives of professions and two students among the 17 members; there also is a 'students' accreditation pool'). Another is the Hungarian HAC, which counts two student representatives among its non-voting [sic] members.

HAC is also exceptional in inviting international confirmation of its accreditation scheme, most thoroughly in its international, external evaluation of 2001, and more permanently in its International Advisory Board. Another exception to the dominance of state and academe is professional bodies with accrediting power in the United Kingdom: here, the accreditation scheme is owned by the profession, i.e. by an organisation of stakeholders. These accreditation processes cover only a small part of well-organised professions and are intended to control the quality of new entrants into the professional practice. They are not linked directly to the main evaluation scheme in the United Kingdom (see next section). Similarly, engineers and some other professions in Portugal are (going to be) involved in accreditation-like schemes for higher education programmes for their respective professions.

The operational control over the process and quite often also over the criteria and standards in a national accreditation scheme lies, as a rule, with a national separate body which, at least in the operational aspects, is independent from both the government and the higher education institutions. These national accreditation agencies are usually located near the ministry of education, formal laws as a rule give accreditation its authority to make or propose binding decisions. The German *Akkreditierungsrat*, which is co-controlled by the rectors' conference and ministerial bodies, may be furthest from the state apparatus in our sample, but even this finds its basis in the Framework Law for higher education at the German federal level. There is a representative of the education trade union (GEW) in the board of trustees. This is an exception, approached but distantly by the consultation of the trade unions by the Netherlands Accreditation Organisation (NAO) in its initiation of frameworks. The co-decision between the Czech Accreditation Commission and the ministry of education processes on the content of decrees controlling the accreditation process may be an example close to the other extreme of little distance between government and accreditation agency.

The actual evaluation processes in accreditation schemes almost invariably involve external visiting teams. In most accreditation schemes, these are made up of academics and are under the control of the national accreditation agency (this is the general Central and Eastern European model). In Germany and the Netherlands, the 'field work' of evaluation is delegated to independent organisations. In Germany, these independent organisations are even given the right to accredit programmes, while the *Akkreditierungsrat* basically limits itself to recognising these accreditation agencies. In the Netherlands, the Netherlands Accreditation Organisation (NAO) retains the right to give final accreditations, and the 'fieldwork' organisations are called 'visiting and judging institutes'. In both cases, these fieldwork organisations can have different make-ups, including representation by stakeholders such as the professions. The more developed German case would show, however, that the academic oligarchy often controls the fieldwork organisations, although the organisations that accredit a single academic area may well be under the control of the profession (explicitly so when they control access to the labour market, as in Portugal or the United Kingdom). Yet even in professions, governmental control is much greater on most of the Continent than in the two cases mentioned. For instance, German lawyers have to pass a *state* examination before being accepted in the labour market.

Formal Rules and Actual Implementation

As a rule, the process of accreditation follows the steps of self-evaluation resulting in a report used by the external review committee that will perform a site visit. The review committee's report will lead to a publication of some sort (van Vught & Westerheijden, 1994). However, in accreditation schemes the publication stage is more complicated. Review teams report to the fieldwork organisation that in turn reports to the national accreditation agency (Germany, the Netherlands), or report to the national accreditation agency directly (Central and Eastern Europe). After further deliberation that may include hearing the evaluated unit's response, the national accreditation agency then publishes its decision (accreditation yes or no – the 'no' often remaining implicit to avoid embarrassment) and in most cases also a more detailed review report.

The validity of an accreditation, once given, stretches from two to ten years. Both extremes are found with British professional bodies. More commonly, validity is four (France), five (NAO for Dutch programmes), or eight years (NAO for Flemish programmes). However, most accreditation schemes are too young to have gone through more than one cycle; therefore it remains to be seen whether the frequencies mentioned will be kept.[18]

---

18 Hämäläinen *et al.* rightly point to programme accreditation as a costly arrangement, and for that reason in the future institutional accreditation may become more common, after a first round of checking all programmes of study (Hämäläinen et al., 2001, pp. 12, 10).

Appeal Procedures

As accreditation, especially state-associated accreditation, may have serious consequences, including closure of existing units of higher education institutions, checks and balances may well be expected to be part of the scheme. One of the ways to achieve this is a two-step process, with an independent vetting of the external review team's judgement by the larger accreditation commission (customary in the US and the Netherlands). In schemes under private law and which are not obligatory, this may be the only checking needed. Another form, which may be more appropriate in cases of official links to governmental decisions, might be appeal to the normal judiciary system. Thirdly, special appeals bodies may be set up to handle complaints (Norway). Finally, incomplete schemes, without checks and balances, may exist as well (as in the Czech Republic, Hungary, Poland).

Consequences of Accreditation

The typical consequences of accreditation, already referred to briefly in the first passage of this section, include the accreditation agency or the government conferring on the higher education institution the status of a certain type of higher education institution, the right to offer a study programme for a certain academic degree as well as the duty for the government to distribute funds for the operation of the programme (often: for a certain number of student places). In the Netherlands, the government's pledge to link its funding to accreditation status is limited to public higher education institutions (in colleges only up to the bachelor's level).

In most countries, the statements made by accreditation agencies are seen officially as advice to the minister of education. However, this advice is not to be taken lightly; in some countries (e.g. the Czech Republic), the minister's rights to diverge from the accreditation committee's advice are delineated in the law on higher education.

For higher education institutions, the funding effect may be seen from two points of view: first, accreditation as a prerequisite, but second, accredited status makes a programme or institution more attractive to students, which in systems where funding depends on student numbers may lead to more funded student places.

From the student's point of view, accreditation means the possibility of obtaining a recognised degree (in the *de jure* or *de facto* controlled professions this may be the only way to enter the labour market) and access to their usual rights (e.g. study grants or loans, free public transport).

Employers (including the public sector) may use the accredited status of a programme or institution as an argument in their decision to recruit one graduate rather than another – in professions with controlled access to the labour market, accreditation may even be a necessity. Similarly, evaluation results may influence employers'

perception of the reputation of programmes or institutions, which again may influence recruitment decisions or decisions to close research or education contracts with
certain higher education institutions. From a research point of view, these are, however, expectations or hypotheses rather than statements undergirded by empirical
research results (Portugal).

Funding and Fees

There are different patterns of covering the costs of accreditations. On the one hand,
there are cases (as in the Czech Republic, Hungary, Poland) where the government
covers all costs. On the other, there are cases where the marginal costs for accreditations must be covered by the higher education institutions while the fixed costs for
maintaining the national accreditation agency are borne by the government (e.g.
Germany, the Netherlands).

Comparison with Accreditation in the United States of America

Accreditation is seen in European higher education as a new phenomenon. Apart
from the 'niches' of specialised accreditation in the United Kingdom (and Portugal
and some other countries), it was only introduced as a main instrument in national
higher education policy, as we saw above, after the fall of communism in 1989. At
that time, however, accreditation had already been in use for a century in the United
States of America. It had greatly changed over the decades. The first national problem to be solved by accreditation was the entrance of students to higher education
institutions: 'At its start, accreditation began with a problem of definition (What is a
high school? A college? A medical school?) and the problem of articulation between
high schools and colleges and between institutions of higher education.' (Young et
al., 1983). With the Higher Education Act of 1952, accreditation started to figure in
federal governmental policies. By 1990, it had become the main instrument by
which 'an institution or its programs are recognised as meeting *minimum acceptable
standards*' (Adelman, 1992). And it continued to change since it influenced developments in Central and Eastern Europe in the early 1990s. But accreditation's principles remained the same, and we now wish to focus on those underlying principles
in order to compare schemes on the two sides of the Atlantic.

First of all, accreditation is voluntary in the U.S.A., in contrast to the obligatory
character it has in most European countries. The voluntary character must be taken
with a pinch of salt, as non-accreditation implies serious consequences for most
higher education institutions, and as states within the U.S.A. often require their public higher education institutions to be accredited, like in Europe. The consequences
of non-accreditation are different for different types of accreditation and in different
fields of study, as will be illustrated below.

There are two types of accreditation in the U.S.A. The most widespread is *institutional accreditation*. This focuses on the characteristics of the institution as a whole, such as educational offerings (and their outcomes – learning outcomes assessment has been an important innovation in U.S. quality assurance in recent decades, instigated by governmental demands), services to students, financial conditions of the institution, and its administrative strength. It is widespread – covering more than 6,400 institutions in 2002 (Eaton, 2003) – because of its consequences, which include eligibility of the institution for certain federal research funds, and eligibility of its students for federal support programmes. There are very few higher education institutions that can afford to let such good income options pass them by. Therefore, it is not just the public higher education institutions that may be required by their state governments to obtain accreditation that undergo this, but also many private higher education institutions, including highly prestigious ones. The category of institutions least accredited includes those that are not research-intensive and that are not dependent on students who are eligible for supports and grants (i.e. full-time students). In other words, the category of institutions that are least accredited includes the teaching-only low-prestige, for-profit[19] private colleges.

Institutional accreditation is operated by six 'regional' agencies that each serve most higher education institutions in a number of states. For specialised institutions, e.g. religious ones, there are institutional accreditation agencies that operate throughout the U.S.A. These accreditation agencies also oversee many for-profit colleges (Eaton, 2003).

The second type is *professional* or *specialised accreditation*. This is accreditation of study programmes against standards of the profession associated with that field and it often secures (easier) access to the profession for graduates of accredited programmes. The specialised accreditation agencies, of which there are about 70, operate nation-wide. In most fields concerned there is a single agency, but in some cases there are two agencies from which programmes might choose. This is the case, for instance, in business studies and for teacher training.

The main contrast between the U.S.A. and Europe is that programme-level evaluation and accreditation in Europe as a rule apply across the board to all fields of knowledge, but that in the U.S.A. (as in the 'old' specialised accreditation in the UK) it is applied only to fields in a strong and organised profession. Examples of such fields include the traditional academic professions such as medicine and law, the younger (para-)medical professions such as nursing, engineering, business administration, social work, etc. Also included are fields with strong state interest in

---

19 Many of the highly prestigious private universities were founded on a not-for-profit, philanthropic basis.

the profession, the prime example of which is teacher training. Not included are the 'pure' academic programmes (e.g. sociology in contrast to social work).

Usually, specialised accreditation will only analyse programmes in higher education institutions that have already been accredited institutionally. Implicit in the professional character of specialised accreditation is that criteria and standards are strongly influenced by the profession, rather than by academic interests. This is not to say that in the voluntary associations that co-ordinate and operate the accreditation activities, academics are not represented, but the outlook of the whole process is the functioning of practitioners in the non-academic labour market. This contrasts with the strong academic influence in most accreditation schemes in Europe, especially in university sectors of higher education systems, where the main thrust of programme accreditation seems to be acceptance of students for further academic studies (especially in the transition from bachelor to master level), even though the Bologna Declaration introduced 'employability' into the equation.

We already emphasised that accreditation in the U.S.A. is, in principle, voluntary. Hence the organisations that co-ordinate and operate the accreditation activities are basically membership organisations made up of – and paid by (Adelman, 1992) – academics and professionals (the latter are predominant in the case of specialised accreditation) and higher education institutions (in the case of institutional accreditation).

Voluntary organisation implies that the recognition of accreditation agencies is less straightforward than the foundation in law, which is the principal model in Europe. There are two recognition schemes in the U.S.A. First, recognition by the umbrella body of accreditation organisations, the Council for Higher Education Accreditation (CHEA). This is important for accreditation agencies to reassure the public that it follows accepted standards of good practice in accreditation. The genesis of the national umbrella organisations that were CHEA's predecessors, starting in 1949, shows many parallels with discussions after 1998 in Europe around the membership of ENQA (Chambers, 1983).

Second, there is recognition by the federal government. This is very important for most accreditation agencies, as only governmental recognition counts to make students eligible for federal support. The lists of agencies recognised by CHEA and by the U.S. federal government correlate strongly, but not completely: some of the circa 80 agencies are recognised by only one of the two.

Because they are membership organisations, accountable firstly to their members, each accreditation agency defines its own procedures and criteria. Some tendencies towards uniformity result from the self-regulatory co-ordination among the agencies and from the indirect influence of the federal government's criteria to gain its recognition. Institutional accreditation criteria focus on the institution's resources and on its processes, including quality assurance processes. In quality assurance, the institution's focus on student learning outcomes has been emphasised since the early 1990s, especially since the federal government began to demand such information (Eaton, 2003). Specialised accreditation also collects information on whether student learning outcomes relate to the requirements of the profession. The criteria concerning the programmes reviewed tended to be based on curriculum requirements. Since the announcement of the 'ABET 2000' criteria that focus on student learning outcomes while leaving the curriculum definition mostly to the individual engineering programmes, this has also been the main thrust of development, in teacher training and some other areas. This has a European parallel in the focus on outcomes in terms of graduate competences in a number of European accreditation systems which are based on what we have called the 'Dublin Descriptors' and the 'Tuning' project outcomes.

1.3.3 Evaluation in More Detail

Coverage

As mentioned above (§ 1.2), the beginnings of quality assurance in Western Europe were in the area of evaluation, not accreditation. Because of the different policy interests, but also considerations of institutional autonomy, the emphases were different. In many cases, the programme level was targeted for evaluation ('quality assessment'), as it would give the most detailed information, whether for accountability or for improvement purposes. To stress the higher education institution's responsibility for quality as an expression of its autonomy, in some cases quality audits of the institution were the main mechanism of evaluation in Sweden and the United Kingdom (for some periods). In the United Kingdom, the size of the higher education system, and hence the costs of a programme level evaluation scheme, may have been another reason for the initial focus on the institutional level. In 2001, the 'evaluation fatigue' that spurred the 'revolt' of the higher education institutions against the QAA schemes of the late 1990s clearly focused on the costs (in terms of money and manpower) of programme level assessments for the universities.

Where higher education institutions as a whole are evaluated, there is a tendency to analyse the institutions' arrangements for quality assurance rather than their teaching or research directly (although this was the aim of the 'total evaluations' in Finland). Such 'quality audits' were the mainstay of evaluation in Sweden (before 2001), Ireland (university sector, from 2003 onwards),[20] and in the United Kingdom (espe-

---

20 In 2003, the HEA announced it would begin to audit the universities' quality assurance arrangements (Conference of Heads of Irish Universities, 2003).

cially England, since Scotland has its own arrangements) in the periods mentioned in the table.

Table 7. Unit of judgement in evaluation schemes

Programme of study	Higher education institution
FR (sometimes), NL (pre-2003), PT, SE (after 2001), GB (1992–2002)	FI, FR (regular case), SE (pre-2001), GB (before 1997 + since 2002), IR (as from 2003)

Geographically, the aim of all countries' governments seems to be to cover all parts of the country. In federal states, therefore, a set of regional evaluation agencies is aimed at (Spain), although in Germany until bachelor's and master's programmes become universal (cf. Schwarz-Hahn & Rehburg, 2004), most of the country will not be covered by formal evaluation activities (main exception: Lower Saxony with ZEvA).

As a rule, government-initiated or government-supported evaluation schemes cover all public higher education institutions or programmes. In Flanders and in the Netherlands, separate evaluation schemes existed for universities and for colleges (before the introduction of accreditation in 2003).

Actors and Ownership

In the sub-section on actors and ownership in accreditation schemes (see § 1.3.2), we mentioned that co-operation between state and academe was not very close. The 'ideal type' of this would be the development of evaluation schemes in the United Kingdom under the Thatcher government, which was a clear example of evaluation as an instrument which showed a dramatic lack of trust in the performance of the (university part of) the higher education system (Trow, 1994, 1996), while ostensibly maintaining the institutions' autonomy.

A logical prerequisite for any quality assurance scheme (accreditation or evaluation) to function properly is the existence of an internal quality assurance system within the higher education institutions. While this is not the focus of our study, it is interesting to note that internal quality assurance is mentioned explicitly in higher education laws in Hungary and Norway.

The evaluators, i.e. the members of review teams, mainly come from the academic world. However, involving a minority representation of other stakeholders (professions, employers) is widespread practice (Flanders, France, the Netherlands pre-2003, Norway, Portugal, Sweden). In fewer cases, student representatives also take part in the external review teams (the Netherlands pre-2003, Sweden).

Formal Rules and Actual Implementation

The total duration of evaluation processes is about one year. This was also the approximate duration of evaluation activities (Flanders, France, the Netherlands pre-2003[21]), although exceptions exist in many higher education systems for different reasons.

Consequences of Evaluation

Consequences of evaluation depended heavily on the functions for which it was introduced. If accountability was the main aim, and if governments stopped short of official recognition decisions (which would transform the evaluation scheme into accreditation), there may have been few direct consequences.

If quality improvement was a main aim, giving consequences to evaluation was normally in the hands of the higher education institutions being evaluated. After all, it is within the higher education institution that quality of education is 'produced'; paraphrasing Dill: quality cannot be 'inspected in' from the outside (Dill, 1995). One might equally question whether collecting officially required data – even setting up special *observatoires* for that purpose (France, Italy) – gives an impetus to the higher education institution's desire to engage in quality management, or whether it is seen as just another bureaucratic burden to be executed, bearing as little connection to the 'inner life' of the higher education institution as possible? (Higher education institutions have been known as 'loosely coupled' organisations anyway (Weick, 1976), but this could add to the looseness.)

In some countries, different official arrangements to monitor – and in that way ensure – follow-up were introduced (e.g. Flanders, the United Kingdom, the Netherlands pre-2003, Sweden) (Scheele et al., 1998). Research led to the conclusion, however, that 'really poor teaching' (as it was characterised in the United Kingdom) may have been weeded out but above the actual threshold level of quality (i.e. as long as one does not get too heavy criticism from the review teams) the impetus for quality improvement from external evaluations remained rare (Jeliazkova & Westerheijden, 2000; Jeliazkova & Westerheijden, 2002).

To the extent that information was aimed at through evaluation, the proof of the pudding would be that students made more informed choices in selecting their location of study. Actual empirical research on this question was not mentioned in the reports underlying the present study. Anecdotal evidence seems to suggest that for prospective students in well-provided public higher education systems such as in

---

21 This period was the rule in the Netherlands for the universities; with the substantially larger number of study programmes to be reviewed in the colleges, review processes from initiation to publication of the national report could take up to two years for the HBO Council.

North-Western Europe, other arguments were more important in their choice than perceived quality differences (e.g. where did friends go to study, distance from the parents' home).

With regard to the consequences of evaluation for government decision-making, opinions still remain divided on the paradoxical situation (Westerheijden, 1990) between the standpoint that real consequences, i.e. incremental or decremental funding, are necessary to take evaluation seriously, and the standpoint that attaching real consequences to evaluation turns it into a power game where the results count more than the quality. As a way out of this paradox, many governments have stated that evaluation results may inform funding, but in a non-formulaic way (the United Kingdom, the Netherlands pre -2003), e.g. through contract negotiations (France).

Funding and Fees

In the United Kingdom and the Netherlands (pre-2003), for example, the costs of external evaluation are paid for by the higher education institutions, basically by subscribing to the umbrella body (VSNU, HBO Council) or quality assurance body (QAA). QAA is a hybrid case: most tasks (hence much of its funding) are contracted to it by the Funding Councils for England, Scotland and Wales – i.e. it is indirectly funded by the government.

In most other country cases, evaluation agencies are state agencies, funded by the government budget.

1.3.4 Approval in More Detail

Approval was defined at the outset as granting a programme or unit the right to exist. In principle, this was the way to create new study programmes or (public) higher education institutions, faculties, etc. in state-controlled systems. Traditionally, approval was a task for a minister of education and the decisions were prepared, as all ministerial decisions, by civil servants. While the principles of bureaucratic decision-making (in its value-neutral, Weberian sense) are division of labour and application of expert knowledge, nowadays it is increasingly accepted that civil servants do not possess sufficient expert knowledge for their decisions (technically: proposals for ministerial decisions) to carry legitimacy with the academic community. This may have been one of the reasons for the rise of evaluation and accreditation.

From this arises the issue of the expertise needed for a legitimate approval decision. In other words, where is the borderline between approval and accreditation? In Weber's ideal type analysis, this question had a simple answer. Approval is advice given for a decision made by (permanent) civil servants, within the ministry, based on paper evidence collected either by the ministry or by its agent. This agent could be an intermediary body or a public higher education institution – in the ideal type state hierarchy it is not material where in the chain of command information is collected. At the other extreme, accreditation is performed by academic peers working in (*ad hoc*) committees in a collegial rather than a hierarchical manner (Clark, 1983) on the basis of site visits, including interviews, as much as on paper evidence. However, as Weber wanted to emphasise in introducing ideal type reasoning, the world is not as clear-cut. We find cases where external bodies involving academic reviewers prepare (and pre-judge) ministerial approval decisions on paper evidence without site visits (Lithuania), or with a site visit by quality assessment agency staff (Denmark). In contrast, in a curious mix of traditional bureaucracy, new public management and collegial academic control, we also find cases where civil servants negotiate recurrent contracts with higher education institutions about time-limited approval of study programmes, sometimes advised by experts from different intermediary bodies (France). In sum, it remains impossible to decide once and for all how much 'evaluation' is needed to call 'approval' 'accreditation'. In some cases, it depended on national political sensitivities or on the way the authors of country reports interpreted our definitions whether certain decision-making processes were called 'approval' or 'accreditation'.

Coverage

As a rule, approval is required for all higher education units, and often also for all individual study programmes. The essence of approval, i.e. the ministerial decision to grant programmes or institutions the right to exist, remains a key element in European higher education systems. Especially, as higher education authorities in Europe have made clear time and again that higher education is seen as a public good. Moreover, other actors and stakeholders generally hold the same view: they want government recognition of the degree(s) and government funding of the programme or institution. Yet there are higher education systems in which private institutions can operate without government approval (e.g. Denmark, but not applying for approval implies no funding).

Private funding and private accreditation are generally only seen as equally or more relevant than governmental approval in some areas, such as postgraduate MBA programmes. Hence, the approval decision can be seen as the culmination of approval, accreditation and even some evaluation processes in the countries involved.

Actors and Ownership

The main actor in any approval scheme is, by definition, the top higher education authority in a higher education system. As a rule, this is the national government. Even in federal countries, where regional state governments may share part of the authority (e.g. Spain, Germany), national laws set the framework under which regional states operate. The extreme case of devolution may be Belgium, where the language communities each decide their own legal decrees, which may even include funding arrangements, independently from the national government.

Formal Rules and Actual Implementation

In the country reports, no indications were given of major discrepancies between formal rules regarding approval and their actual implementation. Although this may well be the case, it may also reflect the focus of attention of the country reports. We concentrated on the accreditation and evaluation schemes, taking the approval schemes as a point of departure and did not elaborate much on problems arising from them.

Consequences of Approval

Our definition of 'approval' was that it granted a unit or programme the right to exist. With this key decision invariably come other rights, unless accreditation or evaluation schemes have been introduced to help make those further decisions. These rights include the recognition of degrees (or the autonomy to award degrees), and government funding according to a given process or algorithm.

Funding and Fees

Governmental approval is free of charge in all higher education institutions in the countries under study. In other words, it is paid for by the government authority that performs it.

1.4   Drivers and Dynamics

Actors involved in an evaluation or accreditation scheme learn during its implementation (as one of us stated in Huitema, Jeliazkova, & Westerheijden, 2002). For example, staff and leadership in institutions learn the art of self-evaluation. Learning leads to changes in the way actors in the higher education system behave. This is what is intended: giving greater attention to the quality of teaching is a precondition for quality improvement. However, once the 'easy wins' have been called as a result of a successful first round of evaluations, a second (unchanged) round cannot add as much quality improvement or accountability as the first did. Routine, bureaucratisation and window dressing are dangers lurking behind. To counteract these tendencies, quality assurance systems need to be designed with a built-in facility for positive change. This can be seen as an *internal* drive for dynamism in evaluation and accreditation schemes. Moreover, there is a – loosely hierarchical – scale of perceived problems which quality assurance systems are expected to address. Tackling one problem (a political decision or compromise and a temporal state of affairs, not necessarily an actual solution to the issue) exposes another one. Attempts to address a 'subsequent' problem may be futile before a 'more basic' one has been brought to closure. We single out these changes in the *immediate* context of quality assurance systems as *contextual dynamics*. Both internal and external drives would lead any evaluation scheme to evolve from checking basic quality through accreditation-like processes, through efficiency-enhancing measures, to quality improvement and quality culture enhancing schemes (Campbell & Rozsnyai, 2002; Huitema et al., 2002). But this inherent logic is not visible in most countries' developments, which ostensibly do not follow the progression of phases proposed in that paper. External dynamics are apparently more important. What are the main drivers in the context of higher education policy that influence the dynamics of evaluation, accreditation and approval schemes, according to the country reports?

For Hämäläinen et al., a central question was 'Why has accreditation become a central issue?' They gave three answers (Hämäläinen et al., 2001, pp. 14–17):

- 'Trust and accountability', i.e. the New Public Management agenda;
- 'A common labour market and student mobility requirements', i.e. the Bologna agenda;
- 'Borderless markets for higher education', i.e. the globalisation agenda, leading to 'proliferation of accreditation systems' starting in the USA and even to the rise of some 'trans-national accreditation systems'.

Our findings underscore these earlier answers, even though we focus on the Bologna agenda.

Chronologically, the first main changes to traditional state-centred steering of higher education occurred in some Western European countries during the 1980s. Researchers on higher education have monitored and analysed these developments since (e.g. Neave, 1988, 1994, 1998, 2002; van Vught, 1988). Of course, governments had engaged in restructuring higher education systems before, but in contrast to the big reform projects of the 1960s and 1970s (cf. Cerych & Sabatier, 1986), the 'philosophy' underlying the changes in the 1980s was the rise of New Public Management (amongst many others, cf. McKevitt & Lawton, 1994; Pollitt & Bouckaert, 2000). For higher education, this implied more emphasis on self-regulation, apparently inaugurating a renewed era of institutional autonomy. However, this new autonomy was only given in exchange for increased accountability to (the rest of) government and society, and thus evaluation schemes were introduced in one Western European higher education system after another, as the country reports in this volume show.

The first large-scale appearance of accreditation in the higher education systems of Europe was an immediate consequence of the post-Communist transformation in the Central and Eastern European countries from 1990 onwards (see also § 1.2 above).

As long as higher education was under strict government control, i.e. until 1989 in Central and Eastern European countries, accreditation as an independent check on minimum quality was not necessary for those societies. It was only when the market was opened to private and foreign providers, and in a period when government control was suspect because the transition from Communism was still incomplete, that accreditation surfaced as the option that carried most credibility in society. Its character of independent, non-political, academic expert opinion was highly valued. In theoretical terms, this can be seen as a mixture of the globalisation agenda (foreign providers) and the neo-liberal ideas that were popular in reaction to Communism and underlied the New Public Management agenda (private higher education provision, less government intervention).

Before then, and continuing alongside the large-scale accreditation schemes, some professions in certain countries were already accrediting study programmes. This required two enabling factors: on the one hand a certain level of organisation and self-regulation within the professions, and on the other a certain degree of independence from state control. Hence, the bar association in the United Kingdom and Ireland had developed accreditation procedures, while in Germany and similar countries entry to the legal profession was controlled by the government through a *Staatsexamen*. In this German examination, legal professionals set the standards and take the examinations, but under the authority of the state, not of their own profession. In addition to these enabling factors, a demand factor was needed, as shown by two of the other standard examples: business studies and engineering. These fields have a relatively highly developed international labour market. Demand from employers and students for clear information about the qualities of the study programmes (and their 'typical' graduates) may therefore also be expected to be highly developed. This paragraph, then, points to another aspect of the development of an international or European labour market, which is not clearly encapsulated in the Bologna process, and although encompassing many aspects, remains focused on state-driven and state-oriented evaluation and accreditation schemes, rather than on the independent role of the professions.

It was only with the Sorbonne and Bologna Declarations that a situation arose in Western European countries' higher education systems that was somewhat similar to the one in the Central and Eastern European countries, and led to introduction of the same instrument of accreditation. Although it was an assumption that underlied our entire project, so that we could be accused of being biased, the country reports underline that the Bologna Declaration was a key driver for the change towards accreditation schemes in Western Europe. At the same time, the fact that all the countries in this volume are signatories of the Bologna Declaration implies that it influences all European policies with regard to evaluation and accreditation. Yet, given that the starting positions of the countries were so different, the impact of the Bologna Declaration varies across the countries. In Western Europe, a discussion about accreditation has been launched, leading to reactions ranging from rejection (Denmark) to rapid introduction (above all Germany). In Central and Eastern Europe, the Bologna process occurs in the context of the region's reintegration in Europe and the preparation for membership in the European Union (e.g. Latvian and Polish country reports). Reintegration has been part of the outlook since 1990, so this European dimension may have been strengthened since 1999, but it did not require a very great change of direction in the accreditation schemes.

Its importance at the level of policy-makers does not automatically entail that the Bologna discussion permeates all the European higher education systems. The *Trends III* report notes that, according to its survey:

> In Estonia, Lithuania, Sweden, Germany, Ireland and most strongly the UK, deliberations on institutional Bologna reforms are even less widespread than in the other Bologna signatory countries. (Reichert & Tauch, 2003, p. 9.)

First of all, this implies – in its almost sarcastic phrasing – that the Bologna discussion is not high on the agenda beyond the circles of those who have a professional interest. Second, this finding mingles countries from all over Europe with and without two-cycle study structures as less than averagely interested in the Bologna discussion. Hence, what may be the driving factors for the Bologna discussion being high on the academic community's agenda cannot be found in obvious systemic factors and our country reports do not give insight into this question either. The insights that they do give are the subject of our final section.

1.5 Conclusions

1.5.1 System Dynamics

In Central and Eastern Europe, the main driving force for introducing accreditation was the transformation after 1989. In Western Europe, the Bologna Declaration spurred new design activities with regard to quality assurance, often in the form of accreditation schemes (Germany, the Netherlands, Norway, Spain and most recently Portugal). In some Western countries, the self-organisation of some professions must also be mentioned as a driver for (non-state) accreditation and evaluation schemes (the United Kingdom, Portugal).

Internal politics were among the main driving forces in Germany. The federal system with shared responsibility of higher education between the states (*Länder*) and the federal level (*Bund*) made the higher education system extremely resistant to change. The Sorbonne and Bologna Declarations may thus be interpreted as creating external pressure to overcome internal inertia (van der Wende & Westerheijden, 2001).

An additional impetus to establish or improve quality assurance schemes with an official nature seems to come from the press. University rankings are a major seller for weekly magazines in several countries (e.g. Germany, the Netherlands, Norway, Poland, Sweden, the United Kingdom), and the sometimes scathing methodical comments from higher education institutions or researchers (e.g. Yorke, 1998) and ministerial officials seem to call for an attitude that could be summarised as: 'we had rather do something (better) ourselves'. Partly as a response to this attitude, partly as a driver for magazines to become interested, in many countries ministries of education or umbrella bodies of higher education institutions publish annual 'performance indicator' lists (e.g. France, the United Kingdom, the Netherlands). International agencies also publish regular information often regarded as performance indicators for countries in international competition (OECD's annual *Education at a Glance*, EU's recent 'open co-ordination mechanism').

1.5.2   Development and Reform

The Bologna process is an obvious driver for change with regard to quality in steering mechanisms.[22] Germany, the Netherlands, Norway and Spain are cases where accreditation has been introduced on Bologna-associated arguments. In France, the introduction of a new master's degree has been argued on the same grounds and will be accompanied by some form of accreditation, although the scheme is still being debated. In the United Kingdom, it seems that in a recent policy paper entitled the 'Future of higher education' Bologna and European issues can be glossed over when making reference to international issues.

Already in the 1990s, active 'mimicking' or borrowing of evaluation and accreditation schemes took place on a large scale (Robertson & Waltman, 1992; van Vught, 1996). In some cases, there seemed to be just one obvious example in the world, which explains why in practically all documentation on accreditation schemes the USA plays an important (if often misunderstood) role. In most cases, however, there were several possible role models, but only one was chosen. For instance, Irish arrangements were and still are based on (some parts of) the British example because much of the Irish institutional arrangement for steering higher education was similar to the higher education system in the United Kingdom (the occasion for which cardinal Newman formulated the 'British' higher education philosophy was the opening of a university in Ireland). Accordingly, similar effects could be expected from borrowing new policy instruments, thus increasing the chance of achieving desired aims and decreasing the chance of unintended and undesired consequences. Similar pat-

---

22   In some of these countries, broader changes have been initiated as well, notably in degree structures (e.g. Italy, the Netherlands, to some extent Germany). Ireland is a major case, showing the influence of the European level in the expansion of the higher education system.

terns of cultural and institutional pre-dispositions to turn to a certain model can be found elsewhere – this is the very reason why we are able to recognise certain regions within Europe. On the other hand, some proponents of certain evaluation schemes were active 'sellers' of their model; the popularity of the 'Dutch model' of evaluation in the 1990s can to some extent be explained by this (Flanders, Denmark, Portugal).

However, in borrowing (some elements) of models for evaluation or accreditation from other countries, adaptations have to be made to the new context in which the model is being introduced. This is good policy, as instruments have to be fitted into an existing legal, institutional etc. framework, yet it makes the question of what one higher education system can learn from another much more difficult. Thus, while both Denmark and Portugal claimed to have used the Dutch evaluation as a model, they were rather different from one another as well as from the original. Moreover, some complexities of the American accreditation and evaluation schemes cannot be copied easily in European countries, e.g. those that have to do with the limited influence of the government in the USA and with the differential treatment of professional as against other programmes of study.

The dynamics of quality assurance schemes (evaluation and accreditation alike), explaining how they are connected to social problems/situations to which they are supposed to respond, have been mentioned at the beginning of this chapter. Yet, there are also internal dynamics involved, with 'easy wins' being made in early iterations and dangers of 'bureaucratisation' and 'window dressing' lurking if quality assurance schemes are copied without sufficient modifications (Jeliazkova & Westerheijden, 2002). The importance of internal dynamics and how they relate to the development of evaluation or accreditation schemes can be demonstrated clearly in the United Kingdom as well as in Greece, where after many years of controversial preparation, the establishment of a National Quality Assurance and Evaluation Committee was proposed in March 2003.

Finally, we should remember that in whatever form we put the assurance of quality, quality of higher education is one of the main drivers of the Bologna process:

> ... together with the preparation of graduates for a European labour market, it is the improvement of academic quality which is seen as the most important driving force of the Bologna process, not just at the institutional level but also at the level of governments and rectors conferences. (Reichert & Tauch, 2003, p. 100.)

Seen from that perspective, that is to say looking at our subject from the opposite point of view, accreditation and evaluation schemes are major factors in shaping the European Higher Education Area. Our hope is that readers, arriving at the end of this chapter, may have a clearer picture of where developments are taking us – and where they themselves may take developments.

References

Adelman, C. (1992). Accreditation. In B. R. Clark & G. Neave (Eds.), *The encyclopedia of higher education* (Vol. 1, pp. 1313-1318). Oxford: Pergamon.

Birnbaum, R. (2000). The Life Cycle of Academic Management Fads. *Journal of Higher Education, 71*(1), 1-16.

Brennan, J., & Shah, T. (2000). *Managing quality in higher education: an international perspective on institutional assessment and change.* Buckingham: Open University.

Brignall, S., & Modell, S. (2000). An institutional perspective on performance measurement and management in the 'new public sector'. *Management Accounting Research, 11*(3), 281-306.

Campbell, C., & Rozsnyai, K. (2002). *Quality Assurance and the Development of Course Programmes.* Bucharest: CEPES-UNESCO.

Centre for Quality Assurance and Evaluation of Higher Education (1998). *Evaluation of European Higher Education: A status report prepared for the European Commission, DG XXII.* Copenhagen: Centre for Quality Assurance and Evaluation of Higher Education.

Cerych, L. (1993). Editorial. *European Journal of Education, 28*, 377-378.

Cerych, L., & Sabatier, P. (1986). *Great Expectations and Mixed Performance: The Implementation of Higher Education Reforms in Europe.* Stoke-on-Trent: Trentham.

Chambers, C. M. (1983). Council on Postsecondary Accreditation. In K. E. Young & associates (Eds.), *Understanding Accreditation: contemporary perspectives on issues and practices in evaluating educational quality* (pp. 289-314). San Francisco: Jossey-Bass.

Clark, B. R. (1983). *The Higher Education System: Academic Organization in Cross-National Perspective.* Berkeley: University of California Press.

Conference of Heads of Irish Universities (2003). *A Framework for Quality in Irish Universities.* Dublin: Conference of Heads of Irish Universities.

Danish Evaluation Institute (2003). *Quality Procedures in European Higher Education: An ENQA Survey* (ENQA Occasional Papers 5). Helsinki: European Network for Quality Assurance in Higher Education.

Dill, D. D. (1995). *Through Deming's eyes: A cross-national analysis of quality assurance policies in higher education.* Paper presented at the INQAAHE 3rd meeting, Utrecht.

Eaton, J. (2003). *Is Accreditation Accountable? The Continuing Conversation Between Accreditation and the Federal Government* (CHEA Monograph Series 2003, Number 1). Washington, D.C.: Council for Higher Education Accreditation.

Enders, J. (2002). *Governing the Academic Commons: About blurring boundaries, blistering organisations, and growing demands* (J. File, Trans.). Enschede: Universiteit Twente.

EUA, & ESIB (2002). *EUA and ESIB Joint Declaration: Students and universities: An academic community on the move.* Paris.

Farrington, D. J. (2001). Borderless Higher Education: Challenges to Regulation, Accreditation and Intellectual Property Rights. *Minerva, 39*(1), 63-84.

Hämäläinen, K., Haakstad, J., Kangasniemi, J., Lindeberg, T., & Sjölund, M. (2001). *Quality Assurance in the Nordic Higher Education: Accreditation-like practices* (ENQA Occasional Papers 2). Helsinki: European Network for Quality Assurance in Higher Education.

Haug, G. (1999). *Trends and issues in learning structures in higher education in Europe.* Paper presented at the Confederation of European Rectors' Conferences and European Association of Universities CRE, Genève.

Hendrichová, J. (1998). Typical Features of Education and Higher Education Reforms in Central Europe. In E. Leitner (Ed.), *Educational Research and Higher Education Reform in Central and Eastern Europe* (pp. 75-85). Frankfurt a.d. Main: Peter Lang.

Huitema, D., Jeliazkova, M., & Westerheijden, D. F. (2002). Phases, Levels and Circles in Policy Development: The Cases of Higher Education and Environmental Quality Assurance. *Higher Education Policy, 15*(3-4).

Jeliazkova, M. (2001). Running the maze: interpreting external review recommendations. *Quality in Higher Education, 8*(1), 89-96.

Jeliazkova, M., & Westerheijden, D. F. (2000). *Het zichtbare eindresultaat.* Den Haag: Algemene Rekenkamer.

Jeliazkova, M., & Westerheijden, D. F. (2002). Systemic adaptation to a changing environment: Towards a next generation of quality assurance models. *Higher Education, 44*(3-4), 433-448.

Kern, B. (1998). A European Union Perspective on Follow Up. In J. P. Scheele & P. A. M. Maassen & D. F. Westerheijden (Eds.), *To be continued...: Follow-up of quality assurance in higher education* (pp. 39-63). Maarssen: Elsevier/De Tijdstroom.

Lane, J.-E. (2000). *New public management.* London: Routledge.

Machado dos Santos, S. (2000). *Introduction to the theme of transnational education.* Paper presented at the Conference of the Directors General for Higher Education and Heads of the Rectors' Conferences of the European Union, Aveiro.

Management Group. (1995). *European Pilot Project for the Evaluation of Quality in Higher Education: European report.* [Brussels]: European Commission, DG XXII 'Education, Training and Youth'.

McKevitt, D., & Lawton, A. (Eds.). (1994). *Public sector management: Theory, critique and practice.* London: Sage; Open University Press.

Middlehurst, R. (2001). University Challenges: Borderless Higher Education, Today and Tomorrow. *Minerva, 39*(1), 3-26.

Neacsu, I. (1998). Higher Education in Romania: The Imperatives of Reform - New Paradigms, New Options, New Strategies. In E. Leitner (Ed.), *Educational Research and Higher Education Reform in Central and Eastern Europe* (pp. 207-218). Frankfurt a.d. Main: Peter Lang.

Neave, G. (1988). On the cultivation of quality, efficiency and enterprise: An overview of recent trends in higher education in Western Europe, 1986-1988. *European Journal of Education, 23*(1), 7-23.

Neave, G. (1994). The politics of quality: developments in higher education in Western Europe 1992-1994. *European Journal of Education, 29*(2), 115-133.

Neave, G. (1998). The evaluative state reconsidered. *European Journal of Education, 33*(3), 265-284.

Neave, G. (2002). *On stakeholders, Cheshire Cats and Seers: Changing visions of the University.* Enschede: Universiteit Twente.

Pollitt, C., & Bouckaert, G. (2000). *Public management reform: A comparative analysis.* Oxford: Oxford University Press.

Reichert, S., & Tauch, C. (2003). Trends in Learning Structures in European Higher Education III – Bologna four years after: Steps towards sustainable reform of higher education in Europe; First draft. Graz: European University Association; European Commission.

Robertson, D. B., & Waltman, J. L. (1992). The politics of policy borrowing. *Oxford studies in comparative education, 2*(2), 25-48.

Rowley, J. (1996). Measuring Quality in Higher Education. *Quality in Higher Education, 2*(3), 237-255.

Sadlak, J. (1995). In Search of the "Post-Communist" University – The Background and Scenario of the Transformation of Higher Education in Central and Eastern Europe. In K. Hüfner (Ed.), *Higher Education Reform Processes in Central and Eastern Europe* (pp. 43-62). Frankfurt a.d. Main: Peter Lang.

Scheele, J. P. , Maassen, P. A. M., & Westerheijden, D. F. (Eds.). (1998). *To be Continued... : Follow-Up of Quality Assurance in Higher Education.* Maarssen: Elsevier/De Tijdstroom.

Schwarz, S. (Ed.) (2003). *Universities of the Future: Transatlantischer Dialog; Universities of the Future: Research, Knowledge Acquisition, Corporate Identity, and Management Strategies. Transatlantic Conference, Bonn, June 2002.* Dok&Mat, 45/46. Bonn: DAAD.

Schwarz-Hahn, S., & Rehburg, M. (2004). Bachelor and master degrees in Germany: A true reform or just partial changes? Summary of a national empirical study. Kassel: Centre for Research on Higher Education and Work (unpublished).

Schwarz-Hahn, S., & Rehburg, M. (2004). *Bachelor und Master in Deutschland: Empirische Befunde zur Studienstrukturreform.* Münster: Waxmann.

Sursock, A. (2001). *Towards Accreditation Schemes for Higher Education in Europe? Final project report*. Geneva, Switzerland: CRE Association of European Universities.

Teichler, U. (1998). The Role of the European Union in the Internationalization of Higher Education. In P. Scott (Ed.), *The Globalization of Higher Education* (pp. 88-99). Buckingham: SRHE and Open University Press.

Teichler, U. (1998). Towards a European University? In P. Baggen, A. Tellings, & W. van Haaften (Eds.), *The University and the Knowledge Society* (pp. 75-86). Bemmel, London and Paris: Concore.

Teichler, U. (1999). Internationalisation as a Challenge to Higher Education in Europe. *Tertiary Education and Management, 5*(1), 5-23.

Teichler U. (2003). *Master-Level-Programmes and Degrees in Europe: Problems and Opportunities*. Keynote Speech. Bologna Process: International Conference on Master-Level-Degrees. Helsinki, March 14-15, 2003.

Towards the European Higher Education Area: Communiqué of the meeting of European Ministers in charge of Higher Education in Prague on May 19th 2001 (2001). Prague.

Trow, M. (1994). *Academic Reviews and the Culture of Excellence*. Stockholm: Högskoleverket.

Trow, M. (1996). Trust, markets and accountability in higher education: A comparative perspective. *Higher Education Policy, 9*, 309-324.

Tsaoussis, D. G. (Ed.). (1999). *Non-Official Higher Education in the European Union*. Athens: Gutenberg Publications.

Uvalic-Tumbic, S. (Ed.). (2002). *Globalization and the Market in Higher Education: Quality, Accreditation and Qualifications*. London; Paris; Geneva: Economica.

Vroeijenstijn, A. I. (1989). *Autonomy and assurance of quality: two sides of one coin*. Paper presented at the International Conference on Assessing Quality in HE, Cambridge.

Vroeijenstijn, T. I. (2003). *Similarities and Differences in Accreditation: Looking for a common framework* (Document prepared for the workshop on the establishment of a European Consortium for Accreditation (ECA)). Den Haag: Netherlands Accreditation Organisation (NAO).

van Vught, F. A. (1988). A New Autonomy in European Higher Education? An Exploration and Analysis of the Strategy of Self-Regulation in Higher Education Governance. *International Journal Institutional Management in Higher Education, 12*.

van Vught, F. A. (1994). Intrinsic and Extrinsic Aspects of Quality Assessment in Higher Education. In D. F. Westerheijden & J. Brennan & P. A. M. Maassen (Eds.), *Changing Contexts of Quality Assessment: Recent Trends in West European Higher Education* (pp. 31-50). Utrecht: Lemma.

van Vught, F. A. (1996). Isomorphism in higher education? Towards a theory of differentiation and diversity in higher education systems. In V. L. Meek & L. C. J. Goedegebuure & O. Kivinen & R. Rinne (Eds.), *The mockers and mocked: Comparative perspectives on differentiation, convergence and diversity in higher education* (pp. 42-58). Oxford: Pergamon.

van Vught, F. A. (Ed.). (1989). *Governmental strategies and innovation in higher education*. London: Jessica Kingsley.

van Vught, F. A., van der Wende, M. C., & Westerheijden, D. F. (2002). Globalization and Internationalization: Policy Agendas Compared. In O. Fulton & J. Enders (Eds.), *Higher Education in a Globalizing World. International Trends and Mutual Observations* (pp. 103-120). Dordrecht: Kluwer.

van Vught, F. A., & Westerheijden, D. F. (1994). Towards a general model of quality assessment in higher education. *Higher Education, 28*, 355-371.

Weick, K. F. (1976). Educational Organizations as Loosely Coupled Systems. *Administrative Science Quarterly, 21*.

van der Wende, M. C., & Westerheijden, D. F. (2001). International aspects of quality assurance with a special focus on European higher education. *Quality in Higher Education, 7*(3), 233-245.

Westerheijden, D. F. (1990). Peers, Performance, and Power: Quality assessment in the Netherlands. In L. C. J. Goedegebuure & P. A. M. Maassen & D. F. Westerheijden (Eds.), *Peer Review and Performance Indicators: Quality assessment in British and Dutch higher education* (pp. 183-207). Utrecht: Lemma.

Westerheijden, D. F., & Leegwater, M. (Eds.). (2003). *Working on the European Dimension of Quality: Report of the conference on quality assurance in higher education as part of the Bologna process, Amsterdam, 12-13 March 2002*. Zoetermeer: Ministerie van Onderwijs, Cultuur en Wetenschappen.

Westerheijden, D. F., & Sorensen, K. (1999). People on a Bridge: Central European higher education institutions in a storm of reform. In B. W. A. Jongbloed & P. A. M. Maassen & G. Neave (Eds.), *From the Eye of the storm: Higher education's changing institution* (pp. 13-38). Dordrecht: Kluwer Academic Publishers.

Weusthof, P. J. M., & Frederiks, M. M. H. (1997). De functies van het stelsel van kwaliteitszorg heroverwogen. *Tijdschrift voor Hoger Onderwijs, 15*, 318-338.

Wnuk-Lipinska, E. (1998). Academic Staff Facing a Changing University. In E. Leitner (Ed.), *Educational Research and Higher Education Reform in Central and Eastern Europe* (pp. 111-122). Frankfurt a.d. Main: Peter Lang.

Yorke, M. (1998). *The Times'* league table of universities, 1997: A statistical appraisal. *Quality Assurance in Education, 6*(1), 58.

Young, K. E., Chambers, C. M., Kells, H. R., & Associates (1983). *Understanding accreditation: contemporary perspectives on issues and practices in evaluating educational quality*. San Francisco: Jossey-Bass.

2 Accreditation and Differentiation: A Policy to Establish New Sectors in Austrian Higher Education

HANS PECHAR & CORNELIA KLEPP

2.1 The Characteristics of the Austrian Higher Education System

2.1.1 Main Components and Size of the System

Austria has 18 public universities, twelve of which are research universities (*Wissenschaftliche Universitäten*) and six are universities of arts *(Universitäten der Künste)*. Since 1999, private universities have been authorised. By 2003, six (very small) private universities – all not-for-profit – had been accredited. 177,000 students were enrolled in the research universities, and 7,500 in the universities for arts, in 2001-02, but no figures were available for the private universities. At present, there is no division into undergraduate and graduate studies. There are only a small number of bachelor's (*Bakk.*) programmes.

The most important and dynamic part of the non-university sector is the *Fachhochschulen* (colleges), established in 1993. Colleges are 'hybrid' institutions: they have private legal status, but public bodies dominate the associations or, when colleges are organised as companies, public bodies are the main shareholders; about 95 % of their funding comes from public sources. At present, there are 19 providers (*Erhalter*), offering a total of 125 study courses. The college sector offers programmes in economics (including administration), technology (including engineering, telecommunication), tourism and now also humanities (e.g. social work).

In addition, there are teacher training colleges (*Pädagogische Akademien*), which only train teachers for compulsory schools, since *Gymnasia* teachers are trained at universities. The teacher training colleges are not considered part of the higher education system. However, it is planned to upgrade these institutions by 2005. There are also colleges for social workers (*Sozialakademien)* and schools for the paramedical professions (*MTD-Schulen*) which have a similar status. They are all public institutions.

Student enrolments for 2001/02 in the non-university sector represented 14,000 in *Fachhochschulen* and in the teacher training colleges, and about 4,000 in the schools for social work and the paramedical professions.

S. Schwarz and D.F. Westerheijden (eds.),
Accreditation and Evaluation in the European Higher Education Area, 43–64.
© 2004 *Kluwer Academic Publishers. Printed in the Netherlands.*

All universities are based on the principle of the 'unity of research and teaching'; teaching and (basic) research are supposed to have roughly equal importance. In colleges (*Fachhochschulen*), the emphasis is on teaching, but they also play a role in applied research. The teacher training colleges, the schools for social workers and the paramedical professions are pure teaching institutions.

2.1.2 Name and Length of Degrees Offered in Each Sector

For all the institutions mentioned above, the entry requirement is to pass the final upper secondary school examination (*Matura*); as an alternative, students may pass the vocational *Berufsreifeprüfung* (which basically has the same requirements as the Matura). At present, some 40 % of the age group meet one of these entry requirements.

The traditional first degrees at universities are the *Magister* and *Diplom Ingenieur* (at Technical Universities), after four, in some disciplines five, years of study. This degree is considered to be equivalent with a master's degree.

At *Fachhochschulen* the first and only degree used to be the *Magister (FH)* after three or four years of study. Academic job-oriented education is the aim of these programmes. Degree programmes are accredited by the College Council, as will be explained below, for at most five years. The programmes take on average eight semesters (240 ECTS), with at least one semester of practical professional training.

Since Austria has joined the Bologna process, universities and *Fachhochschulen* are free to change their degree structure and to introduce *Bakkalaureats* (three or four years) and (a new type of) *Magister* (one or two years) programmes. The first bachelor's and master's programmes began in the academic year 2003/04. The development of new curricula in the *Fachhochschule* sector is decentralised and the College Act and the College Council regulate the procedure.

Only universities have the right to offer doctoral programmes (*Doktoratsstudien*) (two years). College graduates are entitled to enrol in doctoral studies at a university (Ph.D.). This is an important 'bridge' to the Austrian university system. Yet when college graduates decide to take their Ph.D., they have to fulfil additional requirements.

2.1.3 Institutional Governance Structures in Universities

The decision-making structure is in transition, since the legal basis for universities will change in 2005 when the law that was passed in 2002 (UG 2002) will be implemented. The present context is based on the previous law, the UOG 1993:

- Rectors (who are joined by one to four vice-rectors) are the university executive. However, they have only limited executive powers, since universities are state agencies. Rectors are elected by the university assembly (based on a proposal made by the Academic Senate).
- The Academic Senate has the main responsibility for academic matters at the level of the university and mainly consists of representatives of professors and a minority of junior faculty and student representatives.
- The university assembly (*Universitätsversammlung*) consists of senior academics (25 %), junior academics (25 %), students (25 %), and non-academic staff (25 %). It elects the vice-rectors (the rector makes a proposal), and it can recall the rector.
- The Faculty Senate (*Fakultätskollegium*) consists of representatives of senior academic staff (50 %), junior academic staff (25 %), and students (25 %) in a broad academic area. The Faculty is run by a Dean who is elected by the Faculty Senate.
- Institutes are the main disciplinary units. The Institutes Council (*Institutskonferenz*) mainly consists of senior academic staff and representatives of junior academic staff and students. The Council elects the Head of the Institutes. Compared with the departments of Anglo-Saxon universities, most institutes are quite small.
- An Advisory Board (*Universitätsbeirat*) consists of representatives from business, the region, and university graduates and only has an advisory function.

The most important changes of the new law (UG 2002) are that a University Board (*Universitätsbeirat*) will be introduced as a decision-making body, a kind of supervisory board, which appoints the rector (out of three candidates nominated by the Academic Senate) and the vice-rectors. Second, rectors will become the employers of all university staff, they will have full authority over the university budget, which, in future, will be a lump sum budget. Third, the number of junior academic staff and student representatives in most collegial bodies will be reduced. Furthermore, at present the Faculty Senate elects the dean. In future, the organisational structure of each university will be a matter of university statutes; the rector will appoint the heads of all organisational units (whatever their name).

2.2 Accreditation Schemes and Other Types of Evaluation Activities

For some years now, the issues of accreditation and evaluation have ranked highly on the higher education policy agenda. Austria only has a brief history in accreditation and evaluation in specific areas of higher education. Nevertheless, Austria has a highly elaborated form of quality assurance mechanisms. Public universities are still searching for their position concerning quality assurance, but the *Fachhochschul-*

sector and the private universities have developed internationally recognised forms of accreditation and evaluation schemes, and continue to develop them further.

2.2.1   Accreditation by the Austrian College Council

The Range of Activities

The accreditation scheme of the Austrian *Fachhochschulen* (college sector) only applies to degree programmes of Austrian *Fachhochschulen*. Every college institution that wants to offer degree programmes must have recognition by successfully completing the accreditation procedure. A politically independent council – the College Council – oversees the whole Austrian territory. The accreditation procedure encompasses both teaching and research.

The Actors

The organisations in charge of accreditation are the Ministry of Education, Science and Culture and the College Council. On October 1, 1993, the College Studies Act (*Fachhochschul-Studiengesetz*, or *FHStG*) came into force. In it, the Federal Ministry of Education, Science and Culture laid the cornerstone for the creation of the accreditation scheme. The new sector in Austrian higher education was to be characterised by decentralisation and deregulation. Colleges were privately organised, just as companies with limited liabilities, associations or non-profit organisations. The state competence was restricted to co-financing and quality assurance. Regarding finance, the attitude of the Austrian government differed fundamentally from the usual form of higher education funding. The government decided not to pay a huge sum every year, but to finance the costs of an agreed number of study places.

For quality assurance, the politically independent *Fachhochschulrat* (College Council) was established. It is responsible for initial accreditation, evaluation and re-accreditation of college degree programmes. The creation of the College Council as a 'quality-guard' over the college institutions was a novelty in the history of Austrian higher education. All members of the college council are appointed by the Federal Ministry of Education, Science and Culture. The College Council does not receive instructions, but the ministry can overrule its decisions, for example when they are in opposition to the ideas of the state or the government. Concerning financial affairs, the whole college sector is controlled by an official body called *Rechnungshof* (court of accounts), which ensures compliance with the principle that the college sector must operate economically, efficiently and functionally.

The College Council comprises 16 members. Half have an academic background and are qualified as university lecturers (*Habilitation*). The other half are from business or industry. At least four Council members must be women. The term of office for members is three years. The College Council elects its president and vice-president among its sixteen members. The College Council is a member of a number of international quality networks, viz.:

- INQAAHE – International Network for Quality Assurance Agencies in Higher Education (since 1995);
- EURASHE – European Association of Institutions in Higher Education (since 1996);
- ENQA – European Network for Quality Assurance in Higher Education (since 2000);
- DeGEval – Deutsche Gesellschaft für Evaluation (since 1999).

The Austrian government controls the work of the College Council. There is no meta-evaluation. The Ministry of Education, Science and Culture covers all costs of the College Council and its office. All members of the College Council are engaged part-time. They are paid for their participation in meetings; travel and accommodation costs are refunded.

Every applicant for accreditation could be seen as a customer of the accreditation scheme. The main stakeholders in the accreditation scheme are the providers of college courses. Students, their parents, industry and the economy are also potential stakeholders of the accreditation scheme.

The College Council tries to find a balance between evidence and assurance in its fields of work. To achieve this, the office of the College Council invests a great deal of time and probably money in public relations.

Rules, Regulations and Deadlines: Procedures in Accreditation

Confirmation of Government Funds. An important preliminary step before the procedure of accreditation can start is to clarify if the Ministry of Education, Science and Culture intends to co-finance a certain degree programme. To find out, the college institution has to send a summary[1] of the application to the College Council. The annual deadline for the summary is October 1. The summary is the basis for the decision as to whether co-financing will be approved or not. Each member of the Council rank-orders the applications. The College Council then transmits the results of its consultations to the Ministry. Based on the results of the College Council and

---

1   The summary has to include inter alia: the name of the college-degree programme; the number of study places; the form of delivery (part-time, full-time or both); the thematic orientation of the programme; its innovativeness; a description of the professional field and a brief assessment of how the future needs of the labour market will be met; a profile of graduates; the place of the programme in the already existing offer of college education; applied research and development (R&D); planned composition of the development team.

on inner ministerial discussions, the Ministry decides which programmes will be financed and which will not. The Ministry informs the colleges before the end of the year. Accordingly, this step takes about three months.

Application. Once the Ministry guarantees co-financing, the college must engage in more preparatory work. Every applicant (every course providing body) has to fulfil a number of guidelines defined by the Law. To support applicants, the College Council publishes a brochure on the topic.[2] An application for approval of a college degree programme has to contain the following sections:

- One of the first stages for the application is the composition of the development team. The team consists of at least four persons – two qualifying as university lecturer (*Habilitation*) and two with a background in a field that is relevant to the proposed college programme. Members of the development team must be mentioned by name in the application. The priority assignment of the development team is to design a new degree programme that fulfils all legal rules.

- The development team has to elaborate a detailed description of the professional field, the curriculum and examination regulations. This is one of the crucial parts of the application.

- The description has to demonstrate reflection on the teaching methods to be used to ensure academically sound, practice-oriented professional higher education, providing graduates with the required professional skills.

- It has to include an analysis of the courses offered in the post-secondary sector relating to the proposed college degree programme.

- One high-ranking aim of the college sector is to offer alternative ways for students to gain admission to higher education. Hence, the admission regulations have to be described and the criteria for selection of applicants in case the number of applicants exceeds the number of study places have to be explained.

- A relevant point is the demand and access survey. This survey should answer the question as to whether a sustainable pool of applicants is available for the proposed degree programme and whether there is a sustainable demand for graduates on the part of business, society or industry. When first accrediting a degree programme, this study has to be made by an appropriate and independent institution.

- In the application, the composition and the development of the teaching staff and their academic, professional and teaching qualification profiles must be indicated. A minimum of four members of the development team is legally required. They have to be named in the application.

- The measures for programme-specific applied research and development have to be described.

---

2   The brochure can be found at www.fhr.ac.at.

- Regarding financing of the applied college degree programme, each application must contain a financial plan, detailing how the costs will be covered for the duration of the approval period (the state only co-finances college programmes). Furthermore, a calculation of costs per study place must be included. Another important point is the existence of sufficient teaching facilities (rooms and equipment).
- Concerning the involvement of students, measures to obtain their evaluation of teaching have to be presented. It has to be indicated in which way the results of the students' evaluations will be used to further develop the programme pedagogically.

An application consists of approximately 120 to 180 pages. Persons who will assume leading positions in the college degree programme must also be named. In addition, a short (not longer than four pages) statement of why the institution wants to launch a programme must be included. The short presentation must also describe the medium and long-term conceptions of the programme.

Accreditation. The complete application has to be submitted to the College Council before the 1st of July. The office of the College Council checks the completeness and correctness of the documents and seeks to make the applicant remedy deficiencies. Every member of the College Council is presented with a copy of the application. In brief, the accreditation by the College Council is its procedure to verify the compliance with given and published requirements that ends in a positive or negative decision. A positive decision, to be made by the plenary College Council, is only possible when the application fulfils all legal requirements and when the Council is convinced that the proposed programme enriches the college landscape. The College Council informs the respective college institutions about its decisions by the end of the year.

In the next step, the office of the College Council forwards all applications (including negative decisions) to the Ministry of Education, Science and Culture. When the Ministry agrees with the decisions of the College Council and confirms its co-financing, the accreditation is valid for a maximum of five years. The College Council has to send the positive or negative replies to the colleges concerned before the end of March. All in all the College Council and the Ministry of Education, Science and Culture have nine months to take a decision as to whether the application is approved or not. The period of approval for new degree programmes starts on 1st August every year.

After receiving a positive accreditation decision, the college is responsible for implementing the new degree programme and for assurance of its quality.

One year before the first approval phase expires, the degree programme will be evaluated, because an application for re-accreditation requires the submission of an evaluation report.

To sum up, the Austrian college sector is still developing and is currently searching for a stable position in the Austrian and European higher education landscape. In the academic year 1994/95, college studies started with ten degree programmes. In 2003, 19 colleges offered 124 degree programmes.[3] 22 more colleges have applied for accreditation for the academic year 2003/04.

The fact that the College Council accredits while the Federal Ministry approves each application could lead to problems. Upon closer inspection it seems that the autonomy of the 'politically independent' and 'free from order' College Council is reduced through this arrangement.

Tasks of the College Council after Initial Accreditation

The evaluation concept of the College Council is based on international standards, combining internal evaluation by the college, external evaluation by a peer review team, a comment of the evaluated college leadership on the external evaluation report, a follow up process and the publication of the results of the evaluation.

One year before expiration of the accreditation period the college has to make an internal evaluation of the programme's quality. The main aim of the self-evaluation is to improve the quality of the courses offered. 'Fitness for purpose' is the basic concept of quality in these evaluations. The internal evaluation report must be about 30 to 40 pages. The College Council prescribes that self-evaluation reports describe, analyse and assess the programme as implemented (summarised in a SWOT analysis), and list improvement suggestions and planned measures.

The college submits the self-evaluation report to the College Council. The College Council then appoints a review team, consisting of three or four persons with relevant academic and professional qualifications and at least one foreign member, plus an assistant. Site visits last two to four days. On the basis of the internal evaluation report and discussions with management, staff and perhaps with students the peer review team forms its opinion. The review team's report and the statements of the college in response to the team's findings are presented to the quality committee of the College Council.

The College Council deals in detail with the results of both evaluations in a plenary session. It decides about the measures needed to improve the quality of the programme. If the college is not able to remedy the deficiencies, the College Council

---

3   Data can be downloaded from the College Council web site: www.fhr.ac.at.

decides to let the recognition expire. If the college institution remedies all deficiencies the College Council proposes to prolong the approval period.

In the next step, the College Council sends its decisions to the Ministry of Education, Science and Culture, which decides whether the financial support will be prolonged for the next approval period. If this decision is positive, the college can formally apply for re-accreditation. The application must include the evaluation report and be submitted at least six months before expiration of the approval period. The final step in the procedure of re-accreditation is the approval of the application by the Ministry of Education, Science and Culture.

In addition to the programme-based evaluation as described above, the College Council also wants to implement an institution-based evaluation as from the year 2003 to increase quality demands of the sector.

Other Quality-Relevant Activities

Beyond accreditation and evaluation processes the college sector is committed to ensure its quality as follows:

- annual statistical analysis by the College Council;
- observation of final examinations by members of the College Council;
- evaluation in the form of interviews;
- students' assessments of pedagogical training in the academic subjects;
- implementation of an internal quality management system in every college.

2.2.2 Accreditation by the Austrian Accreditation Council

The Range of Activities

The realm of activities of the Austrian Accreditation Council (AAC) is confined to private universities. Whoever wishes to run a private university with the right to confer academic degrees must obtain state recognition in the form of accreditation by the AAC. Accreditation by the AAC covers both the teaching and the research functions of private universities. There is no limitation with respect to subjects and disciplines.

The Actors

The AAC was established in 1999 by the Austrian Parliament. The main aim was to open the university sector to private suppliers. The AAC is not an advisory committee, but an independent body with full decision-making powers concerning accreditation of private universities and is not subject to directives from any other actor.

Legal supervision of the AAC is the responsibility of the Federal Minister who has jurisdiction over higher education (at present: Minister of Education). The AAC must submit an annual report of its activities to parliament through the responsible Federal Minister. Upon request, the Council is also obliged to supply the Minister with documents and to allow inspection of its premises. As a public authority, the AAC is subject to legal control by the audit division (*Rechnungshof*) of the Republic of Austria.

The AAC comprises eight members, who are acknowledged experts in the field of international higher education. They are appointed by the federal government. Four are nominated by the Austrian Rectors' Conference. An appropriate number of women must be considered when the AAC is being appointed. The basic period of office for AAC members is five years.

The Minister appoints a president and a vice-president of the Council from among its eight members. The president and the vice-president are appointed for three years. At the end of this period, the Minister can re-appoint the same persons once for another three-year period.

The AAC is not subject to reviews of any other accrediting body ('meta-accreditation'). However, it is a member of various professional networks, in particular:

- The European Network for Quality Assurance in Higher Education (ENQA).
- The International Network for Quality Assurance Agencies in Higher Education (INQAAHE).
- The Network of Central and Eastern European Quality Assurance Agencies in Higher Education (CEE Network).
- A Project to form an accreditation network between German-speaking countries in order to establish procedures for the mutual recognition of accreditation processes.

Potential applicants are customers of the expertise and service of the AAC. An important and useful stage in the run-up to applying is a series of detailed consultations. During preliminary discussions with the applicant, the office attempts to clarify which preconditions an application must fulfil as regards both content and form, as well as a suitable application time scale. In addition, the office is able to offer expertise relating to the elaboration and formulation of the application.

Students and their parents as well as employers are the main stakeholders of the AAC. The AAC provides transparency in a field of endemic uncertainty with enormous cost to obtain sound information. It guarantees reliability with respect to the quality of education and the recognition of degrees.

Rules and Regulations: Procedures in Accreditation

The legal foundation of the AAC is the Federal Act on the Accreditation of Educational Institutions as Private Universities (*University Accreditation Act* or *UniAkkG*). The federal government covers the costs of maintaining the AAC and its office. The applicants for accreditation must reimburse the expenses of the experts involved in the application procedure. This covers travel and accommodation costs, as well as remuneration for the inspection and the production of a report. The total costs to be reimbursed amount to approximately € 6,000.

Before the formal procedure, applicants can consult the AAC and present the planned project at a Council members' meeting. The formal stages of the procedure comprise the following.

Application. The institution seeking accreditation as a private university must apply to the AAC. The application must contain detailed documentation concerning the structure and organisation of the private university, such as a mission statement, information about its legal status, statutes and constitution, organigramme and its administrative and academic decision-making structures. If the applying educational establishment is part of a foreign or an international educational institution or the franchisee of one, further details are required about this institution (including its accreditation) in order to establish the relationship with the applicant institution. The application must also include proof that minimum standards will be fulfilled:

- The institution must have a permanent staff that is contractually bound for at least two years. Permanent staff must be able to cover at least 50 % of the teaching of each study course, and should normally have a doctoral degree. In accordance with international standards, each study course or discipline on offer requires at least three members of permanent staff whose minimum capacity is half-time employment. This minimum is set to ensure academic discussion and exchange.
- The institution must carry out research. The application must list current research projects and contain information about planned projects involving international co-operation in research and teaching. For this purpose too, the institution needs a critical mass to ensure the institutionalised production of knowledge and corresponding feedback from its research into its teaching activities.
- The selection process for all academic staff must be transparent, competitive and quality-based.
- Curricula (in detail) and examination regulations must meet material, specialist and formal requirements in accordance with international standards. The institution's minimum entrance requirements must be in accordance with Austria's general requirements for university admissions.
- Space and material resources will be judged according to international standards for adequate academic resources.

- The institution should be in a position to offer a reasonable range and variety of study courses.
- The institution must be able to prove that its medium and long-term funding is ensured.

The six-month period within which the Council must complete the procedure begins on the date the application arrives at the office. The application is first checked with respect to formal shortcomings.

Inspection by Peers. As a rule, the AAC appoints two to three experts, selected for their professional position, their specialisation, their academic reputation and expertise. The institution making the application will be informed of the names of the experts. The experts will carry out an inspection of the educational institution on the basis of the written documents submitted with the initial application letter. This usually lasts one day. The Council appoints one of its members as an inspector to co-ordinate and monitor the inspection.

Each inspector writes an independent report. Guidelines for the authors of these reports have been set out by the Council in order to guarantee uniformity of method and comparability. The reports are communicated to the applicant institution by the Accreditation Office. The institution has the right to submit a written comment on the reports by a certain date within the framework of a party hearing.

Accreditation. On the basis of the application documents, the inspection, the report and the institution's comments, the inspector prepares a decision proposal for the Council plenary. The Council then makes a decision on the application, which must have a minimum majority of five votes.

The decision is communicated to the applicant institution by means of a written notification. The AAC makes a press release in order to inform the public about success or failure of accreditation. However, no details of the process are made public.

Official notification by the AAC must be approved by the responsible Federal Minister. Approval can be refused if the decision of the AAC is against the interests of national educational policy.

There are no formal links between accreditation and approval of other subsequent decision-making processes. The federal government is prevented by law from financing the establishment of private universities. However, it can purchase individual services from an accredited private university on demand (e.g. the provision of study courses which supplement the range of studies offered by state-funded universities and are of general interest). The ban on public financing of private universities does not apply to provinces (*Bundesländer*) and local authorities.

Accreditation comes into effect as from the date of the official notification. It expires automatically at the end of the period set by the AAC (a minimum of five years) if an application for extension is not made in time.

Tasks of the AAC after Initial Accreditation: Supervision and Re-Accreditation

The AAC has the duty to monitor the quality of accredited private universities. It has the right to inspect the institutions whenever there is cause for concern, and may also demand specific information. The private university is obliged to provide information on all matters and to give access to all its documents and business records.

Furthermore, each academic year, the private university must submit an annual report to the Council. The report must ensure the AAC that the conditions on which accreditation was granted are being fulfilled. Assessments of report results can, in certain cases, lead to checks by the AAC. Minimum requirements for the annual reports include:

- Number of students and graduates for each course.
- List of university teaching staff, detailing their academic or artistic qualifications and achievements, as well as copies of the relevant employment contracts.
- Results of evaluation procedures on the quality of research and teaching. These must be carried out by the institutions at least every two years (description of the evaluation procedure used, follow-up of results of the evaluation procedure).
- Changes in personnel, space and equipment since the last report, or since the application.
- Clear presentation of the development of financial structures.
- Should there be areas that did not yet fulfil the criteria of the University Accreditation Act at the time of accreditation, these will be recorded in the official notification of accreditation and their development must be clearly outlined in the report.
- Description of continuous quality control measures (quality management system).

In any case, accreditation expires after a certain period of time. Extension of accreditation must be granted in an official notification before the period of initial accreditation has expired. Accreditation of a private university can be extended for a further five years after initial accreditation. After ten years, accreditation can be renewed for a further ten years. As in the initial application, when applying for re-accreditation, the institution must document its compliance with all legal requirements. Special emphasis should be put on developments since initial accreditation.

2.2.3   Other Schemes than Accreditation

Strictly speaking, there are no other approval schemes in Austria. Only in a very limited sense can one speak about 'approval' of the Ministry of Education with respect to the study courses of public universities. At present,[4] the rector has to inform the Ministry about the university's decision to start a new study course and provide all relevant information regarding the curriculum. The new study course does not need approval by the Minister. However, the Minister can refuse the new course for two reasons: if the course – or the procedure to establish it – is at variance with the law, and if the necessary resources to implement the course are not available. The Minister has two months to consider the new study course; if it is not rejected within two months, it is legally valid. Obviously, the supervision of the Ministry is limited to a check of formal correctness and legality. This procedure is not an approval extending to issues of quality of the course.

The new organisational act (*UG* 2002) becomes effective as from 2004. With respect to approval of study courses, there will be only minor changes. The role of the Ministry is still limited to check the formal correctness of the new course. The role of the rector is strengthened, and a new actor, the University Board (*Universitätsrat*), plays a significant role. However, under present regulations, this does not add up to a governmental approval of the curriculum and its quality.

With respect to supra-institutional evaluation on a regular basis, in principle, the law allows the Minister to take the necessary steps for an external evaluation either of one university or of the whole system.[5] However, there is no infrastructure for regular supra-institutional evaluations. For some years now, there has been a debate about an 'evaluation agency'; the Ministry has repeatedly announced the establishment of such an agency, but so far it has not been created. System-wide evaluations of single disciplines are occasionally carried out (on average every two or three years). The most recent was of mechanical engineering (see *Österreichisches Universitätenkuratorium* 2001).

As a consequence, quality assurance schemes for the sector of public universities are at present quite loose, although this sector is by far the biggest and most important sector of Austrian higher education. In 1997, the tight ministerial ex-ante control of university studies (*AHStG*, supplemented by a huge number of detailed study laws and decrees) was replaced by a new study law (*UniStG*), which granted a significant degree of autonomy to the universities and their study commissions. The latter are committees that establish and maintain study courses. However, until now this was not balanced by external supra-institutional evaluation.

---

4   The legal basis until the end of 2003 was *UOG* 1993 and *UniStG*.

5   This is the case both under the present and the new laws (*UOG* 1993, § 18 and *UG* 2002, § 14).

2.3 Underlying Patterns and the Logic of Different Accreditation Schemes

During the 1990s, Austrian higher education moved away from the traditional pattern of a homogeneous system and became more diverse. The main route to diversity was the establishment of new sectors[6] (*Fachhochschulen*, private universities) which now complement the still dominant sector of public universities. Obviously, the establishment of different sectors requires that policy makers draw certain lines between them and treat them differently. Assignment of a distinct role and profile to each sector and different treatment according to that profile are an attempt by the government to limit competition between the sectors. By doing so, the government maintains a relatively high steering capacity, even in a liberalised system. In our context, the differences with respect to quality assurance are of particular interest. The federal government has established distinct rules for quality assurance in each sector. So far, there have been no comprehensive procedures for the higher education system as a whole. Each sector has its own logic and deserves a separate description.

2.3.1 The Rationale to Establish the College Council

Compared with other OECD countries, a non-university sector was established relatively late in Austria. The main reason for the creation of *Fachhochschulen* in 1993 was the policy-makers' conviction that Austria could not avoid diversifying the range of educational profiles in higher education. *Fachhochschulen* should offer relatively short study courses with an explicit vocational orientation. However, besides curricular innovation, the *Fachhochschul*-policy was also a deliberate attempt at organisational reform.

It is worth remembering that the legal basis for the *Fachhochschul*-sector, the *FHStG*, was the result of a heated controversy about the organisational structure of the new sector. In a nutshell, there were two opposing concepts. One saw colleges as state agencies, basically a copy of universities (as they were in the early 1990s) in organisational terms, but with just a different curricular profile. The other was to establish colleges as public enterprises with a lump-sum budget, greater institutional management, and – what is most important in our context – greater autonomy in curricular affairs. The latter concept finally prevailed and was incorporated in the 1993 law. During the reform debate of the early 1990s, this concept was labelled the 'accreditation model'. This is a clear indication that the actors involved in the reform process attached much importance to this aspect of the model. Accreditation was a

---

6 In addition to sectoral diversification, one can also observe growing diversity within each sector. Until the late 1980s the policy was to keep differences between institutions of the same kind as small as possible. With the introduction of *UOG* 1993 and in particular with *UG* 2002 universities are expected to develop a distinct profile.

new feature in the Austrian context, which must be linked to the new curricular development in *Fachhochschulen*.

The remarkable degree of room for manoeuvre at *Fachhochschulen* must be compared with the heavy state regulation of universities with respect to curricular affairs. In 1993, when the *FHStG* was passed, universities were still subject to hierarchical regulation of study courses in four stages: two federal laws, one ministerial decree, and finally 'fine-tuning' by the university itself. It goes without saying that this complex procedure did not foster rapid adaptation of study courses to new demands. The *FHStG* was a tremendous step towards a new understanding of quality assurance in higher education.

One important aspect of this change is a new understanding of the appropriate and feasible responsibility of the political system (parliament, government, ministry). Until the early 1990s, political authorities claimed to define the 'one best solution' for each level of education. Of course, it was not always easy to say what exactly was the 'one best solution'. Views on appropriate curricular measures differed widely, due to contradicting expert opinions and political convictions. Policymakers and academics became increasingly unsatisfied with the resulting slowness of curricular reforms.

Step by step a more liberal attitude replaced the paternalistic tradition of quality control. Public opinion leaders, the general public and finally policy-makers no longer believed in the 'one best solution'. It seemed increasingly uncertain that such an 'optimum curriculum' existed at all; and even if it did exist, how could it be identified if experts did not agree? For these reasons it made sense to allow a certain amount of competition between different curricular profiles; instead of over-emphasising an 'ex-ante approach' of quality control it seemed more promising to pay attention to the outcomes of competing profiles and to judge which one proved a success.

However, the main actors promoting this liberal approach to quality control agreed that it would be necessary to protect students against offerings with unacceptably low quality. If institutions obtained a high degree of autonomy to shape the curriculum, study courses needed a 'mark of quality' guaranteeing that they met at least minimum standards. This was the policy context in which a need for accreditation arose. The accreditation model was strongly influenced by the example of the British polytechnics and the Council for National Academic Awards (cf. § 4 below).

2.3.2 The Rationale to Establish the AAC

Until the establishment of the college sector, maintenance of higher education institutions was a monopoly of the federal government. Each university with the right to confer academic degrees was explicitly mentioned in the university organisation act

(UOG 1975, later UOG 1993). *Fachhochschulen* were the first academic institutions that severely undermined the traditional governance patterns in Austrian higher education. However, although, formally, they were privately owned, public bodies still exercised strong influence on their development. This sector could not be regarded as private in a strict sense. Almost all funding for colleges comes from public sources, either from the federal government or from the provinces and municipalities. It makes more sense to regard *Fachhochschulen* as 'public enterprises'.

During the late 1990s the legalisation of private higher education institutions in a narrow sense became a policy issue. Already in the late 1980s the first private university (Webster University) was set up in Austria, but due to the legal position, its degrees were not recognised in Austria. During the late 1990s it became obvious that Webster would not remain an isolated case. There was a growing number of initiatives from inside and from outside the country to establish private universities.

This development must be seen against the background of increasing internationalisation of higher education. From a global perspective, the emergence of transnational student markets was a new phenomenon with strong repercussions on those systems (basically the Anglo-Saxon countries) which had successfully established higher education as a major 'export industry'. Even if Austria – as most European countries – did not participate in this market as an exporter, the new entrepreneurial spirit shaped the dominant policy paradigms, which at least indirectly influenced all nations. In Europe, internationalisation did not have such strongly commercial features. It was mainly driven by the mobility programmes of the European Union. The goal of these programmes was to strengthen European integration, not only in economic terms but also with respect to culture and a 'European identity'.

In any case, internationalisation undermined the capacities and powers of the nation state. It was no longer feasible for national authorities to shape their own education systems without taking into account international trends and developments. The Bologna process is a striking example, because, from a formal point of view, each government is still free to decide sovereignly upon its priorities. Practical constraints, however, secure a high degree of convergence and adjustment.

Austrian authorities had to take into account that in the new framework of a 'European higher education space' it no longer made sense to prohibit private universities. The (non-monetary) cost to legitimise a state monopoly (to the Austrian public and to potential providers who might take legal action against the Austrian government) was much higher than the potential disadvantages of a private sector. In the past, the view on private universities had been ideologically distorted in many cases. Opponents regarded them as a threat to an egalitarian higher education system; proponents advertised them as superior to the public sector. Opponents and advocates alike took it for granted that private universities would constitute an elite sector of the higher education system. More recently, this polarised view gave way to a rather

matter-of-fact assessment of the strengths and weaknesses of a private sector. Policy-makers became aware that – in a comparative perspective – private elite sectors
are the exception rather than the rule (see Geiger 1986), and that in Austria, as in
most European countries, private universities would constitute a 'marginal segment'
which could not seriously challenge the predominance of the public sector.

A new accreditation scheme was regarded as an imperative precondition for the
legalisation of private universities. In designing such a body, the Austrian authorities
could rely on the experience they had gained with the *Fachhochschul*-Council. The
possibility to enhance the range of activities of the College Council instead of creating a new accreditation body was never discussed seriously. One reason was that,
compared with the *Fachhochschul*-sector, accreditation of private universities would
require slightly different criteria. For *Fachhochschulen* it was important to prove
that the study courses applying for accreditation met sufficient demand from the
labour market. Additionally, colleges had to demonstrate that their curriculum did
not duplicate already existing study courses at universities, but created a new educational profile.[7] Accreditation of private universities does not make such demands.
This difference can be explained by the fact that *Fachhochschulen* are predominantly funded by public sources (thus there is an understandable interest of governments in the coherence and effectiveness of the sector), while private universities are
almost exclusively funded by private money.

2.3.3   Consequences of Accreditation for Students

Accreditation of private universities has consequences with respect to the rights of
students and the recognition of examinations and degrees:

*   Students of private universities have the same rights as students of Austrian
    state universities as far as residence permits and study grants are concerned. The
    same laws also apply to students of private and state universities as regards fam-
    ily allowance, health insurance of children and taxation. In addition, students of
    private universities are members of the Austrian Students' Union (*Öster-
    reichische HochschülerInnenschaft, ÖH*). Students of *Fachhochschulen* have
    their own union.
*   Accreditation by the College Council includes the guarantee of an education
    with a degree compatible to the European Union.
*   Examinations taken at private universities are recognised by the state. Should a
    student move from a private university to a state university, then the examina-
    tions already taken at the private university (providing they are of the same
    standard or level) will be recognised by the state university.

---

7   This was the practice during the first six years of the *Fachhochschul*-Council. Since then, this crite-
    rion was relaxed somewhat.

- The degrees and titles awarded by colleges as well as by private universities have the same legal validity as those from Austrian state universities. It is therefore neither necessary nor possible to have these degrees validated at an Austrian state university. The graduates of private universities have the legal right to use the degree title awarded. College graduates are entitled to use the appropriate academic title with the addition of the letters 'FH'.

- Colleges and private universities can only legally award those academic degrees and titles that have been allowed in their accreditation.

2.4 Policy Transfer from the United Kingdom to Austria

The *Fachhochschul*-policy of the Austrian government followed the broad global trends and fashions of the late 1980s and early 1990s, as found in the higher education literature or in the recommendations of international organisations such as the OECD. The OECD played a crucial role in shaping the *Fachhochschul*-policy. Its examination of the Austrian higher education system focusing on the new *Fachhochschule* concept proved very influential. In the spring of 1993, the OECD presented its review, which expressed strong support for this concept (OECD 1995). A few weeks later the *FHStG* was passed by parliament. The policy debate referred increasingly to one particular national model of non-university higher education, i.e. the British polytechnics. To be more precise, it was the idea of accreditation and the role and function of the *Council for National Academic Awards* (CNAA) that attracted the interest of Austrian reformers (see Pechar 2002). There is some irony in the fact that the CNAA served as a kind of role model for Austria at the time when it was abolished by the British government. But it is even more interesting that the CNAA and the British polytechnics should exercise such a strong influence on Austrian higher education policy. This is by no means self-evident; on the contrary. Due to quite different political and legal traditions, policy transfer from Britain to Austria had been very rare until then. In the 1960s and 1970s, when Austrian policy-makers searched for models and examples from abroad, they turned to the European continent, in particular to Germany.

At the level of organisation and technical procedures, a comparison between the CNAA and the College Council (*Fachhochschulrat*) reveals many similarities and some differences. Most obvious are the almost identical functions of the two bodies. The main task of the College Council, laid down in the *FHStG*, is validation of courses, award of degrees, and assurance and maintenance of quality in the new sector of higher education. In both cases, they have the main and final responsibility for quality assurance in the non-university sector.

There are strong similarities with respect to the composition of the two bodies. The College Council consists of 16 members appointed by the Minister of Education. The members of the College Council need a high-ranking theoretical or practical qualification: either a *Habilitation* (second thesis) if they are academics or practical experience of similar rank if they come from the business community. The composition of the bodies reflects that in both cases there was a balance of tasks and functions at stake: both the CNAA and the College Council should represent external demands, but at the same time should also ensure academic strength.

There are equally strong similarities regarding the procedures of approval and validation of courses. *Fachhochschulen* have to submit a precise description of the course, its structure and content, and prove it has sufficient facilities and adequate academic staff. If satisfactory, the course is approved for five years. As with the CNAA, the validation procedures of the College Council are rigorous. Many applicants fail at first submission. It goes without saying that not all applicants took a favourable view of this rigorous approach. But it is equally clear that this insistence on quality is one of the key factors for the success of the *Fachhochschul*-sector.

The most important difference between the CNAA and the College Council regards the size of the body and its co-operation with the external community of experts. The CNAA was a large bureaucracy, with the 25 members being just the core, and many hundreds of experts from higher education and industry involved through boards and panels. The validation procedure was the main responsibility of the boards and panels. The College Council, on the other hand, only occasionally involves outside members. The members of the body undertake the validation procedure themselves, resulting in a permanent overload.

A comparison between CNAA and College Council at the level of political legitimacy is much more difficult. Here, the different constitutional and legal backgrounds in Britain and Austria and the different traditions in public administration and policy become apparent. The accreditation model sought to change some of these traditions. It is not surprising then that it faced a great deal of opposition. Let us just touch on a few of these points before we finally ask why and how the *Fachhochschul*-policy could succeed in spite of this opposition.

A crucial point is the role of the government in higher education in Austria and the UK. Let us first look at the university sectors of both countries before non-university sectors were introduced. They both have traditions of autonomy, although in a very different sense. Austrian universities are state agencies, and academic autonomy is defined as a constitutional right of the individual academic, not of the university as an institution. Rather, the institution is subject to intense legal regulation regarding the design of the curriculum, the admission of students, the employment of academics, the spending of public money, etc. In the British autonomous tradition, there was no 'university law' and no effective legal power to control it.

These different starting points are important if we compare the relationship between the accreditation body and the institutions of the non-university sector in Britain and Austria. Both the CNAA and the College Council were external, non-governmental bodies. In the British case, the validation procedure of the CNAA was a necessary requirement, because the polytechnics were not part of the autonomous tradition and thus were subject to external control. Compared with universities, this was not an increase, but a limitation of autonomy. In Austria, universities never enjoyed the same degree of institutional autonomy as the British ones. In this very different context, the College Council was to relieve the institutions of the non-university sector from legal control by the government. As a result, *Fachhochschulen* in some respects enjoyed more autonomy than universities.[8]

It was clear that *Fachhochschulen* should be subject to external control. But what kind of control? It was probably the most controversial aspect of the *Fachhochschul*-policy that this control was not exercised by the government, but by a non-governmental body of experts. The main issue at stake was: is the College Council a legitimate advocate of public interests? The concept of the College Council was questioned by some on the grounds that it was not democratically legitimised (Mrkvicka & Kaizar 1994). Only a body that resulted directly or at least indirectly from general elections should be allowed to act in the public interest. This was based on the suspicion that all autonomous or intermediate bodies which undermine the clear distinction between the private, self-interested sphere of society and the state as the representation of the general will of the people generally favoured the upper strata of society. Other objections to the College Council were that employers, who were interested in the quality of the graduates, would not trust the judgements of a non-governmental body.

We cannot find a comparable process of policy transfer with respect to the AAC for private universities. In this case, policy-makers used the already existing experience with the first accreditation agency in Austria. Subsequently, we can see a policy transfer in an opposite direction. Many countries are in the process of establishing an accreditation body, and some want to use the Austrian experience. Authorities from countries as different as Switzerland, the Netherlands, Serbia, Macedonia, Canada[9] and Japan have established contacts with the AAC and made inquiries in order to inform their policies.

References

Austria (1999). *Bundesgesetz über die Akkreditierung von Bildungseinrichtungen als Privatuniversitäten* (Universitäts-Akkreditierungsgesetz – UniAkkG). BGBl. I Nr.168/1999.
bm:bwk (2002). *Fachhochschul-Studiengesetz* – FHStG (Stand 2002), Wien: bm:bwk.

---

8   As mentioned, Austrian universities have their own tradition of academic autonomy. The autonomy of the individual academic, as it is embedded in the Humboldtian tradition, is much stronger in universities than in *Fachhochschulen*.

9   At present, Canada does not have an accreditation body for private universities.

Geiger, R. (Ed.) (1986). *Private Sectors in Higher Education. Structure, Function, and Change in Eight Countries*. Ann Arbor: University of Michigan Press.

Mrkvicka, F. & Kaizar, I. (1994). Die Entstehung und Entwicklung von Fachhochschulen in Österreich aus der Sicht der Arbeitnehmer. In S. Höllinger, E. Hackl & C. Brünner (Eds.), *Fachhochschulstudien – unbürokratisch, brauchbar und kurz*. Wien: Passagen.

Pechar, H. (2002). Accreditation in higher education in Britain and Austria: two cultures, two timeframes. In: *Tertiary Education and Management* (8), pp. 231-242.

3 Czech Quality Assurance: The Tasks and Responsibilities of Accreditation and Evaluation

HELENA ŠEBKOVÁ

3.1 The National Higher Education System

Tertiary education in the Czech Republic includes any type of education that is recognised by the state and requires completed secondary education as an entrance condition. Tertiary education is composed of:

- Higher education;
- Tertiary professional education;
- Post-secondary courses (they will be introduced when a new Act on Education is passed; it is in the process of being adopted by Government and Parliament at the time of writing);
- Lifelong learning courses.

We shall concentrate in this chapter on higher education, but a few introductory words on tertiary professional education may be in order to outline the context. Tertiary professional schools developed from vocational secondary schools. They provide educational programmes that are mostly professionally oriented and sometimes very closely associated with graduates' employers. More than 26,800 students were enrolled in 2001/02. Courses last on average for 2.5 to 3 years and lead to a diploma (which is not comparable to a bachelor's degree). The 1998 Act on Higher Education allows tertiary professional schools to provide bachelor study programmes, but only in collaboration with a higher education institution. Tertiary professional schools, mainly those with experience in such joint study programmes, may serve as the basis for the establishment of non-university higher education institutions. This was the case for the majority of private non-university higher education institutions so far.

At the end of 2002, the Czech higher education system included 57 higher education institutions: 24 public institutions, four state and 29 private higher education institutions. The Ministry of Education, Youth and Sports represented the state in relation to higher education institutions. The activities of the separate state higher education institutions (three military ones and the Police Academy) are partly regulated by the responsible ministry, i.e. the Ministry of Defence and the Ministry of the Interior.

S. Schwarz and D.F. Westerheijden (eds.),
Accreditation and Evaluation in the European Higher Education Area, 65–86.
© 2004 Kluwer Academic Publishers. Printed in the Netherlands.

Table 1 gives the student numbers, which more than doubled in the last decade. Private higher education institutions currently cater for some 8,000 students, who are mainly enrolled in bachelor's programmes. A significant increase in the number of students in private institutions is not expected, as the sector is considered complementary to the public higher education sector. At the same time, it is considered as a positive challenge and competition for the public institutions.

Table 1. Number of students in higher education

Year	1989/90	1991/92	1993/94	1995/96	1997/98	1999/00	2001/02	2002/03
	110,021	109,219	118,842	152,148	177,723	198,961	223,013	243,756

In the academic year 2002/03, the total number of newly enrolled students in higher education institutions (about 58,000) represented approximately 42 % of the cohort of 19-years olds (136,780 in total). One of the main goals of the governmental policy is to raise the percentage of students enrolled in tertiary education to 50 % by 2005. Lifelong learning, and the broad use of ICT, will be a general trend, in accordance with the vision of the European higher education area.

3.1.1 Types of Higher Education Institutions

University type higher education institutions focus on bachelor's, master's and doctoral study programmes. *Non-university* higher education institutions mainly offer bachelor's programmes. If they meet accreditation requirements, they may provide master's programmes, but they are not entitled to offer doctoral programmes. The Accreditation Commission is responsible for deciding on the type of a higher education institution.

Both types of higher education institutions may be public, state or private. The private higher education institutions are still very new, mostly very small, and only of the non-university type.

3.1.2 Main Types of Study Programmes and Degrees

Higher education is based on three levels of accredited study programmes: bachelor's, master's and doctoral. In accordance with the Bologna process, a bachelor programme should enable graduates to enter the labour market or to continue their studies, either immediately or after some work experience.

Bachelor's programmes last for at least three and at most four years. The *bakalář* (Bc.) degree is awarded following successful completion of the study programme and the passing of a state examination.

The master's programme presents new theoretical findings based on scientific knowledge, research and development. Students are required to master the application of these findings and to develop skills for creative and scientific activities. Master's programmes also include a state final examination and in most cases the presentation of a diploma thesis. The length of a continuing master study programme (after completion of the bachelor's) is one to three years. The 'long' master's programme takes on average five years (six in medicine and veterinary medicine) and does not require a bachelor's degree. The *magistr* (Mgr.) degree is awarded in the fields of humanities, education, social sciences, natural sciences, pharmacy, law, theology and arts. The master's degree is a pre-requisite for the state examination in the field of graduation and a dissertation to acquire the 'doktor' in the relevant field. In technical fields of study, such as economics, agriculture and chemistry, the master's level degree is called *inženýr* (Ing.). Medical and veterinary studies lead to the *doktor medicíny* (MUDr.), and *doktor veterinární medicíny* (MVDr.) respectively.

The doctoral study programme consists of an individual study plan under the guidance of a supervisor; holders of a master's degree can apply. It is aimed at scientific research and independent creative activity. The nominal length of the programme is three years. It ends with the state doctoral examination and the presentation of a dissertation which shows independent research skills, theoretical knowledge or independent theoretical and artistic creativity (in relevant fields). The degree conferred is a Ph.D.

All study programmes may be offered in the form of face-to-face study or by distance education, or a combination of both.

3.1.3 Transition from Higher Education to Work

Employment offices regularly provide monitoring on graduates' employment at the end of April and at the end of September. In general, the rate of employment of higher education graduates has improved in recent years: the percentage of unemployment is lower than for those with lower levels of education. It is not possible to determine the study fields with higher than average unemployment rates because the data change and cannot support any hypothesis.

Graduates at master level are well absorbed by the labour market. This is not the case with bachelors at present. Little is known in society in general and by employers about these programmes and about the skills of bachelor graduates. The situation is improving rapidly, but reliable information remains an urgent necessity.

3.1.4   Governance and Steering of Higher Education

Steering the system is the responsibility of the Ministry of Education, Youth and Sports. Its most important tasks are to allocate funding to individual higher education institutions from the state budget, to monitor its proper use, to arrange favourable conditions for the development of higher education institutions and to coordinate their activities. The Act lists all the duties and responsibilities of the Ministry so as to ensure a proper balance between the autonomy of the higher education institutions and the authority of the state.

The Ministry decides on the accreditation of study programmes, *habilitation* procedures to obtain the *venium docendi*, and procedures to appoint professors. It also awards the state permission for private higher education institutions if a positive expert opinion is issued by the Accreditation Commission (see below).

The Ministry must devise a long-term strategy plan for the development of the higher education system. Similarly, each individual higher education institution must elaborate its own development strategy. Both ministerial and institutional plans should be updated annually and should be available to the public. Negotiations on plans should help to harmonise the system developments, to steer the system by means of the allocation of part of the state budget on the basis of contracts and to contribute to quality, transparency and accountability.

Further, the governance of the sector is influenced by the representation of higher education institutions, through the Council of Higher Education Institutions (composed of the representatives of the Academic Senates of all higher education institutions and their faculties) on the one hand, and the Czech Rector's Conference (composed of rectors of all higher education institutions) on the other. The Ministry is obliged by the Act to discuss all important measures concerning higher education with these bodies.

Finally, the activities of the trade unions (in which there is a special group for higher education) focus on the state budget devoted to education and teachers' salaries. Trade union representatives are invited to the regular meetings of the Council of Higher Education Institutions.

3.2   Quality Assurance and Accreditation

Quality evaluation and assurance are relatively new attributes of Czech higher education. Until 1990, the higher education system was extremely uniform. All institutions were considered to be equal, all provided the same type of education leading to the same types of academic degrees. Quality was not evaluated or even discussed. Indeed, the high quality of education was simply declared. The Higher Education Act of 1990 created the Accreditation Commission with the obligation to express its expert opinion which served as the basis for ministerial decisions regarding doctoral (Ph.D.) studies. In addition, since 1992, the Accreditation Commission has conducted peer reviews and comparative evaluations of faculties in related study fields. The 1998 Higher Education Act brought a number of significant changes to the higher education system, together with new competencies and responsibilities for the Accreditation Commission.

3.2.1 Accreditation Commission

The Accreditation Commission is an expert body composed of 21 members. Members, including the chair and the vice-chair, are appointed for a six-year term by the Czech Government on nomination of the Minister of Education. Prior to this nomination, the Minister asks for references from the representatives of higher education institutions (Council of Higher Education Institutions and Czech Rectors' Conference), the Research and Development Council of the Government of the Czech Republic, and the Academy of Sciences of the Czech Republic, and discusses it with these institutions. Members of the Accreditation Commission should generally enjoy authority as experts. They cannot also be rectors, vice-rectors or deans.

The Accreditation Commission may establish working groups to evaluate specific matters or activities. Working groups are composed of specialists in particular fields, forms and objectives.

The activities of the Accreditation Commission and its working groups are regulated by the Statutes of the Accreditation Commission, which is approved by the Government and made public by the Minister. Material and financial means for the activities of the Accreditation Commission are provided by the Ministry.

The Main Tasks of the Accreditation Commission

According to the Act, the Accreditation Commission is responsible for the quality of higher education. This implies a comprehensive evaluation of all accredited activities and the publication of the evaluation results. The Act also empowers it to elaborate a professional standpoint on other matters concerning higher education which are presented to it by the Minister for consideration.

The Act further requires that the Accreditation Commission issues its expert view in the following cases: application for accreditation of study programmes; application for the right to carry out *habilitation* procedures and procedures for the appointment of professors; application of a legal entity to award state permission to operate as a private higher education institution; establishment, merger, amalgamation, splitting or dissolution of a faculty of a public higher education institution; definition of the type (university or non-university) of a higher education institution.

Legal Regulations

The establishment of the Accreditation Commission, the declaration of its rights and the stipulation of its main tasks are included in the Higher Education Act. The Act, however, limits itself to the main arrangements while some necessary details of the Accreditation Commission are included in its Statutes and the Decree issued by the Ministry.

The Statutes give the Accreditation Commission authority to require the necessary information for its work, obliges it to publish an annual report, and stipulates the scope of authority and responsibilities of its members and working groups. The Statutes also prescribe the Accreditation Commission's activities and specifies its finances, which are under the responsibility of the Ministry, as well as the role of the Accreditation Commission Secretariat.

The Decree on the Content of Application for Study Programme Accreditation

The Higher Education Act requires the Ministry to issue a decree that details the content of the written application for study programme accreditation. The decree should be issued in agreement with the Accreditation Commission.

The basic provision specifies how to apply. The application should include the formal data about the study programme and inform about: the objectives of the studies' profile, study branch specification, graduates' acquired general, professional and special knowledge and abilities, the characteristics of the professions which graduates should be prepared to exercise, other possibilities of their employment and the conditions that students must meet. The application for accreditation also includes evidence of study programme objectives, motivations and provision. Doctoral programmes, being to some extent different from the first and second cycle programmes, are the subject of a separate article of the decree. If the application for study programme accreditation is presented together with an application for state permission, the evidence on the preparation of material, technical and information provisions of study programme is an integral part of it. Specific demands concerning distance or combined study forms, and recommendations to the applicants for accreditation are elaborated in an additional short guide issued by the Accreditation Commission. Application for the extension of study programme accreditation's validity should also follow the decree provisions, but the real procedure focuses on the changes made in the programme.

3.2.2   Accreditation

In general, the accreditation is the yes-or-no decision made by the Ministry. The Ministry can only award the accreditation if the opinion of the Accreditation Commission is positive.

Institutions or Units of the Accreditation Scheme

All types of accreditation, i.e. accreditation of study programmes, of *habilitation* procedures and accreditation of procedures for the appointment of professors, are obligatory for all higher education institutions. The award of the state permission for a private higher education institution may be considered as a specific type of accreditation. The institutions under this scheme are all legal entities domiciled in the Czech Republic that intend to act as private higher education institutions, once they have been granted the state permission.

The accreditation scheme functions at the national level; hence, the procedures described here are valid for all higher education institutions. We would like to observe that accreditation of a study programme may be extended to the tertiary professional schools when they submit an application for accreditation of a bachelor's study programme that is offered jointly with a higher education institution. A similar procedure applies to the institutes of the Academy of Sciences of the Czech Republic. In the latter case, the jointly provided study programmes are preferably at the doctoral level.

Function of Accreditation, Subjects and Disciplines

The main function of accreditation is to ensure the minimum standards of quality of the activities that are accredited. The same applies to the state permission concerning private higher education institutions. All disciplines that fall under these activities (study programmes, procedures of *habilitation* and appointment of professors) are taken into consideration.

The Actors, Ownership, Organisations, Reviewers and Stakeholders

The actors of the accreditation scheme are the higher education institutions and their leaders (rectors or statutory bodies), the Accreditation Commission and its working groups and the Ministry. The Ministry is bound by the Act to respect the view of the Accreditation Commission and has only limited freedom to follow its own point of view (see below). The institutions, as stakeholders of the scheme, are responsible for accepting the decision and its possible consequences. Accreditation is very important for the newly established private higher education institutions. Reviewers are mainly members of the working groups, but sometimes also members of the Accreditation Commission (who sometimes act as working group chairpersons).

Customers and stakeholders are mainly the students, as they are fully dependent on the quality of the study programmes. There is a strong belief that accreditation of a study programme and state permission protect students against low quality teaching and connected research, and the development of private higher education institutions. As the awarded, limited or refused accreditation is a public issue the other stakeholders are the students' parents, employers and other interested social groups.

Concerning *habilitation* procedures and the appointment of professors, the range of stakeholders is more limited. Highly qualified teachers are considered important for the overall quality of studies, and hence for student satisfaction and benefits. Therefore students indirectly remain important stakeholders. The other stakeholders – parents, employers, trade unions, government – may benefit even more indirectly from the advantages of well qualified faculty.

The Ministry is the main decisive actor in the scheme, even if the scope of its decisions is limited by the Act.

Accreditation of a Study Programme

All types of study programmes are subject to accreditation. The Ministry oversees the accreditation of study programmes, which confers state approval to the programme and includes the right to award appropriate academic titles. In the case of non-accredited study programmes, it is impossible to admit applicants, hold lectures or examinations, or award academic degrees.

The Accreditation Commission asks the higher education institution to complete the application if information is missing; in the meantime, the review procedure is halted. It is only if the higher education institution fails to so that the Accreditation Commission issues its standpoint which is based on the original documentation.

The Ministry cannot award accreditation if the Accreditation Commission gives a negative opinion. If the evaluation is positive, the Ministry can refuse to grant accreditation only when:

- the study programme does not comply with requirements listed in the part of the Act devoted to the study programmes,
- insufficient staff, equipment and information provisions are available for the study programme;
- the implementation of the study programme is not supported by sufficient financial, material or technical resources;
- the higher education institution is not deemed capable of providing sufficient guarantees for lecturing;
- the application does not contain data that are deemed crucial for awarding the accreditation.

Accreditation is awarded for a limited period, which is at most twice the standard length of study. In the case of doctoral study programmes, it should not exceed ten years. Accreditation can be extended repeatedly, if the positive aspects of the programme continue to be ensured.

A higher education institution can only cancel an accredited study programme if it provides students with an option to continue their studies in the same or a similar study programme at the same or another higher education institution.

To promote higher education studies in non-traditional institutions, the Act stipulates that any legal entity dealing with educational, research, developmental, artistic or other creative activity may ask for accreditation together with a higher education institution. A request for accreditation should be supplemented by a contract for mutual co-operation and should outline a joint study programme. The origin of this regulation was to invite the Academy of Sciences to be active in doctoral study programmes. At the same time, this provision facilitates collaboration between higher education institutions and tertiary professional schools.

Accreditation of Procedures for *Habilitation* and for the Appointment of Professors

Higher education institutions or their units can obtain the right to carry out procedures for academics to be conferred the *venium docendi* (*habilitation*) and for the appointment of professors based on accreditation. The procedure is similar to that for study programmes. It is described in the Act. The decision of the Ministry is bound by the Act and there is a list of conditions whereby it may refuse to award the accreditation.

State Permission

Obtaining state permission is obligatory for any legal entity wanting to function as a private higher education institution. Private higher education is a new element in the Czech system; hence, the procedure is specified by the Act. The application should be submitted to the Ministry and should contain all the formal data, including the legal form of the responsible entity and its statutory body. Furthermore, it should provide information on the following:

- long-term intention of providing education together with research, developmental or other creative activity;
- financial, material, personnel and information resources for the activities;
- design of study programmes;
- design of internal regulations, including organisation, activities and the status of the academic community members.

The Ministry evaluates the application and if there are potential insufficiencies it asks the applicant to overcome them in due course. It has the right to check the information given in the application (for instance by the site visit of facilities). Simultaneously, the Ministry asks the Accreditation Commission to formulate its stand-point on the design of study programmes. The Ministry takes its decision based on the view of the Accreditation Commission and its own evaluation of the application. It is bound by the Act not to grant state permission in the following cases:

- the standpoint of the Accreditation Commission is negative,
- there is not enough evidence that a higher education institution is capable of providing sufficient guarantees for its educational and associated activities,
- the design of internal regulations conflicts with applicable acts or other legal regulations.

The Ministry not only grants state permission, but also decides about the accredita-tion of the submitted study programmes. The private higher education institution should begin the study programmes within two years, otherwise the state permission becomes ineffective.

Type of a Higher Education Institution, Establishment of a Faculty

The Act declares that a higher education institution provides the accredited study programmes (bachelor, master, or doctoral) as well as lifelong learning programmes. The type of the higher education institution is determined by the type of accredited study programmes provided, which is stated in the statutes of the institution. The definition must comply with the opinion of the Accreditation Commission.

The Academic Senate of a higher education institution makes decisions concerning the establishment, merging, amalgamating, splitting or dissolving of individual parts of the institution on proposal of the Rector. If the unit is a faculty, the Rector's deci-sion is subject to affirmation by the Accreditation Commission.

The procedure to apply to the Accreditation Commission is not precisely defined by the Act or any decree. It is up to the institution's and faculty's leadership to explain the reason for creating the faculty and to provide evidence of its necessity.

Possible Consequences of Accreditation

The Accreditation Commission may require improvement within a specified period if it finds shortcomings in an accredited activity. If there are serious shortcomings in a study programme, it may propose relevant restrictions to the Ministry. Ministerial restrictions can consist of 1) a ban on admission of new applicants or 2) termination of the accreditation. This means a ban on students taking part in state examinations and on the award of academic degrees, or even complete withdrawal of the accredi-tation. If the reason for restriction is eliminated (with the exception of withdrawal of the accreditation) the Accreditation Commission invites the Ministry to cancel the measures taken. In the event of temporary termination or withdrawal of the accreditation, the higher education institution must provide students with the possibility to continue their studies in the same or a similar study programme at the same or another higher education institution. The restrictions have direct implications for the institutional budget. A significant part of the budget is allocated on the basis of the number of students. If a study programme is no longer accredited, it cannot admit students and consequently the budget is significantly reduced.

3.2.3   Evaluation of Quality

In the Czech higher education system, there are two types of quality evaluation; both are obligatory according to the Act. The first is external evaluation, which is the responsibility of the Accreditation Commission. The second is self-evaluation (see below).

External Evaluation

The Accreditation Commission has been evaluating the quality of higher education since it was established, even if this obligation was stipulated later by the 1998 Act. The evaluation scheme focuses on institutions as such and involves all higher education institutions in the country. The process is preferably improvement oriented.

Actors and Stakeholders. The actors are higher education institutions, usually their main parts (i.e. faculties), the Accreditation Commission and its (special) working groups. The Accreditation Commission is the owner of the process (e.g. in terms of know-how), whilst the leaders of the evaluated institutions are the main stakeholders. The other stakeholders are students, employers, the state and society. All can use the results of quality evaluation in accordance with their specific needs.

The Process of External Evaluation. While the obligation to carry out evaluation comes from the Act, the necessary extensional description is included in the Accreditation Commission's Statutes. The Accreditation Commission usually selects one or several institutions with similar accredited study programmes. The evaluation focuses on the overall activity of the institution and the conditions under which it is provided. The rules for the evaluation procedure are as follows:

- The evaluation usually lasts for a year and a half.
- The Accreditation Commission determines the institution or the group of institutions of similar study fields and the member of the Accreditation Commission responsible for the evaluation process.
- A special working group is established by the Accreditation Commission.
- The rector or another 'officer' of the institution is informed about the Accreditation Commission's intention and is asked to collaborate.
- The institutional leadership is requested to prepare the self-evaluation report.

- Collected information and other additional documentation are elaborated by the special working group of the Accreditation Commission.
- The 'officer' of the evaluated institution is invited to express an opinion on the composition of the special working group.
- The visiting team to each institution is composed of at least three members of the special working group.
- The special working group elaborates the recommendations and conclusions.
- A discussion is organised with the leadership of the evaluated institutions on the draft report that includes preliminary results.
- Final recommendations and conclusions are submitted to the Accreditation Commission.
- The Accreditation Commission may accept the recommendations and conclusions after a discussion with the leadership of the evaluated institution.
- The conclusions and recommendations, together with the references of the evaluated institution, are presented to the Ministry and published.

Possible Consequences. The evaluation is, in principle, an improvement-oriented process which does not lead to any concrete consequences from either the Accreditation Commission or the state. The results of the evaluation are public. It is assumed that evaluation of quality (its results) is very important:

- For the institution itself, (1) it may serve as marketing promotion in the case of positive results, and (2) it may incite the leadership and the staff to find ways of improvement in the case of negative results,
- as comprehensive and reliable information about the activities of the institution for all other stakeholders including (potential) students and employers,
- for the state.

Internal Evaluation

The Act requires that each higher education institution should organise regular internal evaluation and make its results public. An additional requirement is that higher education institutions must elaborate the evaluation procedures in more detail in their internal regulations but it is left to the institution to design this internal evaluation and how to use its results.

International Evaluation

Czech higher education institutions have undertaken a number of evaluations initiated by international bodies or by foreign institutions. Examples include:

- institutional quality audit by CRE (Czech Technical University in Prague, Palacky University in Olomouc, Silesian University in Opava);

- evaluation by the European Association for Veterinary Education (Veterinary and Pharmaceutical University in Brno);
- evaluation by a prestigious foreign university (Czech Agricultural University evaluated by the Agricultural University in Wageningen);
- FEANI accreditation (obtained by 25 Czech faculties of technology);
- IGIP accreditation (obtained by four higher education institutions);
- NCFMEA (National Committee on Foreign Medical Education and Accreditation) accreditation (obtained by all Czech medical faculties).

The evaluated institutions usually declared that the knowledge obtained and recommendations received were useful and led to the expected improvements. These evaluations also contribute to a better understanding of the importance of evaluation and offer new observations on different evaluating mechanisms and approaches.

3.2.4 Implementation of the Formal Rules

Accreditation of Study Programmes

The 1998 Act required all already established study programmes to be accredited within four years, i.e. by the end of 2003. A total of 1,471 study programmes of all types, offered by various higher education institutions (i.e. 4,380 study branches – branches being the main components of study programmes) received accreditation before the beginning of 2003. Of these, 244 were not evaluated positively. Another 144 were given limited accreditation (i.e. for a short period, and with necessary improvements). In case of failure in the accreditation process (one such case is currently under debate), the situation of students should be solved individually. They should be given the opportunity to finish their studies in a similar study programme provided by another higher education institution.

Accreditation of the *Habilitation* and of the Procedure for the Appointment of Professors

Just over 10 % of all *habilitation* and professorial appointment procedures (out of 879 applications) did not receive accreditation. The applicants were asked to make improvements and submit their application anew.

Evaluation of Quality

The general evaluation of institutional quality was reduced to the strict minimum in recent years, as the Accreditation Commission was fully engaged in the process of accreditation. The aim for the near future is to continue the evaluation scheme as described above and to begin with several private higher education institutions to see how far their mission and goals in the application for state permission have been achieved.

State Permission

Numbers concerning state permission are shown in the following table.

Table 2. State permission procedures

Year	1999	2000	2001	2002	2003*	Total
Number of requests for state permission	13	20	19	19	1	72
Number of private HEIs with state permission	5	9	11	2	–	27
Number of rejected state permissions	8	11	8	14	–	41
Number of requests in process in Accreditation Commission or Ministry of Education				3	1	4

* Data for 2003 available until 1 March.

3.3 Accreditation, Evaluation and other Processes in the Country

3.3.1 Driving Forces for the Establishment of the Accreditation and Evaluation Schemes

The main driving force behind the accreditation scheme and the establishment of quality evaluation was the fear that the quality of higher education was under heavy pressure, mainly for the following reasons:

1. the very high degree of autonomy and self-governance of the institutions, combined with the limited power of the state (1990 Act, approval of the situation by the 1998 Act),
2. the rapid increase in the number of students in higher education,
3. the freedom to establish private higher education institutions.

First, with regard to the autonomy of higher education institutions, the 1990 Act changed the situation dramatically. It gave back their academic rights to the institutions, together with a high degree of self-governance and autonomy from the state. At the same time, it greatly limited the power of the state and changed its role from strict control to indirect steering through budget allocation and the co-ordination of higher education development. Decentralisation was seen as being in line with the overall development in Europe and in the world. The Czech case, however, differed significantly from other European countries at the time, since:

- Starting conditions were very different from those in most Western European countries.
- Central governance was fully subordinated to the political power until 1990, without a realistic decision-making base.
- The change from centralised to extremely decentralised conditions was extremely quick (the first higher education law was passed in Parliament within six months of the change in the regime, much quicker than in most other countries in the region).

The new legal rules (1998), which introduced obligatory accreditation and evaluation of quality, were both a general response to the satisfactory decentralisation of state power and the way to ensure the quality of higher education.

Secondly, the high proportion of the relevant population now entering higher education called for the diversification of the study offer to give students a chance to study in accordance with their abilities and needs. Thus, diversification would improve the overall quality of higher education. The quality of the wide spectrum of study possibilities should be checked. This was another reason to create the Accreditation Commission.

Thirdly, the developing private sector in higher education was considered as a positive motivation and competition for the public sector. The rapid growth in the number of private higher education institutions in most Central and Eastern European countries, however, created a lack of adequately qualified teachers and researchers, insufficient financial means and facilities, etc. This could be a risk for students who were not accustomed to this higher education market. To prevent such a situation, the obligation to obtain state permission for all newly- established private higher education institutions was introduced.

The initiator of the preparation of the legal rules and the adoption of the Act in 1990 was mainly the academic community itself. This 'revolutionary' situation was quite quickly followed by a more evolutionary stage, when the main initiator of the debate on the new Act was the state represented by the Ministry. The debate which resulted in the adoption of the Act in 1998 involved a broad spectrum of stakeholders: representatives of the state, of the academic community, higher education governance, students, members of Parliament, etc.

3.3.2 Political and Social Consequences of the Schemes

The temporary or permanent withdrawal of accreditation which can follow from a negative evaluation of study programme by the Accreditation Commission may cause political as well as social problems.

To prevent students from becoming the victim of these problems, the Act obliges the higher education institutions concerned to provide students with a satisfactory substitution. In theory, it seems that students are safe. In practice, this is not always the case. With programmes that are not widespread, it may be difficult to find an institution which is able (and also willing) to let the students continue their studies. Even such details as a different sequence of study subjects or courses may cause problems. There may be unpleasant psychological barriers due to the unexpected change of location, of teachers, of form of study, of social conditions, etc. The additional pressure on limited student accommodation or the need to travel are costly or time-consuming, or both.

Political problems may ensue if it proves impossible to find a proper institution, or if there are too many non-accredited study programmes in an institution or if there are significant social problems of the kind mentioned in the previous paragraph.

3.3.3   Relationships between Accreditation and Evaluation Schemes

Both accreditation and evaluation schemes were developing without a clear idea of their relationship. During the first years of the evaluation scheme, knowledge gathered from different, fragmented experiences from abroad was used rather than a conceptually composed evaluation scheme. The activity of the Accreditation Commission at that time was not obligatory for higher education institutions. The idea was to encourage a certain type of 'benchmarking'. An institution was willing to undertake the evaluation because it could compare itself with other institutions and meet the aims of the Accreditation Commission, which quite quickly enjoyed high prestige. The process developed step-by-step, using both national and foreign experiences, including the results of the international evaluations listed above.

The obligatory accreditation scheme was introduced in 1998. The accreditation focuses on the study programme (the other types of accreditation are very specific and not important for this section) while the evaluation focuses on the institution. Non-accreditation leads to a reduction of the institutional budget and has a very negative influence on the prestige of the institution. Evaluation, on the contrary, does not lead directly to any decisive result. It is assumed that the published results are a satisfactory tool to oblige the institution to take the measures in accordance with the recommendations.

3.3.4   Relations with Approval Schemes

The Czech higher education system is very decentralised. The only approval scheme, besides accreditation, is related to the allocation of the state budget. The decision-making power in this matter is in the hands of the state, even if the rules of allocation and final decision on it should be discussed with the representation of higher education institutions (see section 3.1.4); in most cases an agreement or compromise has been found. The relation between accreditation and fund allocation schemes appears in the case of a non-accredited study programme, since if students cannot be enrolled, the share of the budget based on the number of students cannot be received.

3.3.5   Current Situation and Possible Projection for the Future

In recent years, attention focused on the accreditation of all study programmes and on the high number of private higher education providers wanting to obtain state permission. The workload of the Accreditation Commission increased. Hence, the evaluation activities were reduced to the strict minimum. The positive side was that the actors of both schemes started to think about:

- the workload of academics involved in accreditation and evaluation;
- the workload of the Accreditation Commission;
- the fact that the expert opinion of the Accreditation Commission needed for accreditation is expressed after the specific evaluation;
- the possibility to incorporate the results of accreditation in the evaluation scheme, i.e. to build on the fact that the study programme has been accredited and to focus the evaluation activity on other elements of institutional performance;
- the amendment of the Decree in connection with the above;
- the reasons why the Accreditation Commission is responsible for both schemes, and what are the positive and negative consequences of this arrangement,
- the arguments for improvements or changes in both schemes,
- the need to co-ordinate both activities very carefully to prevent overload on both sides (i.e. the higher education institutions and the Accreditation Commission).

The short-term objective of the Accreditation Commission is to finalise the accreditation of all study programmes in accordance with the Act and then focus on re-accreditation, accreditation of new programmes, and evaluation. It is not easy to predict the development in the field of private higher education. It is estimated that the submission of applications for state permission – hence the high workload for the Accreditation Commission – will continue. A debate between the Accreditation Commission, the Ministry and the academic community is expected on further improvements of the process and on the question of how to involve other stakeholders, especially employers.

3.3.6   Consequences of the Accreditation Scheme

Consequences for Higher Education Institutions, Departments and Scholars

Between 1990 and 1998, state higher education institutions were implicitly accredited because they were established by the Act. Hence, they were fully responsible for the study programme content, teaching and research capacity, and facilities, as well as for all changes.

As from 1998, the situation changed. A public higher education institution continues to be fully responsible for everything concerning study programmes. The difference is that before the programme can be publicly announced and offered, the institution must apply for accreditation. The consequence for an institution is that is should think very carefully about the requirements of the Accreditation Commission and the additional demands of the Ministry listed by the Act. It should prepare clear evidence that all requirements are met. The unpleasant side of this is the additional workload.

If weaknesses exist, an institution should overcome them. This is an important difference with the period before 1998. There were perhaps no programmes of poor quality (or at least not frequently), but there was no need to ensure and improve quality. Developing the evaluation scheme (as from 1990) required increasingly responsible behaviour on the part of faculties, as they now had to ensure the general quality of study programmes.

The psychological effect of accreditation is the most important. Loss of reputation and a potential loss of income may have grave consequences. Accreditation of the procedures of *habilitation* and of professors' appointments influences the career of academics. The accreditation allows an institution to recruit either its own candidates or candidates from other institutions for (associate) professors' appointments. Obtaining this right helps to improve the qualifications of the academic staff, as well as the institution's reputation.

The rapid increase in the number of private higher education institutions may be very dangerous from the point of view of quality. It is too soon to judge the real consequences of the obligation to obtain state permission in the Czech Republic. The requirements of the Accreditation Commission are rigorous and objectively comparable with those concerning accreditation in the public sector. Also, the ministerial evaluation of data pertaining to provision of financial, material, personnel and information sources, the long-term plan and all formal duties required by the Act is demanding. Therefore, it is hoped that this procedure will help the country not to repeat the negative experiences of some other countries in this region.

Consequences for Students

The unmet demand of applicants for study places could lead to the creation of programmes in attractive study fields (economics, business, law, arts, computer sciences, etc.) without careful assurance of their content and other inputs (qualified staff, facilities, etc.). Accreditation prevents this, so the consequence for students should be fairly positive. Accreditation cannot ensure that all teachers will take good care of students. Nor can it ensure a development of innovative approaches to the teaching and learning process, in particular the substitution of 'frontal teaching' in classroom by the use of modern teaching materials, of modern channels of communication between students and teachers, etc. Nor does it mean that students will be offered acceptable social conditions. But evaluation seems to be very important for students' satisfaction. Students are quite active in this respect and the attention paid to their recommendations may be very positive.

Consequences for other Stakeholders

The accreditation of study programmes is a general assurance of quality for all stakeholders. *Parents* can be assured that studies in each higher education institution, whether it is a venerably old, prestigious one located in Prague or a brand new one in the region, are of good quality. It is also the assurance that the tuition fee (sometimes very high!) of a private higher education institution will be paid for an acceptable quality of study. *Employers* are assured that graduates will be provided with good academic knowledge. It does not mean, however, that the content of the study programme will meet their practice-driven requirements. This is a weak point of the Czech accreditation scheme so far; the composition of the Accreditation Commission is too academic, and evaluation of study programmes from the point of view of employers is almost missing. It seems very difficult to reach a consensus on how to improve this weak point, and even solving it only partly will take time. The accreditation is also assurance for the *state* (Ministry) that the funds granted to the institution are used properly, not for bad programmes.

3.3.7   Other Processes in the Country

There are no other processes of quality evaluation or accreditation in the country that are officially required or organised at the national level. Czech institutions have been active in international evaluation schemes which were generally considered useful. But at least two weak points should be mentioned.

The first results from the significant introversion of institutions about their 'own life' and the lack of inter-institutional collaboration. This causes a lack of shared experience, a lack of use of examples of good practice, and a lack of use of information about possible difficulties which may occur from the different international evaluation processes. To overcome these problems needs time.

The second weak point is conditioned by the institutional funding and the limited possibilities to use government grants for purposes that are not earmarked. The institutional budget is always quite tight and the evaluation procedures offered by the different international bodies or agencies are very expensive for Czech institutions. For this reason, even if some international evaluations would be attractive (e.g. the Institutional Review Programme of the EAU, or the Internationalisation Quality Review offered jointly by the OECD/IMHE, ACA and EAU), they are not used frequently. For instance, the OECD/IMHE evaluation costs about € 19,000, which represents about two year salaries of quite well-paid young teachers in a Czech higher education institution. Evaluation by an international agency requires needs extra funds; for example, the evaluation of Czech Technical University in Prague by CRE (now EUA) was sponsored by the TEMPUS project.

The tertiary professional programmes are approved by the Ministry, but this is just an administrative process. 'Evaluation' of these programmes is the responsibility of the School Inspection. It may be characterised as administration and has very little to do with real quality evaluation. However, a pilot project in quality assurance was launched in early 2003. It is expected that the results will influence the accreditation mechanism at the level of bachelor study programmes and the evaluation of non-university higher education institutions, as the contemporary methods are often criticised because they are too academic.

Any lifelong learning course can be subject to the evaluation process if it is provided by a higher education institution. It is not subject to accreditation as it is considered implicitly that the provider, i.e. a higher education institution, is a sufficient guarantee for its quality. Other lifelong learning courses may be accredited by a special Accreditation Commission established by the Ministry for this purpose.[1] Accreditation is not obligatory, but, as a rule, a provider will ask for accreditation if nationwide acceptation of the course is aimed at.

3.4   Influence of the Bologna Process and of International Examples

3.4.1   The Bologna Process

Both evaluation and accreditation schemes were established in the Czech Republic before the process of the harmonisation of the European higher education studies

---

1   Unfortunately, its name is also Accreditation Commission, although it is a completely different body from the Accreditation Commission for 'normal' higher education

was initiated. So, in theory, the Czech Republic can easily accept the call of both Bologna Declaration and Prague Communiqué for the urgent need for quality evaluation and accreditation schemes.

In practice, though, it will be necessary to pay attention to the weak points of our schemes. The need to pay special attention to the interrelation of evaluation and accreditation schemes was explained in the previous section. Another serious difficulty is the need to devote attention to international developments. There is a strong tendency to focus on home problems and on our ideas of how they are to be solved.

The current driving forces for the Accreditation Commission and for the decision-making and research bodies are the results of activities since Bologna, e.g. the Salamanca Convention (the invitation to create a European platform for discussion and exchange of experience is highly acceptable) and the Prague Communiqué.

The ten years of the Czech Accreditation Commission's experience is longer and in many aspects broader than in many other countries, including those of the EU. Accordingly, it may contribute significantly to the common knowledge of all partners in ENQA. But the Accreditation Commission would benefit considerably from the experience of others and from their comments and recommendations.

The common European Higher Education Area would enable students to move freely across the whole continent, but this is conditioned by the recognition of mutually acceptable levels of quality of studies. The first step at the European level would be the mutual recognition of national evaluation and accreditation schemes, which requires the following:

- To have as much reliable information about the national schemes of quality evaluation and accreditation as possible.
- To have very clear information in order to prevent mistakes.
- To trust each other on the basis of the above two statements.
- To take into consideration the Lisbon Convention which asks us to avoid the former approach based on the equivalence of studies and to accept the recognition approach, as long as significant differences do not exist.

The last statement will play a significant role. The difficulty in our country to recognise studies obtained at different Czech higher education institutions points to the need for mutual trust and a common debate.

3.4.2   Transnational Education

Transnational education has not been a very common issue in the Czech Republic. It is very easy for a foreign higher education provider to act in the Czech Republic as a private higher education institution, to offer study programmes and to award foreign degrees. In this case, however, there is not enough knowledge about the quality of studies, so that the recognition of the academic degree may cause problems. The competent authorities are the Czech higher education institutions and their decisions concerning recognition (or not) may create (unwanted?) precedents. A foreign higher education provider may ask for accreditation. If successful, accreditation means approval of quality, and the permission to award Czech academic degrees. Several providers obtained accreditation.

The Czech Republic does not export higher education at present. However, the exchange of students is developing very rapidly. The debate on the concept of the quality of transnational education is at an early stage, as is that on GATS and education.

3.4.3   International Examples

It is usually stressed that, even if models work smoothly in other countries, they cannot be transferred to different contexts. But there were many comparative investigations that stressed that important elements of quality assurance schemes could be found in other forms in almost every country. The Czech experience can support both views.

We are a society that does not easily accept changes, so we do not like to look for models abroad. On the other hand, we sometimes accept what seems to be modern and very necessary – often without a proper analysis and therefore with questionable results. In this context, we had the opportunity to evaluate the entire higher education system in the framework of a review by OECD. The whole process (it started in 1991) was successful. The final report was presented and discussed in Prague. The reason for the choice of this location was to enable a wide spectrum of stakeholders to take part. The impact was quite strong, the recommendations were the topic of very serious debate and they influenced the development of the higher education system significantly. The common elements of current evaluation schemes were incorporated into our evaluation scheme.

There was no such clear model in the case of accreditation. The experience of US accreditation was disseminated in the Czech Republic in several seminars attended by our colleagues from the American Council on Education and Penn State University. There were personal experiences of those Czechs who were able to stay in the USA, etc. Maybe our accreditation scheme was influenced slightly in some aspects. But, in principle, neither models from abroad nor possible models from the field of professional accreditation were fully accepted. The accreditation scheme was established following the agreement of a wide spectrum of higher education stakeholders who participated in the debates and preparation of the Higher Education Act adopted in 1998.

4   Ministerial Approval and Improvement-Oriented Evaluation in Denmark: An Alternative to Accreditation?

DORTE KRISTOFFERSEN

4.1   The Danish Higher Education System

4.1.1   Structure and Steering of Higher Education

The Danish higher education system is a public education system. Higher education institutions are public and state-regulated. All higher education is subject to ministerial approval of new programmes and institutions. The institutions have a high degree of autonomy but must follow general regulations, e.g., concerning teacher qualifications and award structures.

Private institutions can operate without any approval. There are few private institutions of higher education and no private universities. The last few years have seen some examples of transnational education offers where Danish institutions have established agreements with foreign institutions to offer bachelor's degrees. These agreements have primarily been established by colleges offering medium-cycle professional degrees.

The institutions of higher education are divided into two sectors:

- The college sector, i.e. the professionally oriented higher education sector offering short-cycle and medium-cycle professional programmes
- The university sector.

Higher education programmes are divided into short-cycle (18 %), medium-cycle (39 %) and long-cycle (43 %) programmes. The Ministry of Education is responsible for almost all college sector education whereas the universities are part of the responsibility of the Ministry of Science, Technology and Innovation.

Students pay no fees to enter higher education. They may furthermore obtain a state grant for the official time of their studies plus an additional year in case of a wrong choice.

General entrance requirements to higher education are twelve years of education. Admission to many study programmes also depends on the fulfilment of specific entrance requirements. These may either be a specific subject combination, or re-

87

S. Schwarz and D.F. Westerheijden (eds.),
Accreditation and Evaluation in the European Higher Education Area, 87–100.

quirements concerning the subjects taken or the grades obtained. It is also possible for the institutions to formulate more qualitatively oriented criteria for admission, e.g. work experience, travel, or community service. A *numerus clausus* exists for some study programmes.

Figure 1. Higher education in Denmark

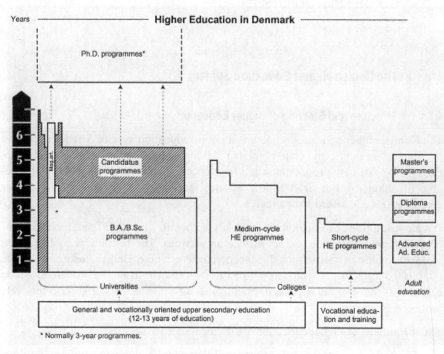

Source: the Ministry of Education website (http://www.uvm.dk)

4.1.2   Size

Danish higher education institutions had an intake of almost 43,100 students in 2001. 44 % of an age group attends one of the three kinds of programmes. The college sector comprises over 150 specialised institutions. One third offers short-cycle programmes and the other two-thirds medium-cycle programmes. As of 2003, there were twelve universities. Five are multi-faculty universities while the rest are specialised in fields such as engineering, information technology and education. All university programmes are research based.

4.1.3 The Main Types of Degrees and Programmes

The degrees offered in the Danish higher education system are organised according to the types of programmes on offer.

Table 1. Types of higher education degrees

Cycle	Degree/Title	Type of institution	Duration
Short-cycle professional qualification	AK[1] 2-year professional degree	College	2 years
Medium-cycle	Professional bachelor degree	College	3 to 4 years
Medium- cycle	Bachelor of arts Bachelor of science	University	3 years
Long-cycle	Master of arts Master of science	University	2 years[2] (awarded after a total of 5 years)
Long-cycle	Mag.art.	University	Bachelor degree + 3 years
Long-cycle	Ph.D. degree	University	3 years (awarded after a total of 8 years)

Source: En Dansk Kvalifikationsnøgle (A Danish Qualification Framework)

There is also an adult education system. It offers Advanced Adult Education, which is comparable to short-cycle higher education. The Diploma programmes are comparable to medium-cycle higher education, and the Master programmes (e.g. MBAs) are comparable to long-cycle higher education. Most programmes consist of two years of part-time study, equivalent to one year of full-time study. Admission requirements are relevant educational qualifications and at least two years of work experience in a relevant profession.

4.1.4 Labour Market Requirements

The labour market in Denmark is unregulated. A degree that is recognised by the government is only required to practise a few professions, e.g. medicine, midwifery, and law. These professions are subject to a formal authorisation process by the relevant authority, e.g. the National Board of Health.

---

1 No official translation is available.
2 The degree in medicine is awarded after a total of 6½ years of study, however.

Table 2. Rates of unemployment (percentage of those holding a degree)

	1997	2001
Short-cycle professional education	6.2 %	3.6 %
Medium-cycle education	3.0 %	2.1 %
Long-cycle education	4.4 %	2.9 %

Source: Statistics Denmark

4.1.5 Governance and Steering of Higher Education

The Danish higher education institutions are governed by various laws, and there are differences in the specific rules for governance and steering. There are a number of principles, however, which apply to all institutions. They are governed by boards with both external members and in most cases members within the institution. For the universities, this principle is introduced with the new university law which is discussed below. The university boards will comprise a majority of external members and the chairman of the board will be chosen among these.

Staff-student study committees are responsible for the planning of the study programmes. They comprise staff and student representatives and sometimes technical and administrative staff.

4.2 Procedures of Accreditation, Approval and Quality Assurance

4.2.1 Accreditation in Denmark

In terms of the definition of an accreditation scheme in this study there are no accreditation schemes in Denmark for public degrees, programmes or institutions. The main reason for this is that all institutions, programmes and degrees are subject to approval by laws and ministerial orders.

As mentioned in the first section, there are no private universities operating in Denmark and only a few private short-cycle higher education programmes. These are subject to accreditation if they want to obtain state educational grants for their students. This type of accreditation was set up to limit the rise in the number of private programmes demanding state educational grants, which took place in the late 1990s. Accreditation is not mandatory for the institutions, but necessary to obtain the state educational grant.

The application for accreditation is sent to the Ministry of Education where it is screened, and it is decided if it should be sent to The Danish Evaluation Institute (EVA) for accreditation. The institutions are asked to prepare a self-study in which they must document how they meet a number of predefined criteria. The self-evaluation is sent to EVA which sets up an internal project team among its staff that is responsible for the accreditation process.

When the self-study is analysed the project team carries out a site visit that has a double purpose. On the one hand, to meet the different groups at the institutions, i.e. students, staff, management and representatives of the external examiners to verify the statements put forward in the self-study. On the other, the site visit offers the team the opportunity to study more carefully the documentation for the statements put forward in the self-study.

In addition to the self-study and the site visit, statistics are prepared that show whether the labour market is favourable for the graduates of the private programmes. It is an important parameter in the accreditation process.

After the site visit the project team draws up a recommendation for accreditation commenting on the strengths and weaknesses in respect of the different criteria. The recommendation may lead to three kinds of decision: unconditional approval, approval on condition and non-approval. If institutions are granted unconditional approval they obtain the right to the state educational grant for four years. In case of approval on condition they typically have to improve certain aspects of their procedures. The typical delay granted to remedy these shortcomings is between six and twelve months. If an institution is not approved it has to reapply for accreditation.

4.2.2   Approval of Higher Education institutions, Programmes and Degrees

General Procedure

The establishment of new institutions, programmes, and degrees is regulated by the relevant ministry, i.e. either the Ministry of Education or the Ministry of Science, Technology and Innovation for the universities. Institutions and programmes under the Ministry of Education are regulated by ministerial orders and subject to approval by the ministry. A proposal for a new university law was presented in Parliament in January 2003. It is part of the proposal that ministerial orders[3] will be replaced by ministerial approval for the establishment and abolishment of institutions and new programmes.

The application to establish new programmes is sent to the relevant ministry. In the case of the Ministry of Education the approval will be decided in relation to the

---

3   Ministerial orders are the written regulations of the institutions of HE in a relation to their various activities. In addition to or on the background of these, various activities or decision can be subject to ministerial approval.

relevant ministerial order. In future, the university programmes will only be subject to ministerial approval and their relevance for society will play an important part in the approval process. Programmes for which special approval procedures exist are presented below. There is no procedure for one type of institution to change status, e.g. for a college to apply to become a university.

Approval of Professional Bachelor Degrees

Following the introduction of the professional bachelor degree in 2001, all medium-cycle higher education programmes were granted the title of professional bachelor degrees (title: bachelor plus the profession). This right is granted by the Ministry of Education on the basis of an assessment of the degree to which the programmes fulfil the requirements set out in the ministerial order for the professional bachelor programmes. The Ministry of Education has furthermore committed itself to carry out a further review of the programmes on the basis of the formal criteria set out in the legislation and a number of criteria defined by EVA to decide whether they can maintain the right to offer the professional bachelor degree. The Minister of Education has not yet decided how this approval procedure will be organised.

Approval of Master Degrees in the Adult Education System

The Ministry of Science, Technology and Innovation approves the establishment of new master's programmes as part of the Adult Education system on the basis of a recommendation made by the Rectors' Conference. An application for approval of a new master degree in the Adult Education system has to include a description of the following points:

- Admission requirements
- The degree of user and labour market influence
- Objectives and content
- Target group and professional profile
- The division of the programme into modules
- Length
- Quality assurance mechanisms
- Placement in the taximeter system (the cash-per-student grant system)
- Relation to the relevant ministerial order.

Approval will be made public on the ministerial website.

If the application cannot be approved, the Ministry contacts the Rectors' Conference to further discuss the application and clarify the criticisms. Depending on the results of this, the application is either rejected or the programme is asked to provide additional information.

Programmes are initially approved for a two-year trial period. After this period, a self-evaluation process is launched and the ministry decides whether the programme should be granted a permanent status, be adjusted or be closed down on the basis of the result.

Programmes within the same academic field will be evaluated together. The evaluation will focus on a number of predefined issues which are known to the programmes beforehand and is the same for all programmes. It will draw on a number of facts about e.g. enrolment and drop-out rates and will include comments from external examiners who were involved in the evaluations and representatives of the labour market for the specific programmes. Furthermore, the judgement of the graduates' competences after graduation by the labour market will also play a role in the evaluation.

4.2.3 The National, Supra-Institutional Evaluation Scheme

EVA's Mandate

The Danish Evaluation Institute (EVA) was established by law in June 1999 with the objective to systematically evaluate all levels of the educational system. Furthermore, EVA must be the centre of expertise concerning educational evaluation in Denmark. Last but not least, EVA can carry out evaluations on request from the Ministry of Education, the Ministry of Science, Technology and Innovation, other ministries responsible for educational activities, school owners or institutions.

EVA is an independent institution under the responsibility of the Ministry of Education. It has its own board and can decide which evaluations to initiate each year. The activities of EVA are presented in annual plans of action which are approved by the minister of education. Participation in the evaluations initiated by EVA is mandatory for the higher education institutions.

EVA can also decide what to evaluate. Between 1992 and 1999, EVA's predecessor, the Center for Evaluation, evaluated all programmes of higher education (both medium and long cycle education) every seven years. With the integration of the Center for Evaluation into EVA it was decided, however, not to continue immediately the round of programme evaluations but to test a number of other types of evaluation, drawing on the experiments in the field of evaluation of higher education in the 1990s. EVA has therefore not decided, for the time being, on one type of evaluation, but carries out follow-up evaluations, programme evaluations, evaluations of faculties and institutions and audits that evaluate the internal quality assurance mechanisms of the institutions.

EVA's Activities and Procedures

According to the law on the Danish Evaluation Institute there are a number of mandatory elements in the evaluations carried out by EVA:

- An evaluation must build on the self-evaluation carried out by the evaluated units
- An external evaluation group is responsible for the recommendations and conclusions in the evaluation report
- EVA staff is responsible for the methodology and the secretariat function
- A public report.

Prior to each evaluation, EVA conducts a preliminary study which encompasses existing material relating to the field of education, e.g. regulations, ministerial orders, study plans and curricula. The preliminary study also often involves a dialogue with the main stakeholders in the evaluated field.

The preliminary study is essential for the preparation of the terms of reference for the evaluation. The Board approves the terms of reference. After their approval, they are sent to the institutions participating in the evaluation and are made available to the public on the EVA website.

EVA is obliged by law to inform the participating institutions about the objectives of the evaluation, the terms of reference, including the time schedule, the methods applied, the composition of the expert group and the institutions' tasks in the evaluation process. EVA also has to inform the evaluated institutions that participation is mandatory, and that they are obliged to provide all the information requested by EVA which is of relevance to the evaluation and must comment on factual and technical errors before the report is made public. All the costs of an evaluation and those of the preparation of the self-evaluation document are covered by EVA. The duration of an evaluation is in general one year between the approval of the terms of reference by the board and the publication of the final report.

As part of the preparation of the terms of reference, members of the external evaluation group are identified by EVA and approved by the board. The external evaluation group is made up of experts in the field evaluated. EVA applies a multi-professional peer concept. As a general rule, the experts are academic experts, representatives of the labour market and general experts in education. It is important for the evaluation process that the experts are external to the institutions or programmes being evaluated. But at the same time great care is taken to find experts who are respected by those being evaluated and who have an understanding and knowledge of the field under evaluation. In order to achieve the necessary level of externality EVA uses a large number of Swedish and Norwegian experts who understand Danish.

The institutions prepare a self-evaluation report on the basis of guidelines for self-evaluation. These are prepared by EVA and commented by the external evaluation group. The guidelines comprise the themes that the institutions must cover in the self-evaluation and sometimes the specific questions that they have to answer. The self-evaluation report serves two purposes. First, it aims at initiating processes of quality improvement within the institutions. Second, it serves as information for the external expert panel. The guidelines also contain advice on how to organise the self-evaluation process. The institutions are encouraged to set up a self-evaluation group comprising members of its management, teachers, students and technical and administrative staff. This group is responsible for drafting the self-evaluation document. EVA always carries out a number of additional surveys, which also form part of the documentation. They can be surveys among labour market representatives and former students, or more statistical surveys e.g. aimed at throwing light on the employment situation of the graduates.

Once the institutions have prepared the self-evaluation report and the surveys are finalised, the external expert panel and the EVA staff visit the institutions for a day. They meet the managers, staff, students, and in some cases external examiners and the self-evaluation group.

Following the site visit, the EVA staff member responsible for the evaluation drafts elaborates the evaluation report on the basis of input from the experts. All reports contain conclusions, e.g. on the strengths of the institutions and specific recommendations as to how quality can be improved. The draft report is sent to the institution for correction of factual mistakes. Furthermore, the institutions can comment on the evaluation process and the methods used. Once the report is finalised, it is printed and made public. All EVA reports are available in Danish (the abstracts will be available in English) on its website (www.eva.dk). Furthermore, they are circulated to a large number of parties, e.g. the evaluated institutions, the relevant ministry and the main stakeholders. The printed reports are also for sale.

Follow-Up to Evaluations

The follow-up to the evaluations of short and medium cycle education carried out by EVA is also regulated by law. It is the responsibility of the Ministry of Education. According to the ministerial order on follow-up, which came into effect in January 2002, an evaluated institution has to plan its follow-up to the evaluation no later than six months after the publication of the report and send it to the Ministry of Education. The Minister of Education has the option to take action if the institution's follow-up is deemed insufficient. The universities are responsible for the follow-up to evaluations.

In May 2002, legislation on transparency and openness was introduced requiring that all educational institutions put the results of both internal and external evaluations on their website.

The Quality System in Short-Cycle Higher Education

Since the year 2000, institutions providing vocational education and short-cycle higher education have been under the obligation to use a system of continuous quality development and a system of assessment of results. Hence, they must have procedures for systematic self-evaluation of central areas of institutional activity. These ensure, for instance, that teaching measures up to the predetermined goals, that appropriate teaching methods are used, that the school or the teachers consult students on their assessment of the instruction provided and of the institution's organisation of the course or programme of study, and the systematic continuing training of teachers. In addition, examination results and any external evaluations must form part of self-evaluation. On the basis of a school's self-evaluation, a follow-up plan must be devised specifying how the pre-determined goals are to be achieved. It is an explicit requirement that teachers, students and the local education committee be involved in this process.

The Examination System

In parallel to the system of external evaluation, there is also a system of external examiners. At least one-third of the exams of higher education programmes must be attended by an external examiner. The external examiners are organised in national boards for the various programmes of study. The national boards of examiners make sure that the examiners are used on a rotating basis at the different institutions offering the same programmes in order to safeguard academic standards across the country.

At least one third of the boards of external examiners should be labour market representatives. The external examiners are nominated by the institutions and approved by the relevant ministry. The course supervisor is responsible for choosing the examiners for each examination.

4.3   The Status of Accreditation in Denmark

4.3.1   Accreditation in the National Context

It has been mentioned above that Denmark does not have an accreditation system of higher education. It is interesting to observe that the discussion of the possible benefits and needs of introducing accreditation has been close to non-existent in Denmark as compared to many other European Union countries. Undoubtedly, the main reason for this is that approval is and has always been centrally managed by the relevant ministries in the form of ministerial orders and ministerial approval. It should be mentioned, however, that the ministries have always been able to use the results of external evaluations to carry out their inspection obligations, e.g. in terms of financing or institutional requirements. But this is not done with an accreditation purpose.

In addition, Denmark has both an efficient evaluation system and a system of external examiners. The evaluation system is a guarantee that the overall quality of higher education is studied at regular intervals, and the system of external examiners checks that the quality of specific subjects and academic standards are maintained and are comparable across institutions and programmes. In sum, these evaluation procedures ensure that Danish higher education activities are evaluated on a regular basis, and regularity has been emphasised in the new university law whereby the universities will also be responsible, through development contracts, for initiating systematic evaluation of teaching and research activities.

Discussions on accreditation have mainly involved the ministries, the advisory system for higher education, the rectors' conferences and EVA. They have not yet involved the staff. The Universities' Rectors' Conference has been the most outspoken. It is not willing to discuss the introduction of accreditation unless the ministries are willing to abolish the ministerial approval system. Ministerial approval and accreditation would imply a double approval system. The discussion of accreditation versus ministerial orders thus goes hand in hand. It has not been challenged further than this, since the system of ministerial approval is still firmly in place.

It could be expected that the professions, e.g. engineering, would be especially active in the debate as national accreditation often paves the way for easier access for students to foreign institutions of higher education. But this has not been the case except for the two business schools which have both participated in the EQUIS accreditation scheme, which covers business schools.

Accreditation is often mentioned as an important steering mechanism in matters of recognition of foreign degrees. During the past year the need for accreditation as a means of controlling offers of foreign degrees or joint degrees has been discussed. There is no doubt that in the long run these types of educational offers will require some kind of control in the form of evaluation or accreditation. To date there are only few examples where these educational offers have caused severe problems and there is at this stage no agreement within and between the ministries as to how seriously this situation should be taken and what measures should be introduced.

As mentioned in 4.2.2, a system for approval of Master degrees in Adult Education has been introduced. It resembles an accreditation system insofar as the criteria are quite specific. Furthermore, the programmes will be evaluated on the basis of a number of pre-defined criteria after a trial period. The same trend can be found in the approval of professional bachelor degrees. The Ministry of Education has announced that the formal approval of these degrees will be on the basis of predefined criteria and will end in a yes or no decision. These schemes have only recently been introduced, and it is too early to say if this is a first step towards the introduction of accreditation. It should be added, however, that neither of the ministries responsible for these degrees are trying to link the introduction of these approval systems to a discussion of accreditation.

It should also be mentioned that EVA has carried out a number of evaluations, both national and international, which are based on specific criteria in the last two years. These evaluations do not lead to accreditation, but they have given both EVA and the participating institutions experience with a type of evaluation that could eventually lead to accreditation.

4.3.2   The Pros and Cons of Accreditation

The national context, and not the international imperative, has decided the fate of accreditation in Denmark. On the basis of the analysis presented above on the concept of evaluation, a number of advantages and disadvantages of accreditation as a national steering mechanism can be identified.

First, accreditation would establish an approval process that is solidly grounded in an evaluation process based on academic judgements of quality. In this way, the judgement of good quality, which would be part of an evaluation process, would be separated from the approval process, which could be part of the ministerial approval responsibility. Second, accreditation based on pre-defined criteria would increase transparency both in terms of the approval process and the quality of the institutions that are subject to accreditation. Third, accreditation could be a means to liberalise higher education by offering a control system in a less regulated market.

But three disadvantages can also been identified. There is a risk that evaluation on the basis of pre-defined criteria will impede the development processes within the institutions as fulfilment of the criteria becomes a goal in itself. Second, the formulation of criteria can be based on or develop a conservative concept of quality and hamper innovation. The third disadvantage is of a financial nature. For accreditation to be efficient it has be to repeated at regular intervals, e.g. five to seven years, to make sure that the quality is always up to current standard. This would involve a large number of resources both within the institutions, at the evaluation institute, and in the ministries.

These arguments do not spring from the Danish discussion, which has not yet reached such an operational level. Apart from the two examples mentioned above, there are no concrete initiatives or signals from the ministries that the situation is about to change. The educational legislation that is being prepared or introduced at the moment follows the same lines of ministerial approval of degrees, programmes and institutions as before.

4.4 The International Dimension of Supra-Institutional Evaluation Schemes

4.4.1 The Influence of Bologna and GATS on Evaluation

In terms of the supra-institutional evaluation schemes, EVA follows the Bologna process very closely and has initiated or is part of a number of projects that attempt to test methods of evaluation that could help to create transparency of the quality of the educational systems and facilitate student mobility and access to foreign higher education institutions.

As part of its 2001 plan of action, EVA carried out an international evaluation of agricultural science in Denmark, the Netherlands, Germany and Ireland. The national evaluations carried out by EVA as a rule take as their starting point the objectives formulated for the evaluated unit, e.g. an institution or a programme. The educational systems in Europe are too different to apply this approach. Therefore the international evaluation took as its starting point a number of predefined criteria. The expert panel in the evaluation consisted of experts from the four countries and a chairman from Norway.

Furthermore, EVA is centrally placed in the Transnational European Evaluation Project (TEEP) of the European Network for Quality Assurance (ENQA) at the request of the European Commission. The project is carried out in co-operation with the quality assurance agencies in England, Catalonia (Spain) and Denmark. It aims to contribute to greater transparency and compatibility in European higher education through the development of a method for transnational evaluation, and it builds directly on the experience of the former European pilot project and the Tuning Institutional Structures in Europe project.

Denmark has been involved in a number of activities aimed at giving evaluation agencies and ministries of education across Europe experience in international evaluations and thus prepare them for future challenges. The most important is the preparation of the 'Dublin' Bachelor- and Master-descriptors. Their value will be tested in an international perspective in TEEP and in a national context in an evaluation of German language at university level in Denmark recently launched by EVA.

Last but not least, the evaluation agencies in the Nordic countries launched a project in 2001 to test a method for mutual recognition of quality assurance agencies. One

of the aims was to decide if the evaluation method helped the two national evaluation agencies in Finland and Denmark, FINHEEC and EVA, to recognise each
other's evaluations and thus accept them as equivalent. Furthermore, it functioned as
a quality assurance project for the two participating agencies.

It is the official position of the Ministry of Education and the Ministry of Science,
Technology and Innovation that there is no need to move beyond the level of liberalisation that currently exists in Europe, i.e. only privately funded education activities are subject to negotiations in GATS. The argument behind this is that the Danish
education market is quite open, giving both publicly funded education and non-
governmental providers of education the possibility to operate. Concerning quality
assurance and evaluation, the ministries consider ENQA to be an important
contribution to the creation of a European platform for quality assurance and
evaluation, but stress that quality assurance remains a national responsibility.

4.4.2   International inspiration

The supra-institutional evaluation procedures have always been inspired by international examples and developments. EVA has always participated in international co-
operation at global, European and Nordic levels. Furthermore, it has been involved
in a number of European projects, e.g. the European pilot project carried out between 1994 and 1995 for which EVA was responsible, together with the French
Comité National d'Évaluation, and the PHARE Multi-Country Project carried out
between 1997 and 1998. They both aimed at giving all countries in Europe an experience with evaluation and methods for quality improvement. International co-
operation and the projects naturally inspired and thus had a positive effect on the
Danish evaluation procedures.

4.5   Other Types of Quality Assessment Activities

For permanent employment, the qualifications of staff at higher education institutions are reviewed by a panel of experts in the field to make sure that the qualifications are of sufficient academic quality. Staff with a research obligation are also
regularly subject to review of their work. These procedures differ according to the
university.

Furthermore, the management responsible for the permanent staff is obliged to carry
out yearly appraisal interviews with staff. The purpose of these interviews is to
evaluate the achievements of the staff members over the last year, give positive and
negative feedback and discuss and plan the personal development activities for the
coming year.

5   Three Rounds of Evaluation and the Idea of Accreditation in Finnish Higher Education

JUSSI VÄLIMAA

5.1   Introduction

This study is based on the analysis of evaluation reports published by the Finnish Higher Education Evaluation Council (FINHEEC) supported by relevant research literature, the higher education databases (KOTA and AMKOTA)[1] maintained by the Ministry of Education, and other statistical data.

The study begins with a discussion on the central concepts of the study. It is followed by a description of the historical layers of Finnish higher education and evaluation to explain the context of accreditation. It then focuses on present day accreditation, evaluation and approval practices. The last sections discuss the nature and social roles of accreditation, approval and evaluation processes in Finnish higher education.

5.1.1   Defining Accreditation, Evaluation and Approval

This section focuses on the processes of accreditation (i.e. approval based on evaluation), evaluation (without approval-like consequences), and approval (without evaluation) in Finnish higher education. These concepts describe both the process where evaluation is related to political decision-making (accreditation) and the evaluation processes in and during which the political dimension is not very evident (evaluation). Approval describes the Finnish traditional administrative way of giving permission to an institution or a degree programme to operate without using any public evaluation or accreditation scheme.

Taking these concepts as intellectual devices, one should reflect shortly on their relationship. According to Scriven (1991) 'the term of "evaluation" refers to the process of determining the merit, worth, value of something, or the product of that process'.[2] Accreditation, in turn, is an evaluation of whether an institution qualifies

---

1   See KOTA database (http://www.csc.fi/kota/nuts.html) and AMKOTA database (http://www.csc.fi/amkota).

2   According to Woodhouse (1996), assessment is, in turn, an evaluation that results in a grade, whether numeric, literal or descriptive. I will use the concept of evaluation because the Finnish word 'arviointi' can be translated as evaluation and because there is no specific Finnish word for assessment. 'Arviointi' (evaluation) is also a rather neutral term in Finland.

S. Schwarz and D.F. Westerheijden (eds.),
Accreditation and Evaluation in the European Higher Education Area, 101–125.
© 2004 *Kluwer Academic Publishers. Printed in the Netherlands.*

for a certain status. Specialised or professional accreditation is, in turn, an evaluation of whether an institution or programme qualifies its graduates for employment in a particular field (Woodhouse, 1999). In addition to these concepts we should also mention audit, which describes the process during which an organisation's claims (explicit or implicit) about itself are checked.[3] All these schemes have been used in the evaluation processes in Finnish higher education. What is challenging about these concepts is that they often coincide in evaluation practices. I will return to this issue in section 5.4.

5.1.2   Finnish Higher Education in an Historical Perspective: Five Historical Layers

Present-day Finnish higher education is a mass higher education system with a 360-year history (Välimaa, 2001). I will outline this historical development by using the idea of historical layers. These should be seen as archaeological layers that were deposited over time. Following the metaphor, earlier layers influence modern practices because the traditions (ideas, norms and practices) have not only provided starting points for new developments but have also given shape to more recent layers.

The basic historical layer in Finnish higher education was laid during the Middle Ages when the Catholic Church sent talented young Finnish men to European universities, especially to the University of Paris. This cultural connection was also one of the factors that made Finland part of the Western European cultural sphere (Nuorteva, 1999).

The second historical layer, and the beginning of the development towards a national system of higher education, was initiated with the foundation of the University of Turku (then named the Royal Academy in Åbo) in 1640. At that time, Finland was part of the Swedish Kingdom and higher education mainly served the purposes of the Lutheran Church by training priests and defending the 'right religion' and of the King by training civil servants. This civil servant function continues to be an important part of Finnish higher education because most university graduates are employed by the public sector.

The third historical layer was added when Finland was an autonomous Grand Duchy which was part of the Russian Empire from 1809 to 1917. This was a period of cultural, political and economic development of Finland and the Finnish nationality. The only university was moved from Turku to the new capital of Helsinki in 1827 and renamed the Imperial Alexander University (later known as the University of

---

3   When an institution states objectives, the purpose of the quality audit is to check whether the institution is achieving its own objectives. When an institution makes explicit claims, audit becomes a validation of those claims (Woodhouse, 1999).

Helsinki). It played a central role in cultural, political and economic processes by creating a basis for the independent nation state which was established during the First World War (Klinge, 1987). The period was also important for the development of the Finnish idea of a university. It is no historical exaggeration to say that the university is considered a national cultural institution. This idea of a cultural institution was rooted in the Humboldtian ideals of a university. University and higher education were considered important aspects of the development of the nation and nation state. It was also realized that access to education – including higher education – was an issue to be decided by politicians, not by academics. These interpretations of the concept of a university continued into the 20th century and the issues they involve have been addressed at different points of time on the basis of a variety of political decisions (Välimaa, 2001).

The fourth historical layer was laid between the two World Wars when Finnish higher education continued to be an elite system. Studying was mainly open to the more prosperous social classes and the number of higher education students remained low. Social exclusion from higher education took place in the school system where one needed money to complete upper secondary school. The lack of public financial aid for students increased the effects of exclusion (Nevala, 1999). Furthermore, university professors belonged to the highest level of Finnish society, and from the 1920s to the 1940s many served as ministers (Klinge, 1992). High social prestige of universities and university degrees is still a reality in Finland.

The fifth historical layer was added with the evolution of Finnish higher education towards a mass higher education system. This development began in the late 1950s. Finnish higher education reached the level of mass higher education in the 1970s, when more than 15 % of the age cohort entered it. The last phase of expansion was the establishment of the polytechnic sector in the 1990s. Following the traditional Finnish reform strategy 'learning by experimenting', the first polytechnics were established as experimental institutions (Välimaa & Westerheijden, 1995). After a certain period of time they were allowed to apply for permanent status.

In 1999, the universities admitted 19,373 students and the polytechnics 25,804 (KOTA). A comparison of these numbers with the size of the relevant age cohort shows that 83 % are offered a place in higher education (Välimaa, 2001, KOTA, 2001, AMKOTA, 2001), even though only about 30 % of the students go on immediately to higher education after having completed secondary education (Havén, 1998).[4]

---

4   An indicator which shows that the proportion of 19-year-olds (the age at which one completes secondary education) who attends universities before the age of 29 is 25 % and those going to polytechnics is 20 % (Havén, 1998, p. 59). This is probably changing, because the indicator shows the situation in the mid-90s when polytechnics still operated mostly on a temporary basis.

The expansion of Finnish higher education was closely related to – and at the same time one of the results of – a welfare-state agenda supported by the major political parties. Creating equal educational opportunities, including equal access to higher education, became one of the most important objectives on this agenda, implemented over a period extending from the 1960s to the 1990s. The expansion of higher education was supported by a regional policy. The founding of a university was seen not only as symbolically but also culturally and economically important for the development of the given region. All major provinces were allowed to establish a university of their own in the 1960s, 1970s, and 1980s (see Välimaa, 2001).

5.1.3   Size, Structure and Degrees of the Present-day Finnish Higher Education System

In 2003, there were 20 universities, located in all parts of Finland. These include ten multi-faculty universities, three technical universities, three schools of economics, and four art academies. All Finnish universities are public institutions in the sense of the traditional continental model (Clark, 1983). They are autonomous institutions but subordinated to the Ministry of Education.[5]

There are 32 polytechnics which are located all over the country. Most of them are multidisciplinary institutions. This non-university sector of higher education was established in the 1990s. Finnish polytechnics (or AMK-institutions) were created by raising the standard of former higher vocational education institutions. As part of this process, institutions were incorporated into multidisciplinary polytechnics. All Finnish polytechnics were established as temporary institutions. Achieving permanent status was based on an approval process based on evaluation, as will be described below. Since August 1st, 2000, all polytechnics have operated on a permanent basis. They are usually local institutions operated by a municipality, a federation of municipalities or a registered Finnish foundation or association.[6] In principle, this means that part of the polytechnics are private institutions because they are run by foundations or associations. In practice, however, they are public institutions because they are funded by public sources - mainly the Ministry of Education (Välimaa, 2001).

---

5   The only exception to the rule is an attempt to establish a private university in Finland when the Preston University established a campus in two villages in Northern Finland at the end of the 20th century. It was not a success.

6   The exceptions to the rule are the Police College (funded by the Ministry of Interior) and Ålands Yrkeshögskola, which is subordinate to the self-governing Åland Islands. The National Defence College is a hybrid between these two higher education sectors, because it has elements of a polytechnic (basic training curricula) and common structures and functions with universities: professors, research activities and the right to grant doctoral degrees (Laine et al., 2001). In this chapter, the National Defence College is included in the polytechnic sector because of its small size (only five professors) and orientation to serve the needs of National Defence rather than those of the academic community.

Finnish universities confer professional degrees, bachelor's degrees, master's degrees, licentiate degrees and doctoral degrees. There are national decrees on the university degree systems for each discipline. They define the broad framework for each degree (length, structure, main objectives), but the universities have full autonomy to decide on the contents of each degree (Higher Education, 2001).

The polytechnics all confer Bachelor level degrees[7] which differ from academic degrees in that they target a particular professional area. In summer 2001, Parliament passed an act on experimental post-graduate polytechnic degrees. According to the Act, holders of a Bachelor's degree who also have at least three years of work experience can complete a 40- to 60-credit (18 months of full-time studies) post-graduate degree (OECD Report, 2002).

Universities and polytechnics select their students, and the competition for study places may be stiff in popular fields of study. All university fields apply a *numerus clausus*, in which entrance examinations are an essential element. Polytechnics also decide on their selection criteria, and in many sectors there is also an entrance examination.

5.1.4   Transition of Students from Higher Education to Work

The change in the social role of higher education from elite universities to mass higher education has changed the pattern of student employment. Holders of Master's degrees are mainly employed in education (34 %), manufacturing, electricity and water supply (14 %), health and social work (13 %), real estate and business (14 %), and also by the public administration and defense (10 %). These sectors employed 84 % of the 1995 graduates in the year 1996. Holders of polytechnics degrees in 1995 had somewhat different patterns of employment. Most (30 %) were employed in health and social work, then came manufacturing, electricity and water supply (14 %), wholesale retail and trade (13 %), public administration and defense (9 %), and real estate and business (78 %) (Havén, 1999). In 1996, these sectors employed 74 % of the 1995 polytechnic graduates.

As a rule, the employment pattern in Finland follows the level of education: the higher the level of education, the less unemployment, as is seen in Table 1.

---

7   These comprise 160 credits (four years of full-time studies) in the sectors of technology, natural resources and culture, and 140 credits (3.5 years) in business and administration, catering and institutional management, health care and social services, and tourism, whereas the degree in music requires 180 credits (4.5 years).

Table 1. Level of education and unemployment, zero, one, five, and ten years after graduation

Educational level	Unemployment rate (%)			
	0 year	1 year	5 years	10 years
Upper secondary/ vocational	51	39	26	21
Vocational college	35	21	12	9
Polytechnic	26	14	7	6
University	13	8	4	4
Doctorate level	4	4	3	2

Source: Havén, 1999

There were also differences between academic fields. The lowest unemployment rates were in medical, engineering and business fields (1-2 %), whereas the highest were amongst fine arts (21 %) and theatre (14 %) graduates in 2000 (KOTA database). The differences between institutions followed the disciplinary structure rather than the geographical location of the institution.

5.1.5   Governance, Steering and Funding of Higher Education

The Finnish Constitution ensures the freedom of the sciences, the arts and the highest level of education. These principles are embedded in the new Universities Act (645/1997), which ensures the autonomy of the universities by prescribing their functions, operation and objectives in general terms only. The new Universities Act is a skeleton law covering all Finnish universities (see Välimaa & Jalkanen, 2001). Within given limits, each university decides on the organisation of its administration and the decision-making power of its administrative bodies (Higher Education Policy, 2001).

According to the Ministry of Education, the steering of Finnish higher education is based on a consultation procedure, called management by results, whereby the Ministry of Education and the institutions jointly set the objectives for each higher education institution and agree on funding levels or number of new students in the case of the polytechnics. The Ministry of Education and each university sign a performance agreement in which both parties commit themselves to certain production objectives (measured by the numbers of degrees) and development projects and level of funding. The agreement is signed for a three-year period but the financial aspects are checked and negotiated every year (Higher Education Policy, 2001).

The change in the structure of funding during the 1990s had a strong impact on higher education. The share of public funding by the Ministry of Education decreased by 21 % between 1990 and 2001 (from 84 % to 63 %), while external funding from both private and public sources grew almost six-fold (KOTA 2001). Hence, the number of academic teaching staff (mainly professors and lecturers) fell from 7,800 to 7,300, whereas the number of other staff on external funding almost doubled (from 5,200 to 9,600) between 1990 and 1999 (Välimaa, 2001b). Together with an increasing student intake, the student per teacher ratio is steadily growing.

Finnish higher education policy objectives reflect the managerial ideas of the New Public Management (Pollit, 1995). The first element was the decentralisation of management authority. This policy is evident in the new Universities Act. The official arguments emphasise that universities have autonomy (in fact, only procedural autonomy) in deciding how to reach the targets (the number of academic degrees) set by the Ministry of Education. The second main trend was the introduction of market or quasi-market mechanisms in Finnish higher education. This led to competition both among and within higher education institutions. In fact, the Ministry of Education uses competition as a national steering instrument in its management by results negotiations with each university (Välimaa & Jalkanen, 2001). In this sense, the social context of Finnish higher education may be described as 'academic capitalism' (Slaughter, 1997). The shift in the funding structures is also related to academic capitalism because it increases the impacts of market-like behaviour, thus changing social dynamics inside universities. The third major trend was the requirement that staff work to performance targets and output objectives. This trend is closely related to the shift in the basis of public employment from permanency and standard national wages and conditions towards term contracts and performance-related wages. In universities, this has led to increasing number of 'project researchers', i.e. academics who have been appointed for a fixed period to carry out a specific research project (Välimaa, 2001).

The account of the five historical layers of Finnish higher education aims to show that the present system has often conflicting understandings of what are its social functions (see also Williams, 1995). From the perspective of accreditation and evaluation this means that there are different and often conflicting expectations concerning higher education and the roles that evaluation may play in its development.

5.2   Evaluation Schemes in Finnish Higher Education

According to the Universities Act (645/1997, § 5), Finnish 'universities are to evaluate their training, research and artistic functioning and the impacts of these activities. Universities also have a duty to participate in external evaluations of their functioning. Universities are to publish the results of their evaluations.' Finnish polytechnics have a similar duty to evaluate and report on their activities. In fact, the same evaluation requirements are repeated at all levels of the Finnish system of education.

The Finnish Higher Education Evaluation Council (FINHEEC) is responsible for the development and organisation of evaluation in Finland. According to the Decree on the Higher Education Evaluation Council (No. 1320/1995) and in its amending decree (465/1998), FINHEEC is responsible for:

- assisting higher education institutions and the Ministry of Education in evaluation;
- conducting evaluation for the accreditation of the polytechnics;
- organising evaluations of the operations and policies of higher education institutions;
- initiating evaluations of higher education and its development;
- engaging international co-operation on evaluation;
- promoting research on the evaluation of higher education, and
- taking responsibility for the evaluation and recording of professional courses offered by institutions of higher education. This last objective was added in 1998.

These tasks show that the national legislation takes evaluation seriously. They also indicate that evaluation is generally understood as a tool for improvement rather than of control. How has this societal understanding developed? In what follows I shall try to answer this question by describing how the Finnish idea of evaluation has developed and what are its consequences.

5.2.1   History of Evaluation in Finnish Higher Education: From Amateurism to Professionalism

Evaluation arrived in Finland on three separate occasions, with varying emphases. The first evaluation projects were carried out at the turn of the 1970s when academic societies (especially the Finnish Physics Society) began to evaluate the scientific level of research in Finland (Suomen, 1981; Marttila, 1971). The history of systematic evaluations began, however, in the 1980s when the Academy of Finland decided to organise the first discipline-specific evaluations (Finnish Academy 13/1981, 7/1983. During this *first round of evaluations* the main aim was to evaluate the level of scientific research in Finland at the beginning of the 1980s (Finnish Academy 13/1981). Inorganic chemistry was the first discipline to be evaluated (Finnish Academy 7/1983). Six institutions out of the seven which were assessed strongly resisted the interpretations (insults were even hurled) by the evaluation team in their published report (Finnish Academy 7/1983). Thus, this evaluation was mainly successful in showing how evaluations should not be carried out: they should not be used to rank individual academics or departments in a given discipline. A positive aspect of this unsuccessful evaluation project was that it helped to prepare the ground to understand that the aim of evaluation should be to encourage development instead of provoking debates on the arguments underlying the findings. This first round of evaluations is still continuing in and through various discipline-specific evaluations.[8] At the beginning of the 21st century the Academy of Finland mainly evaluates the scientific standard of disciplines (Suomen, 2000).

The *second round of evaluations* was launched by the Ministry of Education in the early 1990s. The Ministry supported institutional evaluation projects in two Finnish pilot universities: the University of Oulu and the University of Jyväskylä. At that time it was not clear what kind of national model of evaluation would be adopted, even though it was clear that it should focus on the institutional level. Following the guidelines suggested by the Ministry of Education, the University of Oulu introduced a model based on a wide- scale gathering of information using questionnaires (Oulu Report, 1993). The results of this American style institutional evaluation were not convincing because there was not much commitment to the project within the academic community of the university concerned. Another problem was the fact that, at that time, university central administration had practically no instruments for institutional policy-making. The University of Jyväskylä developed another approach to evaluation based on department self-evaluations. This approach was intended to involve academics in the evaluation process in the basic units. The information was not gathered for institutional purposes but instead the basic units (and the academics themselves) produced it (Jyväskylä report, 1993). This process seemed to lead to a deeper commitment to developing the operations of the basic units (Välimaa, Aittola & Konttinen, 1998) than the Oulu approach.

The Jyväskylä model has influenced the Finnish model of evaluation. A typical feature of all Finnish evaluation projects is a process comprising several or all of the following elements: self-evaluations are produced by the units involved; their self-evaluations are supported by site visits by external evaluators; the external visitors publish an evaluation report that includes their recommendations; and the institution concerned organises a publication or development seminar where the results are discussed and disseminated (Hämäläinen & Liuhanen, 1999).

In addition to these two pilot projects, several other evaluation projects were organised, suggested either by the Ministry of Education or higher education institutions or communities. Institutional evaluation projects were carried out in eight universities. Besides these evaluations which focused on higher education institutions and their functioning, several nation-wide evaluation projects of academic fields were carried out simultaneously with institutional evaluations. These projects included all institutions which organised training in the respective academic field. In total, ten

---

8   Discipline-specific evaluations have been carried out by the Ministry of Education, the Academy of Finland, individual universities, or academic associations (Liuhanen, 1997).

national evaluation projects of academic fields in 16 Finnish universities were organised between 1991 and 1996 (Liuhanen, 1997).

This second round of evaluations introduced higher education institutions and academics to the basic ideas of evaluation. The strategy of implementation promoted a social climate in which evaluation was more or less accepted as part of the activities of a post-modern university (Välimaa, 2000).

The *third round of evaluation* began when the Finnish government decided to establish the Finnish Higher Education Evaluation Council (FINHEEC) in 1995. This decision was made in a context where evaluation had already become one of the regular activities in higher education institutions. The aims of the Higher Education Evaluation Council were defined in ministerial decrees cited above. FINHEEC is funded by the Ministry of Education, but it is not a part of the Ministry. Both in principle and in practice, it is subordinated to the Ministry of Education (like universities and the Academy of Finland), but it has internal autonomy. The Finnish Higher Education Evaluation Council is made up of members appointed by the Ministry of Education for a four-year term. They represent higher education institutions, students and various stakeholders. FINHEEC draws up an annual budget, which is approved by the Department for Education and Science Policy of the Ministry of Education. It is assisted by the Council Secretariat, which is also appointed by the Ministry of Education. According to its brochures, FINHEEC has carried out several tasks (FINHEEC, 2000). Its main responsibility is to organise both institutional evaluations of universities and evaluations to accredit polytechnics. In addition, it has organised subcommittees or subsections to accredit professional courses. It has also made specific proposals in different evaluation projects. Universities and polytechnics have also funded their evaluations from their own budgets. During the first four years of operation, the total sum used by FINHEEC was about € 3 million (FINHEEC, 2000).

5.2.2   Reflections on the Third Round of Evaluation

The development towards 'professionalism of evaluation' seems to be essential in this third round of evaluation, as can be seen from the list of responsibilities of FINHEEC. This professionalism of evaluation is seen in the training of academic staff responsible for evaluations. FINHEEC has also organised study visit to various countries (including the Netherlands, the USA and Australia). Increasing professionalism of evaluation also means the standardisation of evaluation practices through secretarial and project management services to higher education institutions. FINHEEC has also initiated evaluations in higher education institutions and supported uniform reporting of evaluation processes in their publication series. Between 1997 and 2002 FINHEEC published 86 evaluation reports. This is remarkable in a country with 20 universities and 32 polytechnics.

Professionalism of evaluation has not yet created a group of 'managed professions' (Rhoades, 1998). However, there is a strong potential to create a group of experts who will be responsible for various evaluation processes in Finnish higher education institutions because it seems that 'normal academics' have neither the expertise nor the time to 'waste' with various evaluation processes.

5.2.3   Finns Active in ENQA

The members of FINHEEC have actively supported the European Network for Quality Assurance (ENQA). The ENQA secretariat and co-ordinator are located in FINHEEC. The active support of ENQA by the Finns is rational because its objectives coincide with those of FINHEEC. They include training and advisory support, publications in the field of quality assessment and quality assurance (Hämäläinen et al., 2001) and dissemination of information through a website and newsletter.

5.2.4   Other Quality Assessment and Evaluation Activities in Institutions and Units

FINHEEC has been an active expert body responsible for the practical organisation of the evaluations. In the Finnish context this does not mean, however, that it would have a monopoly over all evaluations in higher education. Finnish universities and polytechnics also have their own evaluation projects. For example, an evaluation project at the University of Jyväskylä aimed at improving the quality of teaching by using a method which combines local bench-marking and self-evaluation (Kallio, 2002). This project served local institutional needs and used evaluation as an instrument to improve the university's quality of teaching. Many other similar projects have been organised by Finnish higher education institutions.[9] From a researcher's point of view, it is, however, problematic that these local evaluation and development projects have seldom been documented, especially when they concern basic units. For this reason it is impossible to know the exact number of evaluations. It may safely be stated, however, that evaluation has become one of the regular practices in Finnish higher education institutions. It is used as an instrument to gather and analyse information in order to support improvement and decision-making processes in Finnish higher education institutions.[10]

---

9   E.g., an American teaching evaluation formula was tested at the University of Tampere to improve the quality of teaching (Parjanen, 2002).

10   Teaching development units and offices use various evaluation methods as analytical tools. These units can be found in a large number of Finnish universities.

5.3   Accreditation and Approval Schemes in Finland

An essential element in the increasing professionalism of evaluation was the introduction of accreditation activities in Finnish higher education. Yet, in principle, there are no accreditation agencies or accreditation practices in Finland. Even the concept accreditation (*akkreditointi*) has not been used in higher education policy making. In practice, however, processes can be found which may be called accreditation according to the definition used in this book. Therefore, in what follows I will describe the different processes as they appear in practice. To show the contrast, I shall first describe the two remaining approval processes, and then go on to accreditation.

5.3.1   Approval of New Higher Education Institutions

The main process of approval is that of establishing a new higher education institution. The Finnish government keeps the formal power to grant official approval in the field of higher education. The establishment of a new higher education institution is decided by the Council of State and recognised by law. Higher education institutions can then confer recognised degrees. The founding of a new university automatically means that the institution has the right to grant all traditional university degrees (Bachelors, Masters, Licentiate and Doctor's degrees). As a rule, students do not need additional professional accreditation from a professional body after having successfully completed their studies (Hämäläinen et al., 2001).

5.3.2   Approval of University and Polytechnic Degrees

The Ministry of Education decides on the degrees conferred by a university or a polytechnic. Higher education institutions submit a proposal of their degree programmes for approval by the Ministry of Education. The Ministry's decision states the name of the programme, its extent in credits (especially in polytechnics: the compulsory practical training component in credits), the name of the degree, and the title that the graduate is authorised to use. The higher education institutions, in turn, decide on the curriculum for each programme and how the courses will be organised (Higher education, 2001, OECD, 2002).

5.3.3   Accreditation Scheme for Polytechnics

The decision to establish a polytechnic sector in Finland was taken in the early 1990s. The first polytechnics were established as experimental institutions. The standard of former higher vocational institutions was raised and institutions were incorporated into multidisciplinary polytechnics. After a certain period of time all experimental polytechnics were allowed to apply for permanent status. In this phase of the process there emerged a political and practical need to investigate the standard and quality of the applicant institutions before they were granted the status of permanent institution.

This Finnish accreditation scheme of polytechnics included two separate but interconnected processes. The first consisted in the evaluations organised by FINHEEC in each of the applicant polytechnics after 1995.[11] The second consisted in the political decisions made by the Council of State. It gave the permission to operate to those institutions which had reached a certain level of development. In fact, these two processes amounted to accreditation, even though it was called (and understood as) evaluation in Finland.

In practical terms, FINHEEC established a separate accreditation subcommittee for the accreditation of polytechnics which consisted of the representatives of polytechnics, teachers working in the polytechnics, students and representatives of working life. Polytechnics were evaluated on the basis of applications for the first time in 1995 and 1996 and the process was continued until 1999. Site visits were added to the procedure in 1997. The accreditation subcommittee has compiled public reports of each evaluation which have been published in the publication series of the FINHEEC since 1998 (167 syytä, 1998; Virtanen, 1999). The Accreditation Subcommittee also implemented evaluations if there had been a change in the scope of activities of an accredited polytechnic, or if new institutions were incorporated in it (Hämäläinen et al., 2001).

The criteria used in the accreditation of permanent polytechnics included proven excellence in experimental and development work. Finnish legislation (acts on higher vocational education: 391/91, 392/92, 255/95, 256/95) created one of the decisive starting points of the criteria of assessment. The criteria were developed in discussions involving various partners from polytechnics, regional authorities, students and representatives of industry and commerce. The aim was to agree on minimum standards for permanent polytechnics (Hämäläinen et al., 2001). According to the evaluation of polytechnics in 1998 (167 syytä), the assessment was based on the following criteria:

1. mission, vision, goals and aims
2. curriculum design (up-to-date, programme diversity and co-operation, etc.)
3. strength of the operational plan
4. strengths
5. adequate size in relation to teaching goals and aims
6. the educational level of teachers

---

11 The first nine institutions were given permanent status without a systematic evaluation in 1995. They started as permanent institutions on August 1st, 1996.

7. information and library services
8. co-operation with professional life
9. co-operation with universities, polytechnics, and other educational institutions
10. international co-operation
11. regional training and service functions
12. the organisation of evaluation
13. learning environment
14. working environment.

Items 13 and 14 were recommended by the Ministry of Education. The members of the subcommittee used a five-point Likert scale to rate the institutions. Items 1, 6, 8, 11 and 13 were given double weight compared with other items.

A Case Study on Accreditation: *Kymenlaakso Polytechnic*

I shall describe one of the typical accreditation processes in detail to explain how the accreditation process was implemented. I shall take an example from a typical Finnish polytechnic both in size and structure, Kymenlaakso Polytechnic located 130 km East of Helsinki. Following the genesis of most Finnish polytechnics it was established through a merger in 1992. During this process of change, six educational institutions that were located all over the region and covered various professional fields were merged into one vocational higher education institution.[12] Kymenlaakso Polytechnic is owned by the city of Kotka and the municipalities of the region. By the beginning of the 21st century it grew into an institution with 3500 full-time students and a staff of around 500 persons. There are some 500 part-time students in further education leading to a degree (see: http://www.kyamk.fi/english).

In 1998, Kymenlaakso Polytechnic sent an application for permanent status to FINHEEC. The Accreditation Subcommittee received the application, read the documents and paid a typical one-day site visit to the polytechnic in 1998. Every site visit followed a similar schedule published in the report (see 167 syytä, 1998, Viittä vaille valmis, 1999). According to the procedure, the hosts of the visit opened the day by welcoming the members of the Subcommittee. The Committee then held an organising meeting. The members of the Subcommittee later interviewed the representatives of the students (one representative from each professional field) for. about one hour. Then the members of the committee interviewed the teachers' representatives (three to four persons) for about an hour. The subcommittee then interviewed other staff (three to four persons) for about a quarter of an hour. After the lunch

---

12 The following fields were offered at Kymenlaakso Polytechnic in 1998: arts and crafts, health and social work, business and foreign trade, forestry and agriculture, technical education, and maritime commerce (167 syytä).

break, the afternoon session began with a visit to the library of the institution (30 minutes). Then, the Subcommittee interviewed employers and employees for about an hour, followed by representatives of the owner of the institution (30 minutes). They also interviewed the rector and the heads of the curricula (one hour). The visit ended with a seminar that was open to everybody working or studying at Kymenlaakso Polytechnic (167 syytä, 1998).

Following this visit, which was repeated in all the eight institutions that applied for permanent status in 1998, the Accreditation Subcommittee recommended to the Ministry of Education that Kymenlaakso Polytechnic should be given permanent status, which it did. In the report of these accreditation processes the Accreditation Subcommittee analysed the strengths and weaknesses and the future potentials of each applicant (167 syytä, 1998, Virtanen, 1999).

5.3.4 Accreditation of Professional Courses

The evaluation and accreditation of professional courses have been on the higher education policy agenda since 1996. At that time, public concern arose about the invalid qualifications conferred by a Continuing Education Centre in a certain university. FINHEEC was given the responsibility to register professional courses (Virtanen, 2001). This registration meant that all the courses to be registered were to be evaluated beforehand.[13] In other words, they needed to be accredited. With these activities, the concept of accreditation was introduced in the Finnish education policy field.

The accreditation of professional courses is a process that gives public recognition or registration to professional, non-degree courses that offer good quality educational services. For students, the accreditation ensures that the course is offered on a reliable basis (Hämäläinen et al., 2001).

FINHEEC appointed a subsection (Accreditation Board of Professional Courses, ABPC) to assess professional courses and decide on accreditation. The twelve board members appointed by the Ministry of Education for a three-year term represented universities, polytechnics, students and working life. ABPC started to accredit professional courses by the end of 1998. ABPC has been divided into three committees which concentrate on the following fields of professional training: business training courses, PD-programme courses, social and health care courses (Virtanen, 2001).

ABPC evaluated 49 courses, 33 of which were accepted and registered as guaranteeing sufficient quality during the first two years of its functioning (Hämäläinen et al.,

---

13 According to the act, this accreditation of professional courses is defined as 'evaluation and registration of professional courses'.

2001).[14] 'Sufficient quality' in this context is examined in the accreditation process which contains the following elements:

- the review of relevant documentation (application);
- the visit to the course;
- immediate feedback after the visit.

The application contains background information on the course (organiser, length, target groups), on the training itself (why the training has been organised, what are its aims and structure and the contents of the training given during the course, what are the teaching materials, how is the evaluation and quality assessment organised), on the practical arrangements (who are the teachers and units responsible for teaching, what are the roles of working life and students during the training), and the resources available (teaching facilities, funding).

After receiving the application, ABPC organises a site visit to the course organiser. During the visits, the board members analyse the following aspects: 1) basic requirements, 2) work-orientation, 3) course contents and objectives, 4) the educational process, 5) pedagogical arrangements, 6) practical arrangements, and 7) quality assurance.[15] These criteria were developed by ABPC before it began the accreditation processes. The idea is to develop them continuously with the help of feedback from the field. The criteria can also be found on the Internet (http://www.minedu.fi /asiant/kka/docs/Criteria.html).

The final decision is made on a registered/not registered (yes/no) basis. Feedback and recommendations for the course are given after the registration decision is made. The site visit is participative and constructive (Hämäläinen et al., 2001). The registration of accredited courses is valid for four years, and the register is available on FINHEEC's website (www.minedu.fi/asiant/kka/docs/rekister.htm). If the professional course fails to meet the criteria, the institute may continue to run the course, even though it often leads to immediate further self-development and improvement. Normally, the process is seen as a useful tool to obtain an outside view of the course or institute (Hämäläinen et al., 2001).

It is important for this process of accreditation that the institutions themselves apply accreditation for the professional courses on a voluntary basis. In a market-like situation this helps to maintain or reach a good reputation in a competitive market of professional courses.

---

14 The number of registered professional courses was 42 in 2003. Two-thirds (27 courses) are offered by Finnish polytechnics.

15 Additional criteria are applied to courses taught in a foreign language, and to virtual courses.

The Accreditation Board of Professional Courses adopted the role of adviser and developer rather than of controller during the first years of its functioning. This is in line with the policy of FINHEEC which aims to develop Finnish higher education with the help of evaluation. The purpose of accreditation is to credit the programmes on the basis of their capacity to offer good quality educational services instead of just meeting the minimum standards. Following the principles of accreditation and those of FINHEEC, it is up to the institutions to look for the best way to meet the criteria.

The emphasis on development with the help of evaluation makes sense in the Finnish context where citizens traditionally trust public authorities. The challenge to improve and develop functioning as expressed by public authorities such as FINHEEC or ABPC has a significant potential influence on higher education institutions. In the Finnish cultural context it is natural that institutions and academics take the suggestions seriously. These suggestions are, therefore, a rather significant political act in promoting improvements and change.

5.3.5   International Accreditation

International accreditation is more of an exception than a rule in Finnish higher education, because evaluations are usually carried out by the higher education institutions and FINHEEC. Only in two cases did the evaluation (or accreditation) involve a foreign partner. The EQUIS (The European Quality Improvement System) accreditations were organised by the European Foundation for Management Development in two universities of Business Administration and Economics with financial support from FINHEEC (Quality Label, 1998, Hämäläinen et al., 2001). The accreditation process is based on a comprehensive self-assessment report followed by a site visit by four international members. In addition to EQUIS, the Helsinki School of Economics was accredited by AMBA (Association of MBAs in Britain). It was the first business management programme in Finland and Nordic countries to receive AMBA accreditation (see http://www.hkkk.fi/english/default.asp).

Some polytechnics have independently acquired international accreditation for their quality system from *Norske Veritas*. The European Foundation for the Accreditation of Hotel School Programmes has accredited (recognised) Bachelor of Science programmes in Hotel, Restaurant and Tourism Management in one polytechnic (Hämäläinen et al., 2001).

5.3.6   Discussion on the Nature of Accreditation Processes

In Finland, it is supposed that national degrees are comparable and of equally high standard. Therefore, their aims, scope and general structure are prescribed by law. The State protects, in turn, the value and quality of degrees by controlling which institutions can award them and which educational programmes can qualify for them (Hämäläinen et al., 2001). In Finland, higher education institutions enjoy great institutional autonomy, which is ensured by law (Universities Act 645/1997). In this context, it is only natural that the institutions themselves take full responsibility for the standard and quality of the educational services they provide. It is also natural that the national government uses expert bodies to conduct evaluation projects because it lacks expertise in this domain. In short, both higher education institutions and the Finnish government trust the expertise of FINHEEC to organise evaluations and accreditations (Välimaa & Mollis, 2003).

As for the accreditation of polytechnics, the fact that feedback was given to each applicant is more important than its actual contents. Thus, the idea behind this feedback suggests that the aim of the evaluation process was to develop the institutions more than just give ratings. In this sense, this process of evaluation was both accreditation and development of the institutions. However, it was not accreditation in the sense that it gave a permanent licence to function to all those institutions, even though some of the polytechnics were given a recommendation to develop some evaluated areas within a fixed period of time (normally two years). It should also be added that normally all institutions which applied for a permanent status obtained it, even though it sometimes took several applications. In some cases, the Council of States even gave permanent status to a polytechnic which was not recommended by FINHEEC (Antikainen, 2002). These examples suggest, in turn, that the invisible political processes behind these visible accreditation processes usually lead to a positive outcome. The creation of a polytechnic in a region was normally supported by regional political activities linked with national political actors (Salminen, 2001; Antikainen, 2002). It has also been suggested that the creation of polytechnics was supported by national employer organisations, regions and communities, together with professional interest groups and vocational educational institutions and their teachers (Rinne, 2002). Thus, the denial of permanent status would have increased political confrontations between and inside political parties represented in the Council of State. Furthermore, it would have been very difficult to deny the value of the development if the institutions were able to show it. Therefore, one of the political aims of the accreditation process was to force the institutions to develop their activities. In this sense, both the national level and the institutional level used the accreditation process to advance their own purposes (Antikainen, 2002). On the basis of international evaluation it also seems that polytechnic reform has achieved its national goals (OECD report, 2002).

I have explained the process of evaluation, which led to a political decision to establish a new permanent institution to show that it was essentially a process of accreditation. The analysis of the documents combined with a site visit to the institutions concerned laid a credible basis for political decision-making. My detailed description also aimed to show that the members of the Accreditation Subcommittee had opportunities to become familiar with the standard and quality of the applicant institution, even though it is not possible to know how insightful they were in their analyses on the basis of published reports.

5.3.7   The Role of FINHEEC in National Higher Education Policy-Making

FINHEEC has an important role in the steering of Finnish higher education for two reasons. The first steering mechanism functions through the evaluation of high-quality education units in universities and polytechnics organised by FINHEEC (see reports: Huttula, 2000, 2001, 2002; Liuhanen, 2000; Moitus, 2000; Yliopistokoulu-tuksen laatuyksiköt, 1998). These evaluations are related to the funding of higher education institutions because each high-quality education unit is rewarded with a certain sum in management by results negotiations.

The second steering function is more indirect. FINHEEC organises system-wide evaluations in Finnish higher education on various subjects, e.g. the evaluation of vocational teacher training (Lämsä & Saari, 2000), or the evaluation of student admissions in universities (Sajavaara et al., 2002). The evaluation outcomes may and have been used in political decision-making processes.

These evaluations have a technical advisory role in the sense that FINHEEC organises the processes according to the outlines set by political decision-makers. However, the importance of the evaluations organised by FINHEEC is more than technical, because the organisation and co-ordination of the processes help to influence the contents and outcomes of the processes. For this reason FINHEEC is one of the actors in the field of Finnish higher education policymaking even though it has the role of an expert organisation.

5.4   Analysing Evaluation and Accreditation Processes in Finland

5.4.1   Actors, Purposes and Processes

The relationship between the concepts and social phenomena of accreditation, evaluation and approval should be approached from the perspectives of actors, purposes and processes.

When accreditation is analysed from *the perspective of actors* we are interested in who gives institutions and programmes the permission to operate and who does the actual evaluation work. The Ministry of Education is the main actor in field of evaluation in Finland because it funds the higher education institutions and evaluation activities. FINHEEC organises the evaluation projects, but the Council of State continues to keep formal power to grant official approval (of institutions, programmes and degrees) in the field of higher education. This power of approval has not been changed. Traditionally (i.e. by the end of 20th century), it was not called accreditation.

From the *perspective of purposes of accreditation and evaluation* one is interested in knowing the social functions of accreditation and evaluation. First, accreditation and evaluation aim to improve the quality of the Finnish higher education system. In this context, they have the role of quality assurance in the national system of higher education. Secondly, these processes aim to link higher education institutions to the national innovation system. In this sense, the purpose of evaluation is to make the national system of higher education more efficient and more relevant to the nation state.

However, when accreditation and evaluation are approached from *the perspective of processes* one should ask who does what, when and how. FINHEEC does the actual work of evaluation by organising the teams of experts. They use various methods to evaluate, audit and assess institutions and/or programmes. The Finnish government does not evaluate the institutions or programmes but uses the outcomes of experts' evaluations. From the perspective of processes, accreditation, evaluation and approval unite in practical activities even though they serve different purposes and the actors may vary from process to process.

In the context of this comparative project, it is tempting to define the Finnish government as an accreditation agency. However, it is not. It is rather an 'approval agency'. The Council of State has always had and continues to keep the formal power to grant official approval to institutions, degrees and programmes. As a rule, this power of approval has not been called accreditation, even though it contains elements that relate it to evaluation and accreditation. A clear example is the approval of university and polytechnic degrees, which is in the hands of the Ministry of Education with no public evaluation scheme related to it.

5.4.2   Social Spaces Related to Accreditation and Evaluation

These perspectives on accreditation, evaluation and approval can also be approached from a sociological angle. Three different social spaces can be found in which the social functions of evaluation and accreditation appear differently when we take into account the historical layers and the three rounds of evaluation in Finnish higher education. In each of the social spaces, evaluation and accreditation play somewhat different roles because they are related to different processes in higher education. Bourdieu (1988) coined the term social space to capture the idea that they consist not only of actors (persons and institutions) but also of shared or contested understandings of the goals of higher education. This way they create a discursive space in which certain basic assumptions are shared by the actors, even though they may have contradictory interpretations of them (Herranen, 2003). These social spaces do not exist in hierarchical relationship with each other but simultaneously as 'social fields of action', as described by Bleiklie (2000), that interact and influence each other.

The Defence of the Nation-State

In this first social space, the role of evaluation and accreditation is linked to the making and defence of the nation state. In this context, FINHEEC functions as an expert organisation in the national steering system of higher education. FINHEEC has increased the level of professionalism in higher education evaluations. Accreditation practices have also been introduced by and through it. The ethos of evaluation and accreditation in this social space is to improve and develop the functioning of the national higher education system with the help of higher education institutions? Hence, evaluation and accreditation will help higher education to become part of the national innovation strategy, as has also been argued in official policy documents (Tiedon, 1993; Miettinen, 2002).

Quality Assurance System

The second social space is closely related to the previous one. In the social context of mass higher education, evaluation and accreditation also serve the needs of higher education institutions. They aim to improve the quality in the 'production process' of academic degrees. A national policy goal is to disseminate quality assurance practices in the system of higher education. As a quality assurance system it may serve not only the needs of the national system, but also those of students and institutions.

Humboldtian Values in Danger

The last social space consists of the traditional values of continental Western higher education, often defined as the Humboldtian university ideal, with emphasis on academic freedom and institutional autonomy (Clark, 1983; Huusko & Muhonen, 2003). In this social space, evaluation and accreditation are a potential threat to the traditional values of a university because they try to open the 'black box' of the academic ivory tower. Evaluation and accreditation are not valued as an academic enterprise – perhaps with the exception of discipline-specific evaluations – but are seen as an administrative duty which should be left to evaluation specialists. This way of reasoning points in the direction of managed professionals responsible for matters of evaluation and accreditation.

5.5   Conclusion

The 'accreditation' concept was not used in Finnish higher education before the 21st century. There has been no social need to define certain evaluation processes as accreditation or approval of institutions or degrees other than as approval. Therefore, one should ask: what does the introduction of the concept of accreditation bring to higher education? Does it mean that processes which combine evaluation activities with (political) decision-making will become more popular? If this is the case, a crucial question seems to be: Should we increase the professional level of accreditation to make it more transparent and reliable? After having answered 'yes' to this rhetoric question, the next question is an easy one: Should we create unified criteria and standards for accreditation? The answer is most probably yes. However, one should think further and pay attention to the definitions of the criteria and standards of accreditation. Namely, the question: Who defines the criteria? is easily changed into the question: Who benefits from these criteria?

The processes of defining criteria for accreditation appear differently when one approaches them from the perspective of the Bologna process. The Bologna Process clearly challenges one to develop European criteria for both institutional and professional accreditation. One of the reasons may be the need to resist the American dominance over European higher education. In addition to this political dimension, European ideas and models of higher education are far more diverse than the American model. That is why one could say that Europeans should develop their own criteria, respecting the European variety in higher education. Political, functional and practical reasons can be found to develop European models of accreditation. Therefore, it seems that in the political context of the Bologna process the issue is not whether it should be done but how it should be done.

References

167 syytä korkeakouluksi [167 Reasons for becoming a higher education institution]. Korkeakoulujen arviointineuvoston julkaisuja. Finheec reports 4:1998. Helsinki: Edita.

Bleiklie, I. (2000). Policy and Practice in Higher Education. Reforming Norwegian Universities. Higher Education Policy Series 49. London: Jessica Kingsley.

Clark, B.R. (1983). The Higher Education System. Berkeley: University of California Press.

FINHEEC (2000). Evaluation of Higher Education – the First Four Years. Helsinki: Finnish Higher Education Evaluation Council.

Finnish Academy Publications (1981). Tieteellisen tutkimuksen arviointi [The Evaluation of Scientific Research]. Helsinki: Publications of the Academy of Finland, No. 13.

Finnish Academy Publications (1983). Evaluation of Scientific Research in Finland: Inorganic Chemistry. Helsinki: Publications of the Academy of Finland, No. 7.

Hämäläinen, K. (2001). Akkreditointi kansainvälisessä kentässä [Accreditation in an International Context]. In Vähäpassi, A. (ed.) Erikoistumisopintojen akkreditointi [The Accreditation of professional courses]. Korkeakoulujen arviointineuvoston julkaisuja. Finheec reports 3:2001. Helsinki: Edita, 8-12.

Havén, H. (ed.) (1998). Koulutus Suomessa [Education in Finland]. Helsinki: Official Statistics of Finland: Koulutus:1.

Havén, H. (ed.) (1999). Education in Finland, Statistics and Indicators. Helsinki: Official Statistics of Finland. See also: http://www.stat.fi/tk/he/edufinland/edut.html.

Hämäläinen, K., Haakstad, J., Kangasniemi, J., Lindeberg, T., & Sjölund, M. (2001). Quality Assurance in the Nordic Higher Education. Helsinki: ENQA Occasional Papers 2.

Hämäläinen, K., & Liuhanen, A.-M. (1999). Preface in Five Years of Development. Follow-Up Evaluation of the University of Oulu. Publications of Higher Education Evaluation Council 7:1999. Helsinki: Edita.

Herranen, J. (2003). Ammattikorkeakoulu diskursiivisena tilana. Järjestystä, konflikteja ja kaaosta [Finnish Polytechnic as a Discursive Space. Order, Conflicts and Chaos]. Joensuu: University of Joensuu. Publications in Education No. 85.

Higher Education Policy (2001). Higher Education Policy in Finland. The Ministry of Education. http://www.minedu.fi/minedu/publications/55.html.

Huttula, T. (ed.) (2000). Ammattikorkeakoulujen koulutuksen laatuyksiköt, 2000. Korkeakoulujen arviointineuvoston julkaisuja. Finheec reports 13: 2000. Helsinki: Edita.

Huttula, T. (ed.) (2001). Ammattikorkeakoulujen aluekehitysvaikutuksen huippuyksiköt 2001. Korkeakoulujen arviointineuvoston julkaisuja. Finheec reports 8: 2001. Helsinki: Edita.

Huttula, T. (ed.) (2002). Ammattikorkeakoulujen koulutuksen laatuyksiköt 2002-2003. Korkeakoulujen arviointineuvoston julkaisuja. Finheec reports 12: 2002. Helsinki: Edita.

Huusko, M. & Muhonen, R. (2003). Yliopistojen jännitteiset arvot [Tensions in the values of higher education]. Manuscript.

Jyväskylä Self-Evaluation report (1993). Jyväskylä: University of Jyväskylä (unpublished).

Kallio, E. (2002). Yksilöllisiä heijastuksia. Toimiiko yliopisto-opetuksen paikallinen itsearviointi? [Does local self-evaluation work in developing university teaching?] Finheec Reports 2: 2002. Helsinki: Edita.

Klinge, M. (1987). Kuninkaallinen Turun akatemia 1640-1808 [The Royal Academy at Åbo]. Helsinki: Otava.

Klinge, M. (1989). Keisarillinen Aleksanterin yliopisto 1808-1917 [The Imperial Alexander University]. Helsinki: Otava.

Klinge, M. (1992). Intellectual tradition in Finland. In Kauppi, N., & Sulkunen, P. , Vanguards of Modernity. Jyväskylä: Publications of the Research Unit for Contemporary Culture 32, 33-42.

Lampinen, O. & Savola, M. (1995). Ammattikorkeakoulun syntyvaiheet Suomessa, in Lampinen, O. (ed.), Ammattikorkeakoulut – vaihtoehto yliopistolle? [Polytechnics – an alternative for universities?]. Tampere: Gaudeamus, 26-80.

Laine, I., Kilpinen, A., Lajunen, L., Pennanen, J., Stenius, M., Uronen, P. , & Kekäle, T. (2001). Maanpuolustuskorkeakoulun arviointi [The Evaluation of National Defence College]. Finheec reports 2:2001. Helsinki: Edita.

Lämsä, A., & Saari, S. (ed.) (2000). Portfoliosta koulutuksen kehittämiseen. Ammatillisen opettajankoulutuksen arviointi. Finheec reports 10:2000. Helsinki: Edita.

Liuhanen, A.-M. (1997). Yliopistot arvioivat toimintaansa – mitä opitaan? Korkeakoulujen arviointineuvoston julkaisuja 2/1997.

Liuhanen, A.-M. (2000). Neljä aikuiskoulutuksen laatuyliopistoa. 2001-2003. Korkeakoulujen arviointineuvoston julkaisuja. Finheec reports 7: 2000. Helsinki: Edita.

Marttila, O. (1971). Fysiikan tutkimus Suomessa 1969-1970 [Research of Physics in Finland]. Helsinki: Suomen Fyysikkoseura ry.

Miettinen, R. (2002). National Innovation System. Scientific Concept of Political Rhetoric. Helsinki: Edita.

Moitus, S. (2000). Yliopistokoulutuksen laatuyksiköt 2001-2003. Korkeakoulujen arviointineuvoston julkaisuja. Finheec reports 6: 2000. Helsinki: Edita.

Nevala, A. (1999). Korkeakoulutuksen kasvu, lohkoutuminen ja eriarvoisuus Suomessa [Growth, Fragmentation and Inequality in Higher Education in Finland]. Bibliotheca Historica 43. Helsinki.

Nevala, A. (1991). Mittavat murrokset – pienet muutokset. Korkeakoulupolitiikka ja opiskelijakunnan rakenne Suomessa 1900-luvulla. Suomen historian lisensiaatti-tutkielma Joensuun yliopistossa [Unprinted licensiate thesis: Higher Education Policy and the Structure of Student body in Finland in the 20th century].

Nuorteva, J. (1999). Suomalaisten ulkomainen opinkäynti ennen Turun akatemian perustamista 1640. [Finnish Study Abroad before the Foundation of the Royal Academy of Turku (Academia Aboensis) in 1640]. Societas Historica Finlandiae.Helsinki: Hakapaino.

OECD Report (2002). Background Report: Polytechnic Education in Finland. OECD.

Oulu Report on the Self-Assessment of the University of Oulu (1993). Oulu: University of Oulu (not printed).

Parjanen, M. (2002). Onnistuuko amerikkalainen takaisinsyöttö suomalaisessa yliopistossa? In Honkonen, R. (ed.), Koulutuksen lumo – retoriikka, politiikka, arviointi. Tampere: Tampere University Press, 209-228.

Quality Label? EQUIS Evaluation Report (1998). Helsinki School of Economics and Business Administration. Publications of the Higher Education Council 10:1998. Helsinki: Edita.

Rhoades, G. (1998). Managed Professionals. Unionized Faculty and Restructuring Academic Labour. Albany: State University of New York Press.

Rinne, R. (2002). Binaarimallista Bolognan tielle: erilliset ammattikorkeakoulut tulevat ja menevät [From binary model to Bologna Highway: separate polytechnics come and go]. In Liljander, J.-P. (ed.), Omalla tiellä – ammattikorkeakoulut kymmenen vuotta. Helsinki: Edita. 80-106.

Sajavaara, K., Hakkarainen, K., Henttonen, A., Niinistö, K., Pakkanen, T., Piilonen, A.-R., & Moitus, S. (2002). Yliopistojen opiskelijavalintojen arviointi [Evaluation of Student Admissions in Universities]. Finheec reports 17:2002. Helsinki: Edita.

Salminen, H. (2001). Suomalainen ammattikorkeakoulu-uudistus opetushallinnon prosessina. Koulutussuunnittelu valtion keskushallinnon näkökulmasta. [Finnish AMK-reform as the process of national education administration]. Opetusministeriö: koulutus- ja tiedepolitiikan osaston julkaisusarja. Helsinki.

Scriven, M. (1991). Evaluation Thesaurus. Fourth Edition. Newbury Park: Sage.

Slaughter, S., & Leslie, L. (1997). Academic Capitalism: Politics, Policies and the Entrepreneurial University. Baltimore: Johns Hopkins University Press.

Suomen (1981). Suomen Fysiikan perustutkimus v. 1971-1980 [Research of Physics in Finland]. Helsinki: Suomen Fyysikkoseura ry.

Suomen (2000). Suomen tieteen tila ja taso [The status and standard of Finnish Science]. The Academy of Finland. Helsinki: Suomen akatemian julkaisuja 6:00.

Tiedon (1993). Tiedon ja osaamisen Suomi [Knowledge and Expertise in Finland]. Kehittämisstrategia. Valtion tiede- ja teknologianeuvosto. Helsinki: painatuskeskus.

Vähäpassi, A. (ed.) (2001). Erikoistumisopintojen akkreditointi [The Accreditation of professional courses]. Korkeakoulujen arviointineuvoston julkaisuja.Finheec reports 3:2001. Helsinki: Edita.

Välimaa, J. (2000). Ulkoinen itsearviointi ja käyttötypologiat [On external self-evaluation and practical typologies]. In Honkimäki, S., & Jalkanen, H. (eds.), Innovatiivinen yliopisto? Jyväskylä: Koulutuksen tutkimuslaitos, 70-81.

Välimaa, J. (2001). A Historical Introduction to Finnish Higher Education. In Välimaa, J. (ed.), Finnish Higher Education in Transition. Perspectives on Massification and Globalisation. Jyväskylä: Institute for Educational Research, 13-54.

Välimaa, J. (2001b). The Changing Nature of Academic Employment in Finnish Higher Education. In Enders, J. (ed.), Academic Staff in Europe: Changing Contexts and Conditions. Westport (Conn.): Greenwood Publishing Group, 67-90.

Välimaa, J., Aittola, T., & Konttinen, R. (1998). Impacts of Quality Assessment: The Case of Jyväskylä University, Higher Education Management, Vol. 10, No. 2, pp 7-29.

Välimaa, J., & Jalkanen, H. (2001). Strategic Flow and Finnish Universities. In Välimaa, J. (ed.), Finnish Higher Education in Transition. Perspectives on Massification and Globalisation. Jyväskylä: Institute for Educational Research, 185-202.

Välimaa, J., & Mollis, M. (2003). Social Functions of Evaluation in Finnish and Argentinean Higher Education (Manuscript).

Välimaa, J., & Westerheijden, D. F. (1995). Two discourses: Researchers and policy-making in higher education. Higher Education, 29, 385-403.

Virtanen, I. (2001). Erikoistumisopintojen rekisteröinti: akkreditoinnin suomalainen sovellus. In Vähäpassi, A. (ed.), Erikoistumisopintojen akkreditointi [The Accreditation of professional courses]. Korkeakoulujen arviointineuvoston julkaisuja. Finheec reports 3:2001. Helsinki: Edita.

Virtanen, A. (ed.) (1999). Viittä vaille valmis? Ammattikorkeakouluhakemusten arviointi 1999 [Almost ready? The evaluation of the applications of polytechnics]. Korkeakoulujen arviointineuvoston julkaisuja. Finheec publications 1:1999.

Williams, G. (1995). The marketization of higher education: reforms and potential reforms in higher education finance. In Dill, D.D., & Sporn, B. (eds.), Emerging Patterns of Social Demand and University Reform: Through a Glass Darkly. Trowbridge: IAU Press & Pergamon.

Woodhouse, D. (1999). Quality and Quality Assurance, in Quality and Internationalisation in Higher Education. OECD.

Yliopistokoulutuksen laatuyksiköt (1998). Arviointineuvoston esitys korkealaatuisen koulutuksen yksiköiksi vuosille 1999-2000. Korkeakoulujen arviointineuvoston julkaisuja. Finheec reports 5: 1998. Helsinki: Edita.

6 Quality Assurance and Accreditation in the Flemish Community of Belgium

DIRK VAN DAMME

6.1 Introduction

6.1.1 Some Preliminary Remarks

Two important preliminary remarks must be made for the European readers of this national report. Since education became an autonomous competence of the three Belgian communities (Flemish Community, French-speaking Community and German-speaking Community) in 1988, the development of educational policies went in separate directions. But in this 'national' report, we shall only focus on the developments in the Flemish community of Belgium.

In 2003, a new comprehensive law[1] was in the making in Flanders, implementing the Bologna Declaration by transforming the degree structure into a bachelor–master system, introducing a system of accreditation and redefining the relationships between universities and *hogescholen*[2] as 'associations'. As a rule, a number of *hogescholen* will have to be established. This law's implementation, i.e. the launch of bachelor–master-types of programmes, is foreseen for the 1st of October 2004. In this report, we shall take into account its policies and developments. Where appropriate, a clear distinction will be made between the present *ex ante* context and the *ex post* context which will be in place once the new law is passed.

6.1.2 A Note on Definitions

Despite the growth of practices and systems and the increasing public interest in this issue, there is not yet a generally accepted set of concepts and definitions at the international level. Even in Europe such concepts and terms as quality assurance, assessment, accreditation, evaluation, etc. are used in a different way. In this paper, we shall use these concepts as follows. *Evaluation* is a very broad, generic term that

---

1 A law of a community of region in Belgium is called a 'decree'. We shall use the two terms interchangeably.

2 Since there is no satisfactory English translation, we shall use the Dutch term *hogescholen* to define the Flemish non-university higher education institutions, which can be compared to their Dutch homologues or the German *Fachhochschule*.

S. Schwarz and D.F. Westerheijden (eds.),
Accreditation and Evaluation in the European Higher Education Area, 127–157.
© 2004 *Kluwer Academic Publishers. Printed in the Netherlands.*

refers to a broad range of practices whereby the performance of students, professors, programmes, departments, institutions and even systems is measured and appreciated. *Quality assurance* refers to practices and schemes that aim at assessing, monitoring, guaranteeing, maintaining and/or improving quality in higher education institutions and programmes. They have the functions of accountability (including information provision) and improvement. Usually, we make a distinction between internal quality assurance practices within programmes and institutions and external quality assurance schemes that operate at a system level. By *assessment,* we mean the processes of reviewing and judging quality aspects in programmes or institutions. In internal quality assurance, this is done through self-evaluation and in external quality assurance schemes by means of evaluation activities of panels who carry out peer review and site visits. That is why we shall also call the external quality assurance schemes 'visitation schemes', a literal translation of the Flemish term. Finally, *accreditation* is defined here – in line with the definition given in this book – as a formal approval by responsible authorities of an institution or programme that meets predetermined and agreed standards through a process of evaluation. In the Flemish system, just like in the Netherlands, the established quality assurance schemes provide the evaluation input for the accreditation system.

In Flanders, all processes and schemes of quality assurance and accreditation concern programmes. There is no public system of institutional evaluation or accreditation. Flemish institutions participate in other, mostly international, schemes of institutional evaluation, such as the CRE/EUA institutional evaluation programme or the specialised accreditation schemes of bodies such as ABET or EQUIS, but these activities are voluntary. They fall outside the scope of this report, which only deals with public, i.e. state-controlled or recognised, schemes.

In Flanders, higher education institutions and programmes are recognised by law. This means that the institutions and their disciplines are listed in the higher education laws. Only institutions in that list can call themselves 'universities' and no other institutions can award officially recognised degrees or diplomas. This kind of *ex ante* 'licensing' (approval, in terms of this book) of institutions and programmes is not (yet) linked to a system of quality assurance. Under the current legal provisions, the government can take sanctions after a negative quality assessment and remove the programme from the recognised list, but, in practice, this has not yet happened. The introduction of accreditation will change this, as we shall see in the section on this issue.

The new higher education law also includes a system of registration of non-recognised institutions. Providers that are recognised outside the state will be able to be registered and, under certain conditions, ask for accreditation. Positive accreditation will lead to the recognition of their programmes and degrees in the bachelor–master degree system, without however influencing funding.

6.2   The Flemish Higher Education System

6.2.1   Institutions

Flanders has a binary system of higher education and chooses to keep this divide for institutions and to a certain extent for programmes. In Flanders, which has a population of nearly 6 million, there are six universities: two – Ghent and Leuven – comprehensive, fully-fledged universities with approximately 25,000 students, another two – Brussels and Antwerp[3] – medium-sized universities with some 10,000 students, a small university – the University Centre of Limburg – and a very small university college in Brussels. In line with the Humboldtian tradition that prevails on the European continent, Flemish universities integrate teaching and research. Research, especially fundamental research, is assigned to the universities and, except for a few specialised institutions, there are no major public research institutes outside the universities.

After a major operation of mergers in the mid-1990s, there are now some 23 *hogescholen* in Flanders, but mergers are continuing. The size of these *hogescholen* varies from a few thousand to 11,000 students. Their mission is to offer more professionally- and vocationally-oriented programmes than those at universities, but they are also active in applied research and development. Outside the higher education sector, some adult education centres organise part-time programmes and award degrees that are similar to those of *hogescholen*, but a debate is going on concerning their status and integration in the higher education sector.

All higher education institutions are recognised by the government. Their educational and degree-awarding capacities are defined by law and are therefore restricted. In general, however, they have a relatively high degree of autonomy in the framework of the legislation enacted in the 1990s. Although their legal position varies from 'public' – i.e. established by public authorities – to 'private' – i.e. established by private bodies such as the Church – with some mixed forms in between, all institutions are treated equally by law, are funded according to the same principles and rules and have equal degree-awarding capacities. They mainly differ in their philosophical backgrounds. They are developing their own profile and have a restricted territorial capacity and therefore a regional identity. But, on the whole, differences are less significant than in most other European countries. There are no provisions yet for for-profit institutions or new providers to enter the publicly defined and delineated higher education space in Flanders, although, under the new law, they can have their programmes accredited under certain conditions.

---

3   Antwerp University is the result of a merger of three independent university centres that took place in 2003.

6.2.2   Programmes and Degrees[4]

In the Flemish higher education system, the universities and *hogescholen* recognised by the state are listed in the relevant laws. These laws also list the domains of study in which each institution can offer programmes and award degrees. The actual programmes and degrees are not listed in the law, but in a government act. All state-recognised programmes can therefore award official degrees, which are fully recognised by the state.

Whereas the institutional landscape can be described as binary, that of the programmes is 'ternary'. At present, *hogescholen* can offer three-year professionally- and vocationally-oriented programmes, leading to a '*geaggregeerde*' degree. These 'one cycle' programmes prepare students for middle-rank professions in commerce, nursing, teaching, industry, applied arts, social work, etc. *Hogescholen* also offer four-year, 'two cycle' programmes, which are of a more scientific and academic nature and lead to the '*licentiaat*', which is similar or sometimes equivalent to university degrees.

University programmes are also organised in two cycles, with an intermediate '*kandidatuur*' qualification after two (in some cases three) years of study, and a second cycle of another two or more years of study, leading to a '*licentiaat*' or appropriate disciplinary titles (medical doctor, engineer, pharmacist, etc.). University degrees are therefore obtained after a nominal period of study which ranges from a minimum of four year to a maximum of seven years (medical doctor).

Hogescholen and especially universities also offer post-initial programmes which are of a specialised nature or of a broader, more general nature. Doctoral degrees are only awarded by universities.

According to the new law, higher education programmes will be organised in a bachelor–master degree system as from the academic year 2004/05. After successful completion of a three-year programme (180 ECTS-points), students will be awarded a bachelor degree. A distinction will be made between a professional and an academic bachelor degree, the first being awarded by *hogescholen*, the second by universities and, in the framework of an 'association', also by *hogescholen*. Studies leading to a master degree will take at least one year and will always be academic, integrating scientific education, research and a master's dissertation, but professional objectives can also have their place. Master degrees will be awarded by universities and, in the framework of an 'association', also by *hogescholen*. Thus, 'associations' serve to strengthen the research base in the *hogescholen* for academic bachelor and master programmes by integrating the research activities of *ho-*

---

4   For a detailed list of qualifications and degrees in Flemish higher education, see: Ministerie, 2001.

gescholen into those of universities. Bridging courses will provide opportunities for students with professional bachelor degrees to enter master programmes.

6.2.3   Students, Access, Success and Educational Attainment of the Population

In the academic year 2002/03, the universities and *hogescholen* together enrolled 157,898 students in initial programmes (Ministerie, 2001a, 2002a, 2002b), of which 71,987 were male and 85,911 (54 %) were female. The universities totalled 56,586 students (36 %) and *hogescholen* 101,312 (64 %), of whom 75,451 (48 %) were enrolled in the three-year programmes and 25,861 (16 %) in the 'two-cycle' four-year programmes. The gender distribution ranges from 58 % females in the three-year programmes in *hogescholen* and 55 % in university programmes to 42 % in the four-year *hogeschool* programmes. *Hogescholen*, which hosted 93,976 students in 1996/97, have grown by 8 % in six years.[5] In the same period, university enrolments remained rather stable. Due to demographic factors, the growth of student numbers in higher education seems to be approaching its limits. Seen from a longer-term perspective, however, the growth was enormous: in 1960/61, *hogescholen* totalled 20,624 students and universities 12,195. In forty years, the massification of higher education led to a rise in student numbers of almost 500 % (see Verhoeven, 1995)!

Concerning students who entered higher education for the first time in October 2002 after graduating from secondary school,[6] 26,376 (67 %) were in *hogescholen* and 12,893 (33 %) in universities, i.e. a total of 39,269. More than half (54 %) chose three-year programmes. Between 1996 and 2001, the number of new entrants in universities dropped by 10,8 %, and that in *hogescholen* rose by 5,3 %.

The net entry rate is 70 % (1999) in Flanders, with 64 % for boys and 75 % for girls (OECD, 2002). This is rather high comparatively. Indeed, Flemish higher education is very open and accessible, with no entry restrictions except for medicine, civil engineering and arts, where entry examinations apply. Low entrance fees and study grants for disadvantaged students further increase the accessibility of Flemish *hogescholen* and universities. There is, however, a social divide between the two types of institutions, with lower-class students preferring *hogeschool* programmes. Flemish higher education also witnesses a kind of 'cascade' whereby many students first try university programmes and, if they fail, fall back on *hogeschool* programmes.

The open character of Flemish higher education has its drawback in the massive nature of first-year teaching and the very low success rates in the first year. In *hogescholen* and universities alike, newcomers have an average success rate of approximately 48 %, but there are differences between disciplines. For first-year stu-

---

5   Due to different counting procedures since 1999 there is a very slight error in these data.

6   Called 'generation-students' in Flemish higher education statistics.

dents who repeat their year in the same or another programme, it is higher (approximately 50 %). In the second and further years, it rises to 90 %. In the non-selective system, succeeding in the first year holds the key to a higher education degree. The overall survival rate, as defined by the OECD, in Flanders is 60 % for the tertiary type-A (four-year) programmes and 88 % for the type-B (three-year) programmes, compared to an OECD countries' mean of 70 % and 77 % respectively.

Each year, Flemish universities and *hogescholen* together award some 30,500 initial degrees, more than half of which are for one-cycle programmes. Furthermore, almost 4,000 post-initial degrees are conferred, mostly by universities. According to OECD statistics, Belgium[7] is a country with a highly qualified population (OECD, 2002). Of the 25-64-year olds, 27 % hold a higher education degree (15 % type-B and 12 % type-A or higher), compared to an OECD mean of 23 %. Amongst the 25-34-years olds, this figure is 36 % (19 % and 17 % respectively), against an OECD mean of 28 %.

6.2.4   Qualifications on the Labour Market

In Belgium, as in most continental-European countries, there is no general system of professional accreditation. This means that higher education degrees and qualifications normally give entry to the corresponding professions. Some organised professions, such as medical doctors, medical specialists, accountants or lawyers, have developed specific additional training systems, to which graduates must comply in order to enter the profession. In recent years, this phenomenon became more widespread as more and more professions tended to impose additional requirements for higher education graduates. Recently, this was the case for accountants and psychotherapists.

In general, the labour market position of Flemish higher education graduates is satisfactory to good. There are great differences between the disciplines and the economic conjuncture has a powerful influence on this, but overall the labour market seems to absorb graduates rather well. Especially in the public sector, but to a great extent also in the private sector, the degree system is mirrored in the jobs and wages hierarchy. Because entry to higher education is open and free, there are several disciplines in which there is a mismatch between supply and demand in the skilled labour market. Clear examples of this are engineering, natural sciences in general, or nursing. The oversupply of medical doctors in the 1990s led to the establishment of

---

7   In these figures, OECD makes no differentiation between the Flemish community of Belgium and other parts of the country.

an entrance examination that limited the number of students and, after seven years, the number of graduates.

6.2.5   Governance and Stakeholders

Autonomy, deregulation, decentralisation and quality were the key words of the legislative and policy developments in the 1990s. Quality and autonomy are seen as intrinsically linked. The steering by the Flemish government concentrates mainly on the general regulatory framework, decisions regarding the planning of the supply of programmes by institutions, and funding. The ministry also has a representative in all institutions and monitors the results of quality reviews and the evolution of financial and other quantitative indicators. Finally, the state tries to influence institutional policies with different forms of programmes and incentive funding, for example in the field of innovation of teaching and learning processes. Despite their great autonomy, the state still exerts a strong influence on institutions (Van Heffen et al., 1999). Because of the small size and the nature of Belgian society and polity, which can be characterised as consensual, there are close contacts and dialogues between the institutions and policy-makers.

The institutions join forces in sector associations, namely VLIR (the Flemish inter-university council) and VLHORA (the Flemish council of *hogescholen*). Because of institutional autonomy and the political will to promote co-operation amongst institutions and to control divergences in the system, these associations have a powerful impact on policy-making processes. Governments expect institutions to settle their disputes amongst themselves and propose policies based on a consensus. They also want to protect the exchangeability of courses and programmes and the inter-institutional mobility of students. Hence, these associations act as mediators between the institutions and the state and stakeholders in society. They also function as quality assurance agencies. Besides these sector associations, there are also other organisations with an official advisory capacity, such as VLOR (the general Flemish education council), in which personnel/unions, employers, students and parents are represented, and SERV (the Flemish social and economic council) where social partners are present.

Stakeholders and social pressure groups show great interest in higher education and its development. Access, success and equity are especially high on the agenda of political parties, unions and various organisations in civil society. Politicians and various organisations are also mobilised by the ambitions and aspirations of the institutions in their region. Other important issues regarding higher education in the political and public domain are: funding, internationalisation, quality, flexibility and innovation, and lifelong learning.

6.3   Quality Assurance and Accreditation Systems

In this section, we shall describe the systems of evaluation that apply to higher education in Flanders. First, the quality assurance systems of universities and *hogescholen* will be analysed, followed by the newly developed accreditation system. This will be put in place in the next few years in the framework of the new legislation and in close co-operation with the Netherlands. In fact, these are not two separate systems; the accreditation system builds on the quality assurance schemes already in place.

6.3.1   Quality Assurance of University Programmes: VLIR Quality Assessment Scheme

Origins and Development

From the late 1980s onwards, quality became a central concern in higher education in various countries. The Flemish universities particularly were influenced and challenged by the development of a system of external quality assurance in the Netherlands since 1989. The 'Dutch model' of quality assurance of university programmes, based on self-regulation and improvement, inspired Flemish university leaders. Flemish peers were invited to join Dutch panels, and, from 1990 onwards, Flemish universities occasionally participated in the Dutch 'visitations' organised by VSNU (cf. chapter 15). Plans were made by VLIR to launch a similar system of quality visits by independent teams of peers. In 1992, an agreement between VLIR and VSNU led to joint Flemish-Dutch visitations. In the meantime, the important university decree of 1991 introduced the legal basis and obligation for the Flemish universities to organise an external quality assurance system that is co-ordinated by VLIR. In exchange for autonomy, and based on a negotiated agreement, the state asked the universities to jointly set up a system of external quality assurance of programmes that aimed at both improvement and accountability.

VLIR quality assurance system serves a number of goals:

- Quality improvement: the process of external assessment builds on and reinforces the internal quality assurance mechanisms within institutions and departments; review panels point to the weaknesses of programmes and formulate recommendations to remedy them;
- Accountability: programmes and institutions, which have autonomy, rely on public trust and receive public funding and must be accountable to the state and the general public; accountability is achieved by providing reliable information on the quality of study programmes;

- Information: the quality assurance system provides information to students, families, the press and the general public and promotes the transparency of the system; in the second round, this information is presented in a comparative way in order to further increase transparency;
- Benchmarking: quality assurance is seen as a mechanism to position the programmes and institutions in relation to comparable programmes and to generally accepted standards; in the second round, this benchmarking function is improved by the comparative approach and the use of minimal standards;
- Optimisation of the supply of the higher education system: outcomes of VLIR quality assurance system are not yet used in any other policy device, but play a role in policy debates on the inter-institutional rationalisation of the supply of programmes.

VLIR visitations are assessments of programmes by an independent panel of 'peers'. The universities, through VLIR, decide on the composition of the panels, but certain general rules apply. The visitation builds on the internal quality assurance arrangements within institutions. The basis of the evaluation is the self-assessment report, which each individual programme has to compile from a detailed questionnaire provided by VLIR. During a site visit of several days, the panel critically reviews the programme by questioning the self-assessment report, analysing relevant documentation, and interviewing all relevant actors and stakeholders. The findings of the panel are then published in a visitation report. The responsibility then falls upon the programme directors in the university, who have to follow up the visitation and report on the decisions and actions they take to improve the programme.

This assessment is carried out every eight years, but the first round was carried out over a total period of ten years. Between 1991 and 2001, all university programmes – except the post-initial ones – were reviewed in this system of visitations.

Several evaluations have been made of the quality assurance system of the Flemish universities. In 1995, Flemish tertiary education was evaluated by a team of OECD experts (Ministerie, 1996). The report contained several criticisms of the quality assurance system. In 1996, an international commission instituted by VLIR evaluated internal quality assurance arrangements for scientific research in the Flemish universities. Although it did not focus directly on the system of visitations, the 'Van Duinen Report', named after the chairperson of the commission, greatly encouraged the quality culture in Flemish universities (Ministerie, 1997). In 1997, the department of education set up an international review team, which was chaired by the Dutch inspector-general Mertens. This commission audited the quality assurance system. The commission's report was positive, but it also pointed out some weaknesses (Mertens et al., 1998). Finally, in 1997 VLIR carried out an evaluation of the protocols and methodologies of the quality assurance system itself. The report pointed at a number of elements in the system that could be improved (VLIR, 1998;

Van Lindthout, 1998). An important discussion in the subsequent debates concerned the possibility of quantifying quality indicators. In the framework of a larger process of 'optimisation' of the Flemish universities led by the special commissioner of the minister, Dillemans, a joint working group of government and university representatives proposed a scheme of quantitative indicators that would provide more transparency in the quality reports and also compare programmes on these quality indicators.

On the basis of these evaluations and reports and on the subsequent internal discussions, VLIR drastically changed the visitations system and its protocol. A new handbook was published for the 'second round', which began in 2002. The main changes in the system were:

- The use of quantified quality judgements: each of the 17 quality aspects and indicators are now judged on a scale from 'A' to 'E'; comparative tables are included in the report with the scores of the programmes under review on each of the indicators;
- The 'research base' on which the programmes under review rest is included as one of the quality aspects and indicators.
- The explicit formulation of a frame of reference by the expert panels and its presentation to the programmes that will be assessed.

The establishment of an accreditation system in Flanders came on the agenda when the second round began. The introduction of accreditation in addition to the existing quality assurance arrangements will no doubt lead to further adjustments to the protocols and methodologies of the visitation scheme for the Flemish universities.

In the following section, we shall describe the formal characteristics of the quality assurance scheme for the Flemish universities, co-ordinated by VLIR, using the analytical framework put forward by the project co-ordinators. The present protocol, which is used for the second round of visitations, will be the basis, but when describing new features of the current protocol, discussions and recent changes will be clarified.

Range

Types, subjects & disciplines: According to the law of 1991 and VLIR regulations, all programmes at the Flemish universities leading to first and second cycle diplomas and degrees must be evaluated. In most cases, individual disciplines are the object of the quality assessment, but in some cases disciplines that have many similarities are grouped in one assessment. At present, the programmes of the 'third cycle', i.e. the post-initial programmes, are not included in the scheme, but plans are under way to include them in the future. Nor are the post-initial teacher training programmes, which are followed by students who want to become secondary school teachers after having completed a specific disciplinary degree. But this is also planned.

Geography: The six universities of the Flemish Community of Belgium fall under VLIR scheme. As stated in the law of 1991, they are obliged to assess their programmes on an inter-university basis under the co-ordination of VLIR. There have been several attempts to broaden the quality assurance scheme to a more international approach. In some cases, joint assessments have been set up with the Netherlands, under a VLIR–VSNU agreement. VLIR and VSNU protocols are basically the same or highly compatible, but sometimes some minor adjustments had to be made. In exceptional cases, such as veterinary sciences, participation in an international quality assessment can be used as a substitute for a Flemish visitation. A Flemish physics programmes joined the cross-border quality assessment project together with Dutch and German programmes in 2000.

Functions: Strictly speaking, VLIR visitations scheme only addresses the educational programmes of the Flemish universities; research is not directly evaluated. Reality, however, is a little more complex. In the past few years, the Flemish universities discussed and negotiated specific quality assurance arrangements for their research function (Spruyt, 2002). Emphasis is laid on the internal quality assurance systems within universities, but in several disciplines a bibliometric analysis has been carried out and the research output is increasingly taken into account in several research funding mechanisms. I already referred to the audit of quality assurance mechanisms of research in Flemish universities by the 'Van Duinen' commission in 1996. When evaluating the first round of visitations of programmes in 1997, VLIR discussed the relationship between the quality assurance of programmes and the quality assurance of research. The outcome of this discussion was that, from the second round onwards, the visitation would analyse more closely the degree to which the academic programme was based upon recent scientific research. The 're-search base' of programmes thus became a separate quality aspect that was evaluated in visitations as from the second round which began in 2002. Data concerning the research output of staff involved in programmes, for example, are now integrated in the quality indicators assessed in a visitation.

Actors

Actors and institutions: The *state* has the legal capacity to deal sanctions when a visitation report leads to a negative conclusion. The Flemish government can also carry out a meta-evaluation of the system of internal and external quality assurance in Flemish universities, e.g. the Mertens commission in 1997-98. In its annual reports on the state of higher education, the department of education informs Parliament and the general public on quality assurance of universities and *hogescholen*.

- The *association of universities*, VLIR, is legally responsible for organising and monitoring the quality assurance scheme. VLIR was established by law in 1974, but is a private association. It has the legal capacity to advise public policies and to promote co-operation between universities. Quality assurance is one of its main tasks. It designs the system, develops and updates the protocols and guidelines, appoints the expert panels, receives the reports of the panels, publishes them, etc.

- The *institutions* are each responsible for the quality of their programmes and have the legal obligation to engage in internal quality assurance mechanisms and to participate in external quality assessments. They are also collectively responsible, since they own the system jointly and have to collaborate in VLIR. Each university has what is called an 'institutional co-ordinator' for the visitation system. Finally, the institutions are responsible for the follow-up to a visitation report.

- The *programme directors* within the institutions organise and monitor the programmes of the faculties and departments and are therefore responsible and accountable for their quality. Each university has different ways of organising this, but most have committees consisting of professors and other teaching staff and students who make up the body that is responsible for the organisation and monitoring of a specific programme. These committees are also responsible for the organisation of internal quality assurance. In some universities they are assisted by specific quality co-ordinators at the level of faculties or departments. A responsible co-ordinator is appointed for each self-assessment and visitation. The programme directors also are responsible for the organisation of the follow-up to the visitation report.

Ownership: The ownership of the visitation system is given to the universities collectively and to VLIR. This was a deliberate choice. The idea behind this 'Dutch model' in quality assurance was that external quality assurance is the collective responsibility of the sector and has to be placed in a perspective of self-regulation. When reviewing the newly established accreditation system, we shall evoke recent discussions regarding self-regulation and independence of quality assurance in the institutions and the sector. In the new law, the responsibility for quality assurance is given to the institutions, associated in VLIR.

Organisation: As has been said, the visitation system of the universities is owned and organised by VLIR, the Flemish inter-university council. The following bodies and components of VLIR are relevant:

- The *Council*: all university rectors and a second representative, except for the two small universities, meet regularly in the Council. This is the highest body in VLIR and is responsible for all decisions. In the field of quality assurance, it approves the visitation protocol, decides on the calendar of the visitations, appoints the visitation panels, etc. After a visitation report is completed, the panel hands it to the chairperson of the Council.
- There are several standing *working groups*, with university representatives, who define the protocol of the visitation system, monitor the functioning of the system and discuss its improvement.
- A university professor is appointed as *special administrator* for the management of the visitation system. He inaugurates the visitation panel, instructs it in the visitation protocol, supervises the work of the quality assurance secretariat, etc. He meets regularly with the institutional co-ordinators of the universities.
- The *secretariat* of VLIR, and more especially its quality assurance section, is responsible for the practical organisation of the visitations. One of its staff members is assigned to each panel and is also responsible for editing the visitation report. The reports are published on VLIR website.

Reviewers:

- VLIR nominates a *panel* of independent external experts for the visitations. Normally a panel consists of four peers from the same discipline, including the chairperson and an educational expert. The peers are mainly academics, but someone from the relevant professional field is regularly included. The experts who are invited to join a panel must have a good scientific record, insight into the discipline and the educational design of the disciplinary programmes and a capacity for sound and critical judgement.
- The main *tasks* of the review panel are: (i) to judge the various quality aspects and indicators listed in VLIR protocol; in the new protocol for the second round of visitations, this also implies giving a mark; (ii) to recommend improvements to the programme directors; (iii) to compare the programmes under review by means of descriptive comparisons and comparative tables; (iv) to inform the academic community, students and the general public of their findings and recommendations by publishing the visitation report.
- Certain *rules* must be taken into account when composing the visitation panel. At least one, normally two, experts come from abroad in order to guarantee the international dimension. The chairperson must not have any present or past links with the institutions participating in the review. For the other members, this restriction is less severe, but when a panel member is associated with one of the institutions under review, he does not take part in the visit.

- The composition of the panel is *decided* by consensus in VLIR Council, on the basis of proposals made by the programme directors. According to the nomination procedure, a person who is proposed by one of the institutions can be refuted by another, but, in general, the independence and critical nature of the panel members are guaranteed.

- One of the *critical aspects* of VLIR visitation system, according to several of the evaluations, is the recruitment of reviewers. Although many academics still see participation in a quality assessment panel as part of their professional responsibilities and feel honoured by the invitation, in some areas it becomes increasingly difficult to find experts. Retired academic personnel, who do have the time but lack insight in the latest development of their discipline and the necessary innovations in teaching and learning practices are an issue.

Customers and stakeholders: not only university administrators, academic staff, reviewers and VLIR personnel are involved in the visitation system. The following stakeholders also play an important role:

- *Students and graduates*: In Flemish universities, students play an active role in the management and quality monitoring of study programmes, although their participation in internal quality assurance processes is sometimes problematic. As has been said already, in most universities, students are represented in the committees that are responsible for programmes and their quality assurance. They are included in the panels that have been set up by faculties and departments for self-assessment. During the visitation process, the panel talks with students and graduates. Although this is not systematic, most self-assessments include a survey of graduates, which focuses on their employment and their critical feedback. Student representatives generally incite programme directors and programme committees to take the findings of visitation reports into account.

- *Parents*: Parents are not addressed or affected by internal or external quality assurance processes in Flemish universities.

- *Social partners*: Some self-assessment reports, especially in disciplines that are closely linked to the labour market and professional associations, pay attention to the opinions of socio-economic stakeholders. When this is the case, employers can express their criticisms, demands and expectations regarding the study programmes and their graduates. Trade unions are rarely involved.

Rules and Regulations

General rules and legal regulations: The basic regulatory framework for VLIR visitation system consists of the relevant articles in the law on universities of 12 June 1991, namely articles 122 to 124, and of VLIR decisions and regulations, laid down in a protocol and handbook. In the new law on higher education, the legal framework of quality assurance will basically remain the same, but it is supplemented by accreditation. VLIR guidelines mainly concern the operational management of the assessment process.

Financing: Universities pay for the cost of VLIR quality assurance system. This is not included in the normal funding of VLIR, which consists of a fixed percentage of what universities receive as basic funding from the state. Besides staff costs and operational expenses for the site visits, the remuneration of the experts is the main expenditure.

Stages of the procedure and their duration: There are four main phases in a process of quality assessment in VLIR visitation scheme:

- The first phase can be seen as a preparatory phase, but it is very important. First, the process is planned by VLIR and the review panel is appointed. Then, following the rules and guidelines laid down in VLIR protocol, a questionnaire is designed and answered by the academic, administrative and technical staff, students, graduates and representatives of the labour market and professional stakeholders. The findings and the critical self-analysis of the programme directors are then integrated in a self-assessment report. This report serves three main functions: (i) providing an analysis of the strengths and weaknesses of the programme in order to stimulate the internal quality assurance processes, (ii) preparing all those involved in the management of the programme for the visitation by the review panel, (iii) presenting all necessary information to the review panel. The programme directors are instructed and guided by VLIR staff in the design and editing of the report. Thirdly, the review panel meets several times to prepare the site visits. One of the crucial elements here is to define a common frame of reference which will help the review panel to interpret and critically analyse the information and make its judgements. In general, this phase lasts for one year.

- The second phase is the site visits of the review panel. Normally, a visit takes two-and-a-half days. The panel interviews the personnel and students involved with or affected by the programme under review. The interviews concern topics that the panel finds relevant following its analysis of the self-assessment report and the documentation provided (samples of dissertations, course work, examination questions, etc.). At the end of the visit, the panel gives an oral report to the committee that has prepared the visitation and those involved in the management of the faculty and university. The total duration of this phase depends on the number of programmes under review in one visitation. Normally, visits to the various institutions are planned within a rather short period.

- The third phase consists of the publication of the report. The press is informed and the report is published both on the Internet and on paper. A visitation report includes reports on each of the programmes reviewed and a general, comparative report. The conclusions and recommendations of the panel are given for each of the quality aspects and indicators. The report is usually published about four months after the last visit by the review panel.
- Finally, the fourth phase is that of the follow-up by the institutions. The institution has a legal obligation to reflect on the outcomes and recommendations listed in the report and to give an account of the actions that it has taken.

Rules for objection: There are no formal rules for objection or appeal in the procedures of VLIR visitation system. However, since it is a self-regulated process that is monitored by the universities, there are always opportunities to raise objections. There are also in-built elements in the procedures that prevent formal objections. The review panel is chosen according to the proposals of the various programmes and nominated by VLIR Council by consensus. During its site visit, the review panel devotes a lot of attention to listening to the programme directors and stakeholders involved and only comes to a conclusion after hearing counter-arguments. Drafts of the final report are sent to the programme directors, who can correct mistakes. It is not felt that these practices jeopardise the independent and critical judgements of the review panels, but they do support the acceptance of the results of a visitation by the academic community as a whole and the departments and programmes involved.

Rules for information distribution: the visitation report is published both on paper and on VLIR website. A statement is sent to the press, summarising the main findings and recommendations of the report. All departments and universities involved receive a number of reports, and additional copies can be bought. The report is also sent to the minister and the department of education.

Implementation of Rules and Regulations

Application of rules and regulations: The rules and regulations that govern VLIR visitation scheme are normally applied without major problems. The most frequent practical problems concern the recruitment of reviewers.

Financial constraints: The financial basis of the system is rather limited, because the universities want to control the cost of quality assurance. Rising costs for paying reviewers, who receive only a symbolic remuneration and no 'commercial' fee, put some pressure on the financial basis.

Time frames: Overall, the timing of the various stages of the procedures is well respected. Some prolongation may be due to the final editing of visitation reports.

6.3.2 Quality Assurance of Hogeschool Programmes: VLHORA Quality Assessment Scheme

Origins and Development

The *hogescholen* in the Flemish Community have developed a quality assurance scheme that can be compared to that of the universities and the Dutch *hogescholen*. Because of the many similarities with VLIR scheme, not all of its features will be described extensively.

The Flemish *hogescholen* sector was drastically reformed in the mid-1990s. The 1994 decree not only called for a major process of mergers between institutions, but also an important reorganisation of the management of institutions and the sector itself, which basically followed the example of the university sector. It also introduced a system of self-regulating quality assurance. The council of the *hogescholen*, VLHORA, was given a co-ordinating role. However, there was a period of transition until 2000 during which the previous system of government-driven inspections for the three-year programmes was continued. Historically, these three-year programmes developed from a secondary school context into the higher education system.

In the second half of the 1990s, there were many developments regarding internal and external quality assurance in the Flemish *hogescholen*. Models from the corporate sector, such as the ISO-9000 scheme and EFQM-inspired models, were adapted and implemented. They proved useful instruments, especially for internal quality assurance within the institutions. But, the sector had to develop its own model for the external quality assessment system on the basis of various experiences and influential examples. VLHORA established a working group on quality assurance in 2000, which developed a conceptual framework, a protocol, a set of procedures and a timetable for the visitations that had to be completed by 2008.

As in VLIR system, VLHORA quality assessment scheme focuses on programmes or clusters of programmes. There can be joint visitations of related university and *hogeschool* programmes. Assessments of programmes will be carried out by panels of external experts, who provide a public report of their findings. The panels consist of educational experts and representatives of the professional and labour market stakeholders.[8] The process starts with a self-assessment report. During the site visit, the panel of experts examines the self-assessment report against the reality it faces and the expectations of the professional and social context.

---

8 VLHORA tries to ensure the diversity in gender, age and background of the experts. Because of the number of individual programmes in many review processes, VLHORA tries to create sufficiently large for subgroups of experts to share the visiting of the institutions and programmes.

According to VLHORA, the external quality assurance scheme serves the basic functions of quality control, quality improvement and accountability (Van Dingenen & Van de Velde, 2002). VLHORA also stresses the need for flexibility and rejects uniformity. A protocol has been elaborated on the basis of these starting-points, with a list of quality aspects and indicators, checklists, guidelines for the design of the self-assessment report and procedure, rules for the work of the expert panels, time-tables, etc. The first assessments started in 2001.[9]

6.3.3   Accreditation in Flemish Higher Education

Origins and Development

In the second half of the 1990s, criticisms began to be heard about VLIR quality assurance system. Some policy makers, employers and journalists questioned the vagueness of the visitation reports and the lack of a clear overall conclusion. The general reaction of the academic community to this criticism was that the quality assurance system was meant to serve internal quality improvement functions. However, there was growing awareness of the external functions of quality assurance (Weusthof & Frederiks, 1997). VLIR adjusted its quality assurance scheme for the second round so as to provide more transparent and comparative information on the quality of programmes. In some countries – although not in Flanders – some newspapers and journals published rankings, which apparently satisfied the public need for clear and easily readable information on the quality of study programmes. It was in this context that – starting in the Netherlands and next in Flanders – a debate on accreditation emerged.

Of course, this debate was fuelled by the Bologna Declaration and its demand for transparency, convergence and compatibility of European higher education systems. Co-operation in the field of quality assurance was one of the objectives of the Bologna process. Internationalisation of quality assurance rapidly became one of the main challenges of the higher education systems in Europe and the world (Van Damme, 2000). In the Netherlands, which again was very influential for the developments in Flanders, work began on a system of accreditation of higher education programmes, together with the introduction of bachelor and master qualifications. Germany also introduced accreditation for the new qualifications. These developments were discussed intensively in Flanders.

---

9   The current timetable, ending the first round in 2008, is tight. Many programmes in various locations have to be assessed in a short period of time. Earlier experiences show that there will be a risk of delay.

The new Flemish government that took office in the summer of 1999 included the implementation of the Bologna Declaration in its political programme. This included the introduction of an accreditation scheme. However, there was a growing consensus that the Flemish Community was too small to develop its own accreditation system and that accreditation should be situated at the international level in the context of internationalisation and the Bologna Declaration. VLIR and VLHORA supported this point of view. The Flemish minister of education decided to collaborate with her Dutch colleague. When the Dutch minister set up a commission of 'trailblazers' in November 2000 to develop a proposal for an accreditation system in the Netherlands, some Flemish observers joined the commission. At about the same time, a working group of Flemish higher education experts and representatives started work on a new higher education law. The Netherlands and Flanders also launched the 'Joint Quality Initiative' within the Bologna process to promote international co-operation in quality assurance and accreditation, which was soon followed by several other countries.

In the spring of 2001, the institutions and their sector organisations nurtured the political debate by issuing some policy papers. VLIR issued a statement, asking for an international accreditation scheme which would be independent of the quality assurance system, but would use the results of the visitation reports (VLIR, 2001). According to VLIR, accreditation could fulfil many functions, but priority should be given to guaranteeing the basic quality of programmes. Via these and other policy statements, a consensus on accreditation gradually developed in the Flemish higher education community.

The new legal framework for higher education in the Flemish Community consisted of three main parts:

• The introduction of the bachelor–master degree structure, covering all university and *hogescholen* programmes;
• The introduction of an (international) accreditation system for all programmes;
• The establishment of 'associations', frameworks for close co-operation between a university and several *hogescholen,* in the areas of research, study trajectories for students and quality assurance.

This new legal framework will be implemented soon, because the new bachelor and master degrees will be introduced in the academic year 2004/05. The accreditation system should also start that year.

Regarding accreditation, the new higher education law closely follows the Dutch law, so that reference can be made to the Dutch country report for many aspects. Late 2002, the Dutch government founded the National Accreditation Organisation (NAO). In September 2003, a treaty was signed between Flanders and the Netherlands for formal co-operation, and NAO was renamed the Dutch-Flemish Accreditation Organisation (NVAO). The accreditation system will have slightly different characteristics in both countries, depending on variations in degree systems, specificities of the higher education system, legal conditions, etc., but basically the accreditation system will be the same as far as standards, criteria and protocols are concerned, allowing for comparable and compatible accreditation decisions by one public body.

The main characteristics of the new accreditation system in Flanders will be that:

- All programmes in the new bachelor-master degree system will have to be accredited in order to ensure their basic quality for the students, stakeholders and society.
- Accreditation will follow the bachelor-master degree system. This implies that the binary divide in programmes, which is maintained in the Flemish degree system at bachelor level,[10] will lead to different accreditation standards and criteria.
- Accreditation will be given to programmes if there are sufficient guarantees that they meet the basic standards and criteria.
- Accreditation will be given on the basis of the results of existing quality assurance schemes, co-ordinated by VLIR and VLHORA. Visitation panels will have to comply with the accreditation frameworks. In this sense, accreditation will become a kind of meta-evaluation of existing quality assurance systems.
- Accreditation will have external effects on the public recognition of the programme and its degree. Public institutions cannot offer a non-accredited programme.
- New programmes will have to submit themselves to a specific kind of *ex ante* accreditation procedure, organised by the accreditation organisation.

The characteristics of the new accreditation system will be described in greater depth in the following sections.

Range

Types, subjects & disciplines: Accreditation will be compulsory for all programmes offered by recognised universities and *hogescholen* in the new bachelor-master degree system. Transition to the new degree system will be mandatory. Accreditation will also cover the post-initial programmes, but not the professionally-oriented programmes and continuing education courses offered by universities and *hogescholen*.

---

10 In contrast with the Netherlands, in the Flemish bachelor-master degree system, there are no professional master programmes and degrees. All masters will be academic. The binary divide is therefore limited to the bachelor degree level. *Hogescholen* will be able to award master degrees on condition that they integrate themselves with universities via the 'associations'.

A novelty in the legal framework is that non-traditional providers, such as foreign institutions or for-profit providers operating in Flanders, can also submit their bachelor-master degree programmes for accreditation, provided that they are registered at government level. These institutions and programmes, hitherto operating completely outside any legal context, will not be recognised or funded by the state, but their programmes and degrees can have the same *effectus civilis* as those from recognised institutions if they are accredited by the accreditation organisation.

Geography: Accreditation will be compulsory for all institutions in the Flemish Community of Belgium.

Functions: The accreditation system will only address programmes and will thus cover only the educational functions of universities and *hogescholen*. However, since both VLIR and VLHORA visitation schemes address the other functions of institutions in their impact on teaching and learning processes, there is indirect reference to other functions in the definition of quality. It is clear that the scientific and research base will be an important criterion for accreditation in academic bachelor degree programmes and master programmes.

Actors

Actors and institutions: In the new decree, the *state* has the legal obligation to set up an independent accreditation system and organisation. However, the Flemish Community will not do this on its own; it can only develop accreditation in an international context. The state will also have a meta-evaluative role in the system of quality assurance and accreditation.

* The *accreditation organisation* will be established with the Netherlands by means of a treaty. The agency will have four major tasks: (i) accreditation of existing bachelor-master programmes; (ii) *ex ante* evaluation of new programmes to check whether they meet the basic quality standards; (iii) assessment, on demand of the institution, of specific quality aspects of the programme; and (iv) the promotion of the European and international dimension in Dutch-Flemish accreditation and the development of international contacts in order to achieve co-ordination and collaboration. In this section, we shall focus on the first function, since the differences in procedure between the first and second functions are only minor.

* An accreditation framework with basic quality standards and criteria has been developed (NAO, 2003b). In the Dutch law, the accreditation organisation is competent to develop the accreditation framework, which must subsequently be approved by the minister. In the Flemish context, however, because of the constitutional freedom of education, the basic conditions and criteria must be defined by Parliament and therefore included in the new law.

- The *associations* of *hogescholen* and universities, VLHORA and VLIR, organise and co-ordinate the quality assurance schemes. They will not have direct responsibility in the accreditation system, but the reports of their quality assurance schemes will be fed into the accreditation process. NVAO will not develop its own quality review and assessment schemes, but will base its judgements on the reports of visitation organisations. These will have to comply with the framework and rules of NVAO for their reports to be acceptable for accreditation decisions. The rationale for this delicate relationship between quality assurance and accreditation is that duplication must be avoided as far as possible and that accreditation must be developed in addition to already existing and highly valued quality assurance schemes. In this sense, accreditation becomes a kind of independent approval of the conclusions of the visitation panels.

- VLIR and VLHORA quality assurance schemes will not have the monopoly of accreditation. As in the Netherlands, other agencies may well apply and obtain recognition from the accreditation organisation to act as a visitation organisation, although, legally, VLIR and VLHORA retain their co-ordinating functions.

- In the first instance, the *institutions* will not face major changes in the system of quality assurance. The accreditation system will follow the timetables of the quality assessments already planned by VLIR and VLHORA. In the longer term, there is a risk that the introduction of accreditation will change the attitudes of programmes towards quality assurance. Programmes and institutions will increase their 'window-dressing' activities and perhaps reduce their transparency if faced with highly critical procedures. The accreditation organisation tries to minimise this risk by entering a trust-building dialogue with VLIR and VLHORA.

- Accreditation will be gradually introduced in Flemish higher education. As from 2004, programmes will receive a transitional accreditation until the moment their visitation is planned, according to the timetables of VLIR and VLHORA quality assessments.

Ownership: Formally, the accreditation is 'owned' by the Flemish and Dutch governments and Parliaments that have instituted the legal framework and the organisation. The accreditation organisation must report to the two Parliaments. For the rest, it is autonomous. A close informal partnership is developed with the higher education community, as it is deemed impossible that an accreditation system can operate without the institutions' trust. In reality, there is thus a mixed ownership.

Organisation: The *presidency* of the accreditation organisation consists of a chairperson and two vice-chairpersons. All three are former heads of institutions and represent the higher education community. At first, the presidency was entirely Dutch. A Flemish representative was added to the presidency as an observer at the end of 2002.

Reviewers: the accreditation system will not develop its own quality assessment and visitation activities, but will build upon the existing VLIR and VLHORA schemes.

Rules and Regulations

General rules and legal regulations: The basic rules and regulations are laid down in the new decree on higher education. Compared to the Dutch law, the Flemish decree goes a little further in regulating the procedures and standards of accreditation. Of course, the accreditation organisation itself will also develop and impose its own rules and regulations. NAO issued a draft paper on the basic rules of the accreditation system, which was negotiated with the higher education community and external stakeholders (NAO, 2003a).

Financing: The accreditation organisation is financed by the state. Institutions will have to pay for an accreditation, in addition to the cost of the visitations. The actual cost of an accreditation for institutions is still unclear.

Stages of the procedure and their duration: the process leading to accreditation has the following components:

- An institution asks a quality assessment agency (VLIR, VLHORA or another) to carry out a review and a visitation according to its protocols, which meet the NAO requirements.
- Programmes carry out a self-assessment and produce the self-assessment report that will be transmitted to the review panel.
- The actual external review and site visit take place.
- At least six months before the previous accreditation for a programme comes to an end, the institution submits a request for a new accreditation that includes its self-assessment report and a recent (not more than one year) external quality assessment report.
- The accreditation organisation examines the report and takes a decision within three months following the request. Before the decision is formally confirmed it is presented to the institution, which has two weeks to react.
- The accreditation organisation publishes its decision.

In total, the process will take about a year and a half. In the Flemish higher education law, accreditation is granted to a programme for a period of eight years. This is different from the Netherlands, where it is only valid for six years.

Rules for objection: Institutions have the legal right to object to accreditation decisions in court. In order to limit court cases, certain appeal procedures are included in the Flemish higher education law.

- The procedures in the quality assurance systems that allow programmes and institutions to react to the reports of the review panels still apply.
- The institution does not have to agree with the statements of the visitation panel. There can be fundamental disagreements, resulting from divergent approaches and quality frameworks. In that case, the institution can produce a well-argued reaction to the visitation report and include it in its request for accreditation.
- The accreditation organisation will present a preliminary decision to the institution, which will have two weeks to react.
- In the Flemish higher education law, absence of accreditation does not mean that a programme must automatically be abandoned. The minister can give a temporary recognition to a non-accredited programme for a maximum of three years. The minister can take this decision if programmes are unique, if non-accreditation would endanger the access to education for students, etc. Obviously, this is an emergency clause.

Rules for information distribution: Accreditation decisions will be published. Accredited programmes will be listed in a higher education register.

Implementation of Rules and Regulations

Accreditation is not yet in operation, so it is too early to say anything about the implementation of its rules and regulations.

6.4   Analysis

Above, we analysed actors, driving forces, considerations and rationales behind the three schemes in the Flemish system. It was felt necessary to give a brief description of the origins and development of these schemes to better understand their descriptors. In this section, we shall expand on the analytical questions.

6.4.1   Driving Forces and Rationales Behind the Introduction of Accreditation

The introduction of a system of accreditation of higher education programmes in Flanders was the result of two closely related rationales. On the one hand to continue the existing schemes of external quality assurance, operated by VLIR and VLHORA. The accreditation system in Flanders – following the Netherlands – was designed as a system 'on top of' the existing quality assurance schemes, which were seen as functioning well and of high quality. At the same time, however, accreditation was also seen as an answer to tackle some of the shortcomings of the existing quality assurance schemes, namely their lack of clear conclusions and their limited capacity to make the higher education system more transparent. But accreditation was also introduced to implement the Bologna Declaration. Although it was not mentioned explicitly in the Bologna Declaration, Flemish higher education leaders, from the outset, saw it as a necessary instrument to achieve the ambitions of 'Bologna'. Bologna provided an additional trigger for forces that were already developing in the Flemish higher education policy system.

These two main rationales were especially relevant in the context of the challenge of the Flemish bachelor–master degree system, namely the transformation of the two-cycle four-year programmes of *hogescholen* into master's degrees. These four-year programmes must be incorporated in the academic qualifications by strengthening their research base, a challenge for which the 'associations' between *hogescholen* and universities are designed.

The discussion on quality assurance and accreditation incited various stakeholders to voice other arguments. First, we note the desire of the 'social partners', trade unions and employers' organisations to strengthen their control over higher education programmes. They felt that institutions did not pay enough attention to their legitimate demands.

Moreover, students' associations have taken a positive stance on accreditation. They see it as a necessary instrument for transparency in the Flemish higher education system in a European context and as an information tool.

Finally, the government and the civil servants consider accreditation as a device to recognise programmes in a different manner. In an accreditation system, programmes will no longer be recognised *ex ante* by the state, but will obtain recognition on the basis of an externally guaranteed quality mark.

6.4.2   Relationships Between Quality Assurance and Accreditation Schemes

The accreditation system is designed to follow 'on top of' the existing VLIR/VLHORA schemes. However, the actual relationship between quality assurance and accreditation is still being debated. The accreditation procedure will consist of a marginal assessment of the validity of the judgement in the visiting report. In practice, therefore, the accreditation decisions will be taken by the quality assessment panels in the first instance. To some critical observers, this induces a confusion of responsibilities between quality assurance and accreditation (Van Damme, 2001b). The higher education sector also fears that the improvement function of the existing VLIR and VLHORA quality assurance schemes will be jeopardised. On the other hand, there is the argument that a duplication of quality assessment processes would increase the evaluation burden. A subtle balance will have to be found between quality improvement and supportive functions of quality assurance on the one hand, and external accountability functions and the requirements of accreditation on the other.

In both the Dutch and the Flemish legal frameworks for accreditation, visitation organisations other than those established by the sectors' organisations are allowed. It is believed that this open character will induce competition and prevent existing organisations maintaining a monopoly. In practice, however, many believe that it will be very difficult to compete with the existing quality assurance organisations or to achieve sufficient trust at the level of the institutions and the accreditation organisation. It would also imply duplication for the programmes, since they must participate in VLIR and VLHORA quality assurance schemes anyway.

6.4.3   Consequences of the Introduction of Accreditation

Consequences for Higher Education Institutions

Financial Consequences and the Greater 'Quality Burden'. The introduction of an accreditation system is expected to raise the overall cost of the total quality assurance system for Flemish universities. The rise can be attributed to three elements.

First, the direct cost of accreditation: institutions will have to pay for each accreditation. *Second*, the rising cost of visitations: the protocols will have to be adapted to accreditation demands, which will probably increase the workload of the visiting teams. Moreover, at present, reviewers are not paid much. It is doubtful whether this will be sustainable in a context of accreditation and professionalisation of the quality assurance system. *Third*, the introduction of accreditation will also affect other costs in institutions. Academics will have to spend more time on self-assessments to comply with the higher standards for such documents. They will also be forced to improve the quality of teaching and learning processes and their conditions to meet the accreditation standards. Because of the high quality of Flemish higher education programmes, it is not expected that the introduction of accreditation will require institutions to invest much in quality improvement, but internal quality assurance systems will certainly have to be updated.

All this involves a hidden cost: the time of the academics, the bureaucratic burden in institutions involved in internal quality assurance, and maybe a risk of de-motivation and 'quality fatigue'.

Changes in Attitudes Towards Evaluation. Accreditation will affect the way in which programmes conduct self-assessments. More information will be needed and it will have to be structured differently. The peer review teams will have to arrive at sharper conclusions, so the discriminatory character of the information will have to be increased. This will require diagnostic and analytical competences and a great deal of honesty, self-criticism and open-mindedness on the part of the programme directors.

In a longer-term perspective, many observers expect a change in the attitudes of institutions, departments and programme directors towards external evaluation because of the impact of accreditation. It is anticipated that they will have a less open and self-critical attitude towards their own programmes and will become 'experts in window-dressing'. Counter-arguments to this somewhat pessimistic view are that peer review teams will be able to distinguish between rhetoric and reality, that VLIR and VLHORA visitation systems will continue to have an improvement orientation and a supportive attitude towards programmes, and that accreditation is only concerned with checking the basic quality standards.

Consequences for Students

Referring to many other countries where this is normal practice, students asked for the inclusion of a student in each programme review team. This demand has been met in the new Flemish higher education law. So students will have a direct impact on the accreditation system. They consider this to be an important aspect of their empowerment and an important condition to arouse interest among students in quality-related matters.

Ultimately, students are also interested in strengthening the international recognition of their degrees. Especially in a small country with an international labour market and an open economy, they demand qualifications that are recognised and respected. They expect that accreditation can improve this in the internationalisation context. Students feel that the international basis of the new bachelor–master degrees should be safeguarded in order to protect students and families that invest in studies leading to these degrees.

Consequences for Other Stakeholders and the General Public

The strong political support for the introduction of accreditation in Flemish higher education mirrors the belief that it will lead to more transparency and to qualifications that are better recognised at the international level.

6.5   International Activities and Aspects

6.5.1   International Examples and Role Models

In our description of VLIR quality assurance scheme, we already mentioned the international context in which the universities developed an external quality assurance scheme. In particular, the Netherlands was a very influential model in this. In its operational phase, many forms of co-operation with the Dutch colleagues developed. Dutch influence was also clearly visible in the emergence and development of

VLHORA external quality assurance scheme. VLHORA and the Dutch sister-organisation *HBO-Raad* developed close co-operation in the field.

As has been indicated before, the introduction of the accreditation system in Flanders was greatly influenced by the developments in the Netherlands. There was even an ambition, inspired by the strong will of the Dutch Minister of Education at the time, to take the lead in accreditation within the Bologna group of countries and extend international co-operation. Consequently, in the spring of 2001, Flemish and Dutch civil servants visited other countries in order to study possibilities for co-operation. Visits were undertaken to agencies and policy-makers in the Czech Republic, Catalonia, Sweden, Germany, Italy and Spain and a report was published in April 2001 (Vroeijenstijn & Schreinemakers, 2001). From this report it was clear that some countries expressed great interest in developing co-operation in the field of quality assurance. But it was too early to expect a structural co-operation or integration of accreditation systems between countries in the short run. The Dutch and Flemish governments then agreed to launch a more voluntary co-operation project, the 'Joint Quality Initiative', which held a number of very successful meetings and conferences and produced some interesting output, e.g. the 'Dublin descriptors' for bachelor and master degrees.

NVAO still aspires to broaden the co-operation in the field of accreditation to other European countries in the context of the Bologna process, as can be seen in its initiative to establish a European consortium of accreditation agencies. In June 2003, the founding meeting took place.

6.5.2   The Impact of Bologna and GATS

The VLIR quality assurance scheme was developed in a context in which the Bologna process had not yet been launched. The adaptation of VLIR quality assurance scheme in the late 1990s was decided in quite a different international context. The protocol for the second round in VLIR scheme was certainly influenced by the Sorbonne and Bologna Declarations, without explicitly referring to them.

As has been said already, Bologna was a very powerful policy imperative in the development of accreditation in Flanders. In early 2001, VLIR and VLHORA adopted policy papers that welcomed the Bologna process and indicated the way in which they wanted to see it implemented in the Flemish higher education system. Looking at the passive and active resistance to Bologna in many European countries – including the French-speaking Community of Belgium – there was a very positive stance towards Bologna in Flemish universities and *hogescholen*, as well as amongst policy-makers already at an early stage. The implementation of Bologna was greatly influenced by the sector associations, which were in close contact with the minister and the policy-makers. As from 2001, the general director of VLIR was seconded to the office of the minister to chair a working group that drafted the new law.

The impact of GATS is much less clearly visible in the policy developments regarding accreditation. GATS has not yet been a major topic of debate in Flemish higher education policy because the minister took a firm position in the European debates regarding the public nature of the educational system. However, there is a feeling that the context of transnational and for-profit providers has to been taken into account in the development of an accreditation scheme in Flanders. That is why, in the new law, private – i.e. non-state recognised – providers can be registered and can present themselves for accreditation. When accredited, their degrees can be recognised by the state. A direct impact of GATS in this issue is not perceptible. This arrangement would probably also have been elaborated without GATS.

6.6   Other Evaluation Practices

Some other evaluation practices in Flemish universities and *hogescholen* need to be mentioned. The first is that universities and *hogescholen* are obliged by law to evaluate professors and teaching staff every five years. Each institution is free to develop its own methodology for this. Some universities carry out staff evaluations every two years. Results of these evaluations are included in the person's files and can influence wages and promotion. In some universities, 'tenured' professors have been dismissed as a consequence of consecutive negative evaluations. VLIR has tried to achieve some minimal convergence in the procedures developed in the universities. The institutions are requested to report regularly on how they do this and on the results.

A second practice is that, in the framework of internal quality assurance, procedures have been developed in many institutions for students to evaluate professors and teaching staff. The results of student evaluations, when meeting certain statistical minimum conditions, are included in the personnel files of each professor. The aggregated results are often included as information in self-assessment reports for VLIR and VLHORA visitations.

At present, universities are discussing various systems of research evaluation. Emphasis is laid on the intra-institutional approach, where research councils include evaluations of research teams' and departments' previous work when assessing research proposals. Some institutions invite peer review teams to do research assessments, but this is completely voluntary and autonomous. Increasingly, bibliometric tools are used as indicators in research assessments. At present, the minister has asked VLIR to set up an audit of research evaluations in the institutions. There is no interaction between research assessments and the systems of quality assurance and accreditation for educational programmes, but it is clear that when dealing with topics such as the research base of master programmes, departments and external visitation teams will study these materials and indicators.

References

Bronders, M. (2001). Externe kwaliteitszorg onderwijs: het visitatiestelsel herbekeken, *Universiteit & Beleid*, 15 (3), pp. 8-12.

Bronders, M. (2003). Kwaliteitszorg aan de universiteiten in Vlaanderen, in: *Kwaliteitszorg in het Onderwijs*, Afl. III, maart 2003.

Hoornaert, J. (2002). Onderwijsvisitaties aan de Vlaamse universiteiten: ervaringen en evaluatie van de eerste ronde 1991-2002, *Tijdschrift voor Onderwijsrecht en Onderwijsbeleid*, 2002-2003 (1), pp. 45-52.

Mertens, F.J.H. et al. (1998). *Aandacht voor kwaliteit in de Vlaamse universiteiten. Verslag van de Auditcommissie Kwaliteitszorg in het academisch onderwijs* (Brussel: AHOWO).

Ministerie van de Vlaamse Gemeenschap (1996). *OESO-verslag tertiair onderwijs in Vlaanderen* (Brussel: Departement Onderwijs).

Ministerie van de Vlaamse Gemeenschap (2001a). *Rapport hoger onderwijs 1999-2000* (Brussel: AHOWO).

Ministerie van de Vlaamse Gemeenschap (2001b). *Higher education in Flanders* (Brussel: AHOWO).

Ministerie van de Vlaamse Gemeenschap (2002a). *Rapport hoger onderwijs 2000-2001* (Brussel: AHOWO).

Ministerie van de Vlaamse Gemeenschap (2002b). *Beperkte statistische telling van de studenten in het hoger onderwijs op 31 oktober 2002* (Brussel: AHOWO).

Ministry of the Flemish Community/VLHORA/VLIR (2002). *Changing higher education in Flanders* (Brussels: NARIC/VLHORA/VLIR).

NAO (2003a). *Uitgangspunten accreditatie. Concept* (Den Haag: NAO).

NAO (2003b). *Accreditatiekader bestaande opleidingen hoger onderwijs.*(Den Haag: NAO).

NAO (2003c). *Toetsingskader nieuwe opleidingen hoger onderwijs.* (Den Haag: NAO).

OECD (2002). *Education at a glance. OECD Indicators 2002* (Paris: OECD).

Spruyt, E. (2002). Kwaliteitszorg onderzoek. Proeve van toepassing van een VLIR-advies, *Universiteit & Beleid*, 15 (4), pp. 22-31.

Van Damme, D. (2000). 'Internationalisation and quality assurance: towards worldwide accreditation?', *European Journal for Education Law and Policy*, 4/1, pp. 1-20.

Van Damme, D. (2001a). Van Bologna over Salamanca naar Praag. De Europese hoger-onderwijsruimte en de consequenties voor de Vlaamse universitaire ruimte, *Universiteit & Beleid*, 15 (2), pp. 2-17.

Van Damme, D. (2001b). De drie P's getoetst: Rapport Commissie-Franssen onder de loep genomen', *Tijdschrift voor Hoger Onderwijs & Management*, 9 (5), pp. 19-24.

Van Dingenen, I. & L. Van de Velde (2002). Een beleidsplan voor de kwaliteitszorg in de hogescholen in Vlaanderen, in: *Kwaliteitszorg in het Onderwijs*, Afl. II, december 2002.

Van Duinen, R.J. (1996). *Om de kwaliteit. Een analyse van het beleid van de Vlaamse universiteiten inzake kwaliteitszorg in het wetenschappelijk onderzoek* (Brussel: VLIR).

Van Heffen, O., P. Maassen, J. Verhoeven, F. De Vijlder, K. De Wit (1999). *Overheid, hoger onderwijs en economie. Ontwikkelingen in Nederland en Vlaanderen* (Enschede – Utrecht: CHEPS & Lemma).

Van Lindthout, A. (1998). Optimalisatie van de methodologie van het visitatiestelsel, *Universiteit & Beleid*, 12 (2), pp. 22-31.

Verhoeven, J.C. (1995). *Towards mass tertiary education in Flanders (Belgium)* (Leuven: KULeuven).

VLHORA (2001). *Visitatie van de opleidingen. Handleiding* (Brussel: VLHORA).

VLIR (1998), *Optimalisatie van de methodologie van het visitatiestelsel* (Brussel: VLIR).

VLIR (2001). Handleiding voor de onderwijsvisitaties in de tweede ronde (Brussel: VLIR).

VLIR (2001). *VLIR-advies betreffende de implementatie van de Bolognaverklaring in Vlaanderen* (Brussel: VLIR).

Vroeijenstijn, A.I. & J.F. Schreinemakers (2001). *Naar een Pilot Consortium Internationalisering van Accreditatie* (Amsterdam).

Weusthof, P.J.M. & M.M.H. Frederiks (1997). De functies van het stelsel van kwaliteitszorg heroverwogen, *Tijdschrift voor Hoger Onderwijs*, 15 (4), pp. 318-338.

Relevant websites:

www.jointquality.org
www.nao-ho.nl
www.vlaanderen.be/onderwijs
www.vlhora.be
www.vlir.be

7 The Changing Role of the State in French Higher Education: From Curriculum Control to Programme Accreditation

THIERRY CHEVAILLIER

7.1 Presentation of the Higher Education System

The French higher education system is currently undergoing deep changes in relation to degree structure and accreditation process. In the wake of the Bologna declaration, new state regulations have been introduced since 2000 that aimed at building a degree structure that is common to all higher education institutions. As their implementation will be phased in step by step until 2006, a study of the accreditation processes in operation in France must present both past and future schemes.

7.1.1 Size of the System

In the academic year 2000/01, some 2,160,000 students were enrolled in higher education programmes in France.[1] The French definition of higher education is fairly broad: it comprises all programmes for which the *baccalauréat* (end of secondary education degree) or an equivalent qualification is required for access.

7.1.2 Types of Institutions

Basically, the French higher education system is characterised by a small number of large comprehensive institutions, the universities, accommodating nearly two-thirds of the student population, several hundred smaller specialised institutions with 20 % of total enrolment and a large number of very small two-year programmes offered in secondary education institutions which enrol 15 % of the student population.

Universities and Similar Institutions

The number of universities and similar institutions is: Universities (85), Universities of Technology (3), National Polytechnic Institutes (30). In total, these higher education institutions accommodate 1,404,000 students, i.e. an average of 15,400 students

---

1 For up-to-date statistical data on French higher education, see *Repères et références statistiques*, the statistical yearbook of the Ministry of Education, http://www.education.gouv.fr/stateval/rers/repere.htm#1.

S. Schwarz and D.F. Westerheijden (eds.),
Accreditation and Evaluation in the European Higher Education Area, 159–174.
© 2004 *Kluwer Academic Publishers. Printed in the Netherlands.*

per institution. Their legal framework is that of 'Scientific, cultural and professional public corporations' (EPSCP). Accordingly, they are autonomous but are supervised by the ministry of higher education. There are 19 private universities and university institutes, with 21,000 students, or on average 1,100 students per institution. Then there are the Teacher training institutes (30) (*Instituts universitaires de formation des maîtres*, IUFM), with a total of 84,000 students, for an average size of 2,800 students. They are less autonomous than universities.

Specialised Schools of Higher Education (*Grandes Écoles*)

A typically French category of institution is the specialised schools of higher education *(grandes écoles)*. The majority recruit students who have already studied for two years after graduating from secondary school. Recruitment is competitive and some of these institutions are considered more prestigious than university departments.

Then, there are the independent Engineering schools (153, with 62,000 students, average size: 400 students). These are mostly public institutions, under the responsibility and control of several different ministries (higher education for the majority, but also industry, agriculture, defence, etc.). There are also engineering schools or programmes that are part of universities and that are organised in the same way (90 schools, 33,700 students, average size: less than 400 students).

The 234 business schools are home to 70,300 students (average size 300 students). Mostly private, many are operated by local chambers of commerce and come under the responsibility of the ministry for industry.

There are 252 Schools of Art and Architecture. They enrol 55,800 students, for an average size of 240 students. These schools are under the responsibility of the ministry for cultural affairs and are operated by the state, the regions or some cities.

Other public higher education institutions in this category, of which there are about 200, include various public institutions such as *Écoles normales supérieures* (for teacher training), *Écoles des hautes études en sciences sociales*. These schools are under the responsibility of various ministries (veterinary schools, schools of journalism, schools of administration) with 30,000 students in total, which makes their average size 150 students.

Paramedical and Social Programmes

Nearly 100,000 students are enrolled in 500 schools of paramedical and social programmes, with an average size of less than 200 students. These schools are not part of universities. Most are public and under the responsibility of the ministry of Health and Social Affairs. Some are operated by charities (e.g. the Red Cross).

Short Higher Education Programmes Offered by Upper Secondary Schools

This is a large category in numbers of institutions (2,560). However, with 310,000 students, the average size is only 120 students. Most of these programmes (three-quarters of enrolments) consist in two-year vocational courses (higher technicians courses) that would not be considered higher education in other European countries. The other part comprises very selective preparatory programmes *CPGE* (*Classes préparatoires aux grandes écoles*) leading to prestigious non-university higher education institutions, mostly engineering or business schools.

7.1.3   Main Types of Diplomas and Certification

Traditionally, the state regulates vocational and higher education degrees, diplomas and certificates. It has a monopoly on 'Academic titles and degrees' as well as on 'vocational and professional titles'.

- National diplomas (*Diplômes nationaux*). A large number of diplomas are awarded on behalf of the state by institutions that are formally authorised to do so in a process called 'habilitation'. Some of these institutions also confer degrees and academic titles (*Grades et titres universitaires*).

- Institutions' own diplomas (*Diplômes d'école ou d'université*). Public and private universities and higher schools may award self-accredited diplomas usually called '*Diplôme d'université*' (DU) or '*Diplôme d'établissement*'. Universities are not entitled to recurrent funding from the ministry for higher education for students enrolling in the programmes leading these types of own diplomas. They must fund them out of their own resources, but may charge full fees.

- Professional and vocational qualifications (*Titres professionnels*). These degrees are vocational qualifications that are protected by the state and certify specific training and abilities (e.g. engineer or psychologist). Usually granted on the basis of accredited diplomas.

7.1.4   Types of Programmes, Access, Attrition

Higher education comprises a wide variety of programmes ranging from two-year vocational programmes to eight years or more studies as in the medical sector.

Most programmes are organised in cycles (usually of two years) and in many fields, students are allowed to change tracks or programmes at the end of a cycle. Access to second cycle programmes may be open or competitive. Access to third cycle higher education is always competitive.

As a rule, access to the first year of higher education is open to all secondary school graduates who hold a *baccalauréat*. In practice, this is only true for the general academic programmes offered by universities. In the 'open sector' of higher education (general academic programmes offered by universities) selection takes place during the first years. Access to preparatory programmes for the *grandes écoles* (*CPGE*) is highly competitive, especially for the most selective schools. Access to short vocational programmes, either in university institutes of technology or in secondary school higher technician programmes is on application; the admission procedure is more or less selective according to subject or region.

Access to medical studies is open but there is a competitive examination at the end of the first year. Only 10 to 20 % of the students proceed to the second year. Some of those who fail this exam are admitted to paramedical studies (nursing, osteopathy, speech therapy etc.). The majority, however, turns to other fields of higher education.

In general academic programmes, the rate of failure and drop-out during the first two years is high and students often try a new orientation in another programme. Yet some 30 % of students enrolling in these general academic programmes leave higher education without any degree, diploma or certificate.

Once the first cycle of study is completed (usually the two-year DEUG diploma), students proceed to the second cycle and may leave higher education with a degree at the end of each further year of study successfully completed with a *Licence* degree or a *Maîtrise* degree. Following the *Maîtrise*, a third cycle of study begins, leading to a DESS (*Diplôme d'études supérieures spécialisées*), a one-year professional programme, or a DEA (*Diplôme d'études approfondies*), i.e. the first year of a research track opening the way to three to four years of doctoral studies.

The final and higher diploma is the Habilitation *(Habilitation à diriger les recherches)* which is required for application to permanent academic positions at the professorial level. It is awarded after examination of the research record of the applicant by a board of examiners drawn from several universities or research institutions.

7.1.5   Transition to Work

In recent years, about 60 % of every age group graduated from secondary education, 80 % of whom enrol in a higher education programme, which gives an access rate to higher education which is close to 50 %. More than 20 % of students leave higher education without a degree. One third will leave higher education with a two-year programme diploma (DEUG, DUT, BTS, nursing, etc.). Over 40 % graduate from longer programmes. A recent study by CEREQ provides a comparison of transition to work of all graduates of higher education in France.[2] The unemployment rate

---

2   Giret, Jean-François, Stéphanie Moullet, Gwenaëlle Thomas, CEREQ, décembre 2002. *De l'enseignement supérieur à l'emploi: les trois premières années de vie active de la 'Génération 98'.*

three years after leaving higher education varies according to the qualification. Short programmes in the health care and social sector provide nearly all their graduates with a job (less than 1 % unemployed), but 10 % of students leaving higher education without a degree are unemployed. Concerning long (five-year) programmes, graduates from engineering and business schools are less likely to be unemployed (2 to 3 %) than graduates from university academic programmes (6 to 9 %).

There is a clear hierarchy of programmes in terms of earnings: compared to the median earnings of higher education graduates, engineering and business schools graduates earn two-thirds more and graduates from short general programmes (DEUG) one third less.

7.1.6   Governance

With a few exceptions, higher education is tightly controlled by the state. The ministry in charge of higher education does not supervise the whole of the higher education system. Other ministries control their own higher education systems (Agriculture, Industry, Cultural Affairs) with specific structures, statutes and modes of operation. Non-profit organisations are in charge of most private higher education institutions, especially Catholic universities. The unions, especially teachers unions, play a part in the governance of higher education by having seats on the numerous consultative boards that advise the ministers and their administration.

Institutions are more or less autonomous in the management of their operations. They nearly all have governing boards where faculty, students, industrial representatives and local politicians are represented. Heads of Universities are elected for a single five-year term. School directors are appointed by ministers.

7.2   Accreditation, Approval and Evaluation

Generally, official accreditation and approval schemes involve the state which is represented by the government and more specifically the ministers in charge of the various departments of the government. Ministers must ask the advice or the opinion of specific consultative committees for each type of study programme or institution. For all decisions made at the national level, the opinion of the National Council for Higher Education and Research (CNESER) is required. Consultative committees are partly elected and partly appointed by the minister and they consist of representatives from the education administration, teachers and academics, as well as industry concerned with the programmes to be accredited. CNESER members are elected among students and staff of higher education institutions in a ballot where candidates are presented by unions. A number of representatives of employers and workers in industry, appointed by the government, also sit on this council.

Evaluation of the higher education institutions is conducted by a specialised autonomous agency, the National Evaluation Committee (*Comité national d'évaluation des établissements d'enseignement supérieur*, CNE).

7.2.1   Accreditation Schemes

Official accreditation, in a large majority of cases, is based on degrees or diplomas. An institution is granted the right to award an accredited diploma on the basis of the programmes it offers or plans to offer and the resources it intends to devote to teaching and training.

Accreditation of National Diplomas (*habilitation*)

All national diplomas are accredited by the ministry in charge of higher education after consultation with various consultative bodies. Accreditation is granted to universities following a process that takes place every four years. Universities prepare a development plan, which is submitted to the ministry for higher education. On this basis, a contract is agreed between the ministry and each institution. It includes the list of national diplomas the institution is allowed to award, as well as a commitment of the ministry to fund the institution for the students enrolled in the corresponding programmes. Guidelines on curriculum, course structure of the programme, name of the diploma and regulation of examinations are set by the ministry.

Accreditation is decided after an examination of the organisation of the programme, as well as the number and qualification of the teaching staff of each institution applying for accreditation.[3]

*General Diplomas, Academic Degrees and Titles (*Diplômes Généraux, Grades et Titres Universitaires*).*

*   DEUG (*Diplôme d'études universitaires générales),* intermediary diploma awarded after two years of study in universities.
*   *Licence*, equivalent to a bachelor's degree, one year after DEUG.
*   *Maîtrise*, one year after the *Licence*.
*   *DEA (Diplôme d'études approfondies*), one year after the *maîtrise*. It is a prerequisite to enrol for a Ph.D. The DEA is roughly equivalent to a British research master degree.

---

3   For a description of the internal process in universities and an assessment of the ministerial accreditation, see: F. Kletz & F. Pallez, *L'offre de formation des universités: création de diplômes et stratégie d'établissements*, Juin 2001, see http://www.cpu.fr/Publications/ Publication.asp?Id=138.

*Technological and Professional National Diplomas (*Diplôme de l'Enseignement Technique Supérieur*).* As a rule, these diplomas are accredited by the minister for higher education on the advice of a mixed consultative committee where academics and representative from industry sit in equal numbers.

- BTS (*Brevet de technicien supérieur,* higher technician certificate) a two-year programme.
- DUT (*Diplôme universitaire de technologie,* university technology diploma), two years.
- *'Licence professionnelle'* (vocational bachelor degree), three years.
- Master-engineer qualification awarded by IUP (*Instituts universitaires professionnalisés*), four years.
- DESS (*Diplôme d'études supérieures spécialisées,* specialised higher education diploma), five years.

The New Master Degree. A new type of Master degree, a national degree and diploma, has been introduced in France as a step towards a unified European higher education area. It is to be awarded after an overall period of study of five years to graduates of both professional and general programmes by private as well as public institutions.

The accreditation procedure for this degree is still under discussion. It will have to merge three distinct existing accreditation schemes, one related to general university programmes, one recently introduced for business schools and one longstanding scheme for engineering schools. In the present state of the debate, all programmes leading to master diplomas would be accredited by the ministry of education following screening by panels of experts of the MSTP *(Mission scientifique, technique et pédagogique)* appointed by the minister in charge of higher education. Parallel to that, programmes in engineering and business would be assessed by the Committee for engineering qualifications *(Commission du titre d'ingénieur)* and the Committee for evaluation of management programmes and diplomas (*Commission d'évaluation des formations et diplômes de gestion*) created in 2001.

State Approval of Institutional Diplomas (*Diplômes Visés par l'Etat*)

After five years of operation, a private school of higher education may apply to the ministry for higher education for approval of its diplomas. The programmes and examination procedures are screened by experts of the ministry who advise the minister. The approval is reviewed periodically.

Private External Accreditation of Diplomas

It is not always clear whether an accreditation scheme concerns institutions or diplomas. Private and public schools of higher education have entered a race to 'external accreditation' under the pressure of the labour market. Almost every business school can boast affiliation to a more or less prestigious group or network, very often international or European. Engineering schools are just beginning to consider similar external accreditation.

Networks and Clubs:

* *Conférence des Grandes Écoles*. The French *Conférence des Grandes Écoles* is a select group of schools that co-opt their members to maintain a high level of quality. They 'own' a postgraduate diploma, the '*mastère spécialisé*' (a registered trademark). They are organised in two chapters (*chapitres*), one for engineering schools, the other for business schools. Of the 234 business schools, only 27 belong to the CGE.
* *Networks of excellence and accreditation by foreign or international bodies.* Schools of business and management and, to a lesser extent, schools of engineering, are looking abroad for accrediting bodies, for example: AMBA, a British group for the accreditation of Masters of Business Administration, EQUIS (European Quality Improvement System), or AACSB (American Assembly of Collegiate Schools of Business).

Certification of Professional Diplomas and Qualifications

What used to be called *homologation* is mainly a certification by the state of a given vocational qualification, certificate or diploma awarded at the end of a vocational training programme by including it in a national register, the *répertoire national de qualification professionnelle*. The register, which is made public, gives information on the industrial sector and the level of qualification that is relevant to the programme and certificate.

Programmes and national diplomas that are accredited by the state (*habilité*) are registered without further examination and with no time limit. Higher vocational education institutions or industries may apply to the national committee for vocational certification (*Commission nationale de certification professionnelle*) for inclusion of a training programme and the resulting certificate in the national register for a period of five years.

This scheme applies to vocational, professional and technological diplomas and certificates. For higher education, this means that most of the institutions that are not universities and some of the programmes offered by universities are concerned.

7.2.2 Approval Schemes

Official recognition of higher education institutions takes various forms, from the weakest – the mere administrative authorisation to open a school – to the strongest, i.e. creation of a public corporation for higher education and research.

Creation of Public Corporations in Higher Education

Public corporations are legal entities, specifically created by the state for the purpose of educating and training, that are granted formal autonomy to administer themselves and manage their own resources.

Higher Education Public Corporations. EPSCP (*Etablissement public à caractère scientifique, culturel et professionnel*) are the public universities, the National Polytechnic Institutes and the Technology Universities. The law (Higher Education Act 1984) defines and organises these institutions. Their constitution provides for a federal structure of departments (UFR, schools or institutes),that offer both research and teaching and for an elected executive. They are created by the government after consultation with the National Council for Higher Education and Research (CNESER). Changes in the internal structure of the institutions must be approved by the minister in charge of higher education.

Administrative Public Corporations. The legal framework for administrative public corporations does not only concern higher education institutions but also all sectors of public administration (*établissement public administratif*). Heads of such corporations are appointed by the minister in charge of the government department that controls them (*Ministère de tutelle*), i.e. the minister in charge of higher education for the majority of them. Some institutions, such as the IUFM (teacher training institutes) and some schools of engineering are formally linked to Universities (*rattachés à une université*). Others are autonomous administrative public corporations (most schools of engineering and many other institutions).

Departments of Public Administrations. Some higher education institutions are mere departments of ministries, without any formal autonomy or corporate identity.

State Approval of Private Institutions

Private institutions of higher education must fulfil a number of minimal conditions to be authorised (*autorisé*) by the state. The conditions concern the qualifications of the teaching staff and administrators, premises and facilities, etc.

They may also apply for formal recognition by the state (*reconnaissance par l'État*). A recognised school of higher education may apply for public subsidies, employ faculty seconded from public sector higher education institutions, and attract recurrent grants for themselves and bursaries for their students.

Approval of their degrees by the state confers private institutions a status close to that of public institutions in exchange for a periodical review of their programmes and the obligation to have examination boards that are chaired by a professor from a public higher education institution.

To sum up, private schools are ranked in three classes of increasing prestige according to the extent of state recognition they enjoy: authorised schools, recognised schools (*École reconnue par l'État*), and recognised schools awarding approved diplomas (*École reconnue délivrant un diplôme visé par l'État*).

7.2.3   Evaluation Schemes

Institutional Evaluation

The CNE, the National Council for Evaluation of Universities, was created by the 1984 Higher Education Act. It is an autonomous administrative entity that reports directly to the President of the Republic. The CNE consists of 25 members assisted by administrative staff led by a general delegate. Its members are appointed by the President of the Republic. They represent the academic and research community.

The CNE's mission is to evaluate universities, schools and other institutions in the areas linked to the missions of the higher education public sector, i.e. initial and further education, students' living conditions, research and the use of its results. It also examines the way an institution is governed, its policy and management. However, the CNE is neither entitled to evaluate individuals, nor to accredit programmes nor to apportion state funds. Its reports on individual institutions are published.

The CNE has already conducted institutional evaluations of all French universities and about 50 schools (more than 180 reports have been published so far). It also conducts comparative evaluations of disciplines (e.g. geography, information and communication studies, chemistry, applied mathematics) or of a type of degree course (postgraduate degrees in medical studies, pharmacy courses) across all institutions. And it also advises on national higher education policy issues in its annual report to the President of the Republic.

The institutional evaluation conducted by the CNE includes an internal and an external phase. The evaluated institution prepares an internal evaluation record with the help of guidelines. The external phase is a peer review, consisting of site visits by experts who write confidential reports for the committee. The CNE then builds upon both the internal evaluation and experts' reports to elaborate the evaluation report, which is published.[4] The average duration of the complete evaluation process is about one year.

In its 2002 annual report, the CNE suggested that its institutional evaluations should be synchronised with the development plans of the institutions and the contracts they sign with the ministry.[5]

Programme Evaluation

The accreditation process has increasingly been associated with the evaluation of programmes. Application for accreditation of new programmes and review of existing programmes include information that institutions have to provide: transition to work of the graduates, drop-out rates, time to obtain a degree, etc.

Since 1996, universities are required to conduct an internal evaluation of study programmes which includes student surveys. For this purpose, institutions have developed their own statistical and analytical capacity by creating specialised services called '*observatoires*' in charge of collecting data, conducting surveys and producing local indicators on students and graduates.

Higher Education Indicators

In recent years, the central statistical office of the ministry of education started publishing comparative results of all universities in terms of drop-out and efficiency, especially in the first stages of study at university where open entry is balanced by high attrition. The media also produce sets of indicators and league tables, which are becoming ever more sophisticated and ever less criticised by university officials. They usually draw on data made public by the ministry of education and on surveys conducted with institutions.[6] New legislation is currently being prepared to further increase the autonomy of institutions; this will stimulate the demand for indicators to monitor the evolution of the higher education sector, especially from the parliament.

Quality Assessment in Staff Policy

Training, recruitment and promotion of academic staff can be seen as essential elements of quality assurance in higher education. Recruitment for long time was considered the only instrument for maintaining and improving the quality of teaching and research in France. The main argument for recruiting permanent academic staff

---

4   For further information, see http://www.cne-evaluation.fr.

5   http://www.cne-evaluation.fr/WCNE_pdf/bulletin36.pdf.

6   See, for example, the university league tables (*palmarès des universités*) published by the *Nouvel Observateur* in March 2003.

through national competitive examinations ('*concours*') is that it ensures a high level of scientific quality. Once recruited to a permanent position, they are supposed to maintain the high level demonstrated when recruited. There is no further assessment of teaching and research abilities unless a person applies for promotion.

Promotion is largely based on the scientific record of the candidate, i.e., on his publications and research related activities. Until recently, promotion was decided upon by the same national body that recruits permanent staff, the National Council of Universities for lecturers and professors and the National Committee for Scientific Research (or its equivalent) for researchers. Recently, institutions have been allowed to grant about half the promotions open every year, making it possible to assess and reward different profiles of academic staff.

Recurrent evaluation of teaching performances is fiercely opposed on the basis of the principle of independence of the professoriate, defined in a law and upheld by the administrative courts. A 1997 statute ordered universities to organise the evaluation of teaching but it was prohibited to do it in a way that would resemble an external evaluation of individual faculty members. Although a majority of the academic community seems now to accept or support such an evaluation,[7] the legislative framework still seems to be a hindrance to a wider use of evaluation to assess and ensure the quality of teaching in universities.[8] This situation explains why staff development is almost non-existent for academic staff in French institutions.

7.3   Origin and Consequences of the Schemes of Accreditation and Evaluation

7.3.1   Purpose of Accreditation and Evaluation Schemes

The role of the state in the accreditation of higher education institutions and programmes is a consequence of the monopoly conferred to the state after the French Revolution in order to end the traditional control of the Catholic church over education. The concept of the national diploma reflects this monopoly.

A second function of the state is to improve the information available to potential employers and future employees by certifying and ranking by levels the various diplomas and vocational qualifications issued by all providers of education and training. In addition to the national registry of professional qualifications, the state provides general and specific information on education and training programmes, as

---

7   Rapport Fréville sur *La politique de recrutement et la gestion des enseignants et des chercheurs*, http://www.senat.fr/rap/r01-054/r01-0541.pdf.

8   Rapport Dejean sur *L'évaluation des enseignements dans les universités*, see http://cisad.adc. education.fr/hcee/publications-2002.html.

well as their relation to the labour market. A national agency for information on education programmes and occupations (ONISEP) and a network of local information and guidance centres produce comprehensive and up-to-date information for the benefit of school pupils and students.

A third function of the state is to support education financially, jointly with local governments. Although local governments have come to finance part of the development of universities and other institutions, it is still the responsibility of the state to provide higher education to all young people who are 'willing and able' to study. In this capacity, the national government has to ensure that institutional funding and student financial support are adequately distributed. Only programmes leading to a national diploma entitle higher education institutions to public funding and students are only supported financially if they attend approved institutions ('*Établissements reconnus par l'état*').

Evaluation is required by both funding agencies and institutions as the higher education system has become more diversified and too complex to be directly administered by a central administration. In the 1980s, expansion and diversification of higher education led the Ministry of Education to relinquish the control it was no longer able to exert and to rely increasingly on institutional autonomy to take care of the day to day management of universities. The National Evaluation Committee was created in 1984 when the Ministry was initiating a new relationship with institutions based on institutional development plans and funding contracts signed on the basis of such plans. The introduction of explicit evaluation was clearly triggered by the need for institutions to better understand their operations in order to plan them. At the same time, the Ministry was seeking a more holistic view of institutional performance. The Parliament and other public funding bodies also became aware of the need for assessment of the overall achievements of the higher education system; the financial effort of the nation was greater than ever before because of a policy of widening access to higher education, known in this country as 'democratisation'.

7.3.2   Relations Between Accreditation and Evaluation

Nevertheless, evaluation has never been directly linked with funding. Although accreditation of national diplomas triggers funding of teaching according to a formula linked to the number of students enrolled, no specific financial constraint is imposed on the advisory committees that review the proposals of the universities. They accredit (or propose accreditation) purely on the basis of quality criteria (qualification of the teaching staff and structure of the programme).

In addition to recurrent funding of teaching based on this formula, universities receive additional public grants through a contractual agreement struck every four years with the ministry of education on the basis of specific projects stated in the institution's development plan. Ministry officials stated repeatedly that institutions had a duty to conduct *ex post* evaluations of these state-funded projects. Even if universities did sometimes attempt to do so in the report they produce at the end of each planning period, the ministry has tended to neglect such prescriptions for lack of time and staff. This is why it was recently proposed that the National Evaluation Committee (CNE) should be asked to centre its review of institutions on the achievement of their development plans. This would tie the CNE institutional evaluations to the planning period. As the development plans are for four years, the CNE would assess each university once every four years.

Institutions apply for accreditation of programmes leading to national diplomas as part of their institutional development plan and the ministry accredits the programmes in the contract it signs with each university. In the review process, universities are asked to provide an assessment of the effectiveness of each programme, based on past evidence for renewals and forecasts for innovations. Such assessment takes into account performance indicators such as the time to obtain a degree, ease and speed of transition to jobs for graduates.

7.3.3   Relations Between Accreditation and Approval

As can be seen from the description of the various existing or planned schemes, the approval of institutions and the accreditation of programmes are not necessarily linked. Public institutions, which do not need approval, have to apply periodically for accreditation by the state for each of their programmes to award national diplomas and to receive public funding.

Accreditation is not necessarily granted to all programmes for which the institutions apply. This feature, which has been central to higher education policy for decades, is the consequence of the overwhelming domination of the national diploma in the minds of the French population. Attempts to relinquish it and grant universities self-accrediting powers have always been nipped in the bud. Employers and students alike only trusted the state to guarantee the 'value' of diplomas, even when there was massive evidence that the content and selectivity of national diplomas varied widely from one institution to another. This may be due to the weakness of external evaluation of teaching on which students could rely for their choice of programme and employers for their recruitment policy.

Nevertheless, the process of programme accreditation by the state has been deeply transformed in the last 20 years. As university curricula used to be defined by the ministry, all that was needed was to ensure compliance with the ministerial regulation. This 'conformity check' was carried out in a formal way only for new institutions or when institutions applied for new programmes. Once granted, the 'approval' was not questioned in subsequent reviews. The same held true for engineering schools: their accreditation by the Committee for Engineering Qualification entitled them to permanent approval by the ministry.

As the autonomy of institutions in designing their curricula increased, the need for proper accreditation and periodic review began to be felt. New types of programmes were introduced for which there was no national curriculum, but only a few guidelines provided to the universities and therefore a large diversity in structure and content. This was particularly true for the DESS, which are postgraduate professional programmes, and the IUP, which are professionally oriented university institutes. As it was no longer possible to check the conformity of local programmes with a national model or yardstick, the ministry altered its approval process and created new bodies and new processes for accreditation.

This was made absolutely clear when, in 2002, it was decided to change the whole degree structure following the Bologna Declaration. The ministry allowed universities to propose new programmes leading to the master's degree and the only guidance they would receive was the criteria that the ministry would use for its accreditation decision. This new policy surprised and annoyed a large part of the academic world, especially the teachers and students unions. It was obvious to all that the French higher education system was subject to radical change. A similar change had also been under way for the *grandes écoles*, as an accrediting body was created for business schools and periodical review of accreditation was introduced for engineering schools.

Over the last decades, the French higher education system has greatly evolved and, surprisingly for those who know the country, in a pragmatic and gradual way.

7.4   External Influences on Accreditation and Evaluation

As far as external influences are concerned, the situation is somewhat different for evaluation and for accreditation. Institutional evaluation as conducted by the CNE has been developed with little reference to foreign examples. During the 1990s, the 'French model' of evaluation of higher education was often opposed to the harsher and more inquisitive British and Dutch 'models'.

Accreditation on the basis of national diplomas was established at a time when universities were mainly training judges, teachers and civil servants for the state. The private sector of the economy mainly employed graduates from private engineering or business schools and the national diploma made no great sense. With the expansion of enrolments and the diversification of programmes offered by universities, university graduates started competing with those from private or non-university institutions for the private sector jobs and the whole picture became blurred.

France played a leading part in the design of a European higher education area by organising the first meeting in 1998 at the Sorbonne. The French minister of education of the time saw in this process a powerful instrument to reform the national higher education system. The introduction of a new degree structure in the wake of the Bologna conference led to a complete reshuffling of the cards, which is still taking place on the French scene. The construction of a 'European higher education area' and the threat of competition from graduates from neighbouring countries are pushing all institutions towards a common degree structure and a common accrediting system. For the time being, given the weakness of the organisation of higher education institutions in the country, such a system can only be provided by the state.

Glossary

BTS (*Brevet de technicien supérieur*), higher technician certificate: diploma for two-year vocational programmes organised in secondary education institutions (*lycées*).

CNE (*Comité national d'évaluation des établissements d'enseignement supérieur*), national evaluation committee.

CNESER (*Conseil national de l'enseignement supérieur et de la recherche*), national council for higher education and research.

CPGE (*Classes préparatoires aux grandes écoles*), two-year preparatory programmes prior to access to 'grandes écoles'.

CTI (*Commission du titre d'ingénieur*), committee for engineering qualifications.

DEA (*Diplôme d'études approfondies*), postgraduate diploma, a pre-requisite to enrol for a PhD, roughly equivalent to a British research master degree.

DESS (Diplômes d'études supérieures spécialisées), postgraduate professional diploma.

DEUG (*Diplôme d'études universitaires générales*), intermediary diploma awarded after two years of university studies.

DUT (*Diplôme universitaire de technologie*), university technology diploma, awarded by IUT after a two-year vocational programme.

Licence, equivalent to the bachelor's degree, one year after DEUG (either *Licence professionnelle*, vocational bachelor's degree, or *Licence générale*, academic bachelor's degree).

Maîtrise, one year after *Licence*.

8 Shift of Paradigm in Quality Assurance in Germany: More Autonomy but Multiple Quality Assessment?

ANGELIKA SCHADE

8.1 The National System of Higher Education

8.1.1 Types of Higher Education Institutions

The tertiary sector in Germany includes higher education institutions and other institutions that offer courses which qualify for entry into a profession and that address to students who have completed upper secondary education and obtained a higher education entrance qualification. The state and state-approved higher education institutions are the following:

*   Universities (i.e., *Universitäten, Technische Hochschulen / Technische Universitäten, Pädagogische Hochschulen, Theologische Hochschulen*);
*   Colleges of art and music (*Kunsthochschulen* and *Musikhochschulen*);
*   Universities of applied sciences (*Fachhochschulen*).

Of the 331 higher education institutions (118 universities, 157 universities of applied sciences and 56 colleges of art and music), as of March 2003, 263 are members of the *Hochschulrektorenkonferenz (HRK)*, which is the voluntary association of state and state-recognised universities and other higher education institutions in Germany. According to a provisional statement by the Federal Ministry of Education and Research (*Bundesministerium für Bildung und Forschung)* issued in January 2003, there are 43 private institutions which are not members of the *HRK*.

There are a number of special higher education institutions that only admit certain groups (e.g. higher education institutions of the Federal Armed Forces, of the Police and *Verwaltungsfachhochschulen* – public administration). Holders of a higher education entrance qualification can also choose to enter a *Berufsakademie* as an alternative to higher education. These vocational training institutions combine on-the-job training with academic work and were established in seven of the 16 *Länder* in 1974 (cf. Eurydice: Eurybase).

S. Schwarz and D.F. Westerheijden (eds.),
Accreditation and Evaluation in the European Higher Education Area, 175–196.
© 2004 *Kluwer Academic Publishers. Printed in the Netherlands.*

8.1.2   Size of the Higher Education System

While enrolment numbers follow cyclic variations, there has been a clear trend to-wards growing numbers of student enrolments in the last 25 years. Between the academic years 1975/76 and 2000/01, numbers doubled (cf. HIS-Ergebnisspiegel, 2002, p. 61). Students are distributed by type of institution as in Table 1. The vast majority of students are enrolled in state institutions, which accommodate over 1.8 million (97 %), while private state-approved higher education institutions count 34,000 (2 %) and church state-approved institutions 2,000 (1 %) (Higher Education Compass, January 2003).

Table 1. Students by type of higher education institution

Type of institution	Number of students	Percentage of students
Universities	1,388,812	73 %
Universities of applied sciences	487,286	25 %
Colleges of art and music	32,813	2 %
Total	1,908,911	100 %

Source: Statistical information on higher education institutions from the Higher Education Compass, http://www.higher-education-compass.de (January 2003)

8.1.3   Main Degree Types

The traditional university degree programmes lead to the *Diplom*, the *Magister* and the *Staatsexamen*. The average length of studies to obtain a degree is ten to twelve semesters or five to six years. Universities have the exclusive right to award doctoral degrees. Universities of applied sciences award the *Diplom (FH)*, where studies usually last for eight to nine semesters. The level of equivalence of the old gradua-tion system degrees on the international scale occasionally led to misinterpretations. As the publication of the 'European Glossary on Education' should have made clear, the university *Diplom* in the old graduation system is equivalent to the master's degree in the new graduation system (Tables 2 and 3; cf. Eurydice, 1999).

With the amendments to the German Higher Education Act *(HRG)* of 20 August 1998, Germany's higher education institutions, universities and universities of ap-plied sciences, were given the opportunity – initially for a test phase, and now per-manently – to introduce bachelor's and master's degree courses. The new graduation system only supplements the traditional system of degrees, as can be seen in the numbers of new degree programmes and students enrolled in them (about 3 % in winter 2001). There is, however, a lively discussion about changing the graduation system to bachelor's/master's degree courses, except for parts of the *Staatsexamen* (cf. Wissenschaftsrat, 2002).

Some *Diplom/Magister, Staatsexamen* and *Abschlussprüfung* programmes follow upon a first degree. The vast majority of postgraduate degree programmes, however, is made up of the new master's degree programmes.

Table 2. Main degree types (first-degree – graduate/undergraduate)

Degree type	No. of programmes	In percent
Bachelor/Bakkalaureus	749	8 %
Diplom (mainly in science and engineering)	1,624	17 %
Diplom (FH)	1,700	18 %
Lehramt (teaching degree)	2,972	31 %
Magister (mainly in arts and humanities)	2,044	22 %
Staatsexamen (in state-supervised professions)	168	2 %
Others	78	1 %
Total	9,335	100 %

Source: Statistical information on higher education institutions from the Higher Education Compass, http://www.higher-education-compass.de (January 2003)

Table 3. Main degree types (postgraduate)

Degree type	No. of programmes	In percent
Abschlussprüfung (final exam in art, music)	137	9 %
Diplom	219	14 %
Diplom (FH)	96	6 %
Magister	80	5 %
master's	789	51 %
Staatsexamen	119	8 %
Others	105	7 %
Total	1,545	100 %

Source: Statistical information on higher education institutions from the Higher Education Compass, http://www.higher-education-compass.de (January 2003)

We do not yet have any statistics on the labour market acceptance of the various degrees; there is, however, good reason to assume – as first research results and the recent press show – that the new bachelor's/master's degrees are not well-known by personnel managers (e.g. List, 2000).

8.1.4 Transition of Students from Higher Education to Work

On average, higher education graduates have a relatively better position in the labour market than most other groups, as can be seen in the unemployment data (Table 4).

Table 4. Unemployed persons by level of qualification (data: 2001)

Level of qualification	Number
Persons without vocational training	1,386,000
Persons with vocational training	2,356,000
Persons with a university degree	127,000
Persons with a university of applied sciences degree	53,000
Total	3,742,000

Source: Bundesministerium für Bildung und Forschung, Zahlenbarometer, 2001/2002

The factors that facilitate or hamper transition from higher education to work are complex and difficult to identify (for more information on this, see Kehm, 1999), so they have to be interpreted with caution. The significantly lower number of unemployed amongst academics should not, for example, hide the fact that they can increasingly be found in underqualified jobs, in temporary work, or are avoiding unemployment by entering continuing qualification programmes (for more information see HIS-Ergebnisspiegel, 2002, pp. 247 ff).

Table 5. Number of unemployed persons holding an academic degree by field of study

Subject group	Year 2000	2001
Language and cultural studies	15,785	16,882
Law, economics and social sciences	36,459	37,848
Mathematics and natural sciences	15,177	14,945
Medicine	9,913	9,013
Agriculture, forestry and nutritional sciences	4,513	4,810
Engineering	52,664	52,932
Art, music	7,469	8,365
Teaching	19,329	17,493
Total	176,255	180,399

Source: Bundesministerium für Bildung und Forschung, Zahlenbarometer, 2001/2002

The data show significant differences between the subject groups (Table 5); these differences, however, change cyclically.

8.1.5 Governance and Steering of Higher Education

In the Federal Republic of Germany, responsibility for the education system is determined by the federal structure of the state. Educational legislation and the administration of the education system are primarily the responsibility of the *Länder*. The *Länder* Ministries of Education, Cultural Affairs and Science develop policy guidelines in the fields of education, science and the arts, adopt legal provisions and administrative regulations, co-operate with the highest authorities at national and *Länder* level and supervise the work of authorities under their purview and that of subordinated bodies, institutions and foundations.

The Standing Conference of the Ministers of Education and Cultural Affairs of the *Länder* in the Federal Republic of Germany (*KMK*) brings together the *Länder* ministers and senators who are responsible for education and training, higher education and research, and also, as a rule, cultural affairs. This body works on the basis of an agreement between the *Länder* and deals with policy matters pertaining to education, higher education, research and culture that are of supra-regional importance, with the aim of forming a common viewpoint and a common will, as well as representing common interests. Resolutions of the *KMK* can only be adopted unanimously. They have the status of recommendations – with the political commitment of the competent ministers to transform the recommendations into law – until they are enacted as binding legislation by the parliaments in the *Länder,* implemented in the form of administrative action, ordinances or laws. As a rule, higher education institutions have the status of a public law corporation and are public institutions under the authority of the *Länder*. They have the right to self-administration within the framework of the law. The higher education institutions draw up their own statutes (*Grundordnungen*) which require the approval of the *Land* in which they are situated (cf. Eurydice: Eurybase).

The general principles for the legal position of higher education institutions, including the participation of all members of these institutions in self-administration, are laid down in the federal higher education law (*HRG*). On the basis of these principles, the organisation and administration of higher education institutions are regulated by *Länder* legislation for those institutions that come within the purview of each *Land*. The *Länder*'s and higher education institutions' room for manoeuvre in reforming their organisation and administration has been extended through the 1998 amendment of the *HRG*.

8.2   The Schemes

Whereas quality assurance in teaching in Germany was primarily carried out through ex-ante control (quantitative specification and approval of examination regulations by the state), other countries increasingly pursued it as ex-post control on the basis of evaluation results. Following the international development and with growing quality assurance awareness, evaluation procedures were introduced as from the mid-1990s and accreditation procedures at the end of the 1990s.

8.2.1   Accreditation Scheme for Study Programmes at Public Higher Education Institutions

Paradigm Shift: From Approval to Accreditation as a Precondition for Approval

Responsibility for the contents and organisation of studies and examinations as well as for the quality of higher education lies with the *Länder*. This has been finally implemented by a system of approving programmes and defining exam requirements. Proposals for standards of study courses and degrees as well as for their mutual recognition were made for a long time through framework regulations on studies and examinations (*Rahmenprüfungsordnungen*), which had to be jointly adopted by the *Länder* and the *HRK*. The creation of these framework regulations has proven to be an extraordinarily ponderous procedure, often taking many years and producing results which, when finally adopted, had already become inefficient because of new developments and therefore proved to be counterproductive, especially with regard to study programmes competing in the international market (cf. Akkreditierungsrat, 2002, pp. 1 ff.).

Framework regulations include the quantitative reference data of degree courses, in particular the standard time to obtain a degree *(Regelstudienzeit)*, the amount of hours of teaching in required and elective subjects, the number of credits required for admission to examinations (*Leistungsnachweise*), examination details and the length of time allowed to complete the final dissertation. While accreditation procedures were introduced initially for new bachelor's/master's study courses, they were extended through the new 'organisation statute' issued by the *KMK* (KMK resolution of 24 May 2002 in the currently valid version of 19 September 2002) to all study programmes where there is no valid framework regulation. This means that, in the long run, the former system of framework regulations will be replaced by the new system of accreditation.

The Actors Engaged in the Creation of the Accreditation Scheme

The opening of Germany's higher education system to the developments at European level by introducing bachelor's/master's degree courses specifically aims to:

- increase the flexibility of the range of study opportunities offered,
- improve the international compatibility of German degrees, and thus
- increase student mobility and demand among international students for study places in Germany.

To provide the higher education institutions with the autonomy required for the implementation of the reform, the former system of state control became less widespread. In order to give consideration to the different areas of competence and responsibility of the state and higher education institutions in the establishment of degree courses, the *Länder* ministers of education and culture decided on a functional separation between state approval and accreditation; they also reached an agreement with the *HRK* on the establishment of a cross-*Länder* Accreditation Council (*Akkreditierungsrat*).

The *Akkreditierungsrat* is responsible for the establishment of comparable quality standards for bachelor's and master's degree courses in an essentially decentralised accreditation process, which will be carried out by accreditation agencies. According to its 'organisation statute', as from 1 January 2003, the 17 members of the *Akkreditierungsrat* include four representatives from higher education institutions, four representatives of the *Länder*, five practitioners, two international experts and two students. This shows the social dimension of the education policy restructuring process – all stakeholders should be involved.

The Basis for and Framework of the *Akkreditierungsrat*

The introduction of the accreditation system in Germany is based on resolutions passed by the KMK and the HRK. The *Akkreditierungsrat* was first established for a test period of three years and, following assessment by an international group of experts, was given permanence through the 'organisation statute' adopted by the KMK in 2002. It sets the criteria to accredit accreditation agencies and degree programmes and co-ordinates how these agencies assess the content and quality of degree programmes. The resolutions adopted by the *Akkreditierungsrat*, as well as complementary guidelines, aim to ensure the reliability, comparability and transparency of the procedures. The resolutions include (cf. Akkreditierungsrat, 2002, pp. 31 ff.):

- *Basic Standards for Accrediting Accreditation Agencies.* These standards comprise, *inter alia*, institutional independence, adequate staffing, facility and funding infrastructure, performance of accreditation for all types of higher education institutions and, with respect to all types of programmes and disciplines, national and international competence, evidence of transparency, quality control, documentation and information concerning procedures, and accountability.

- *Criteria for accrediting degree programmes leading to bachelor's and master's degrees.* The rather general set of criteria refers, *inter alia*, to standards concerning the quality and international compatibility of the curriculum, as well as control of student achievement, professional qualification of graduates on the basis of a consistent and coherent programme design, and assessment of the foreseeable developments in potential career fields.

- *Frame of reference for bachelor's/master's study programmes.* As there is no single model for bachelor's and master's programmes, but a large variety of possibilities, the criteria defined by the *Akkreditierungsrat* had to take German academic traditions and expectations into account. Moreover, they had to be in accordance with the declarations and statements made at European level. The *Akkreditierungsrat* therefore developed an open framework for bachelor's and master's degrees which has interfaces with existing European frames.

- *Relation between evaluation and accreditation.* In the *Akkreditierungsrat's* interpretation, evaluation and accreditation serve different purposes and should therefore be dealt with in separate procedures and by different bodies. However, recent evaluation results may be taken into account in an accreditation procedure.

- *Participation of students in the* Akkreditierungsrat, *in accreditation agencies and peer groups.* The *Akkreditierungsrat* considers the participation of students in the organisation and carrying out of accreditation procedures very important. To facilitate such participation, various student organisations set up a 'students accreditation pool' in summer 2000[1] on the initiative of the *Akkreditierungsrat*.

- *Monitoring of accreditation agencies.* The *Akkreditierungsrat* is the 'monitoring authority' that determines whether the standards are respected. It co-ordinates, critically monitors and supports the work of the agencies.

- *Procedure for admission to careers in the public service.* Master's degree courses offered at universities of applied sciences which apply for a decision on admission of their students to careers in the public service have to be accredited through a special procedure which involves a representative of the civil service.

Meta-Accreditation and Scope of Accreditation

A system of meta-accreditation and checks and balances exists, since the *Akkreditierungsrat* accredits agencies and is itself evaluated regularly. Accreditation agencies can be accredited by the *Akkreditierungsrat* when they meet the principles and basic standards listed below.

---

1   For more information cf. www.studentischer-pool.de.

- Accreditation agencies must be institutionally independent of higher education institutions as well as of business, industry and professional associations. The agencies must ensure that higher education institutions and representatives of professional practice are given appropriate opportunities to participate in the accreditation decision-making process.[2]

- Accreditation agencies need to have adequate staffing, facilities, and funding infrastructure, that are reliably ascertained for the medium term. They operate on the principles of efficiency and economy, and will not be profit-oriented.

- Accreditation agencies carry out accreditation for all types of higher education institutions.

- Accreditation agencies must bring together national and international competence. As an essential factor to evaluate the professional qualification of accreditation agencies, such approaches should be reflected, *inter alia*, in the recruitment of experts and in the design of assessment procedures.

- Accreditation agencies must prove that the procedures followed in processes of programme accreditation are comprehensible and transparent. They must provide for internal measures of quality control and suitable documentation and information practices.

- Accreditation agencies are also accountable to the *Akkreditierungsrat* after they have been accredited. In particular, they must inform the *Akkreditierungsrat* without delay of any degree programme for which they have extended accreditation status and submit an annual activity report (Akkreditierungsrat, 2002, pp. 38 f.).

In the course of processing the application from the agency to be reviewed, the *Akkreditierungsrat* produces a review report based on the institutional profile submitted by the applying agency, and on one or several consultations with it. The *Akkreditierungsrat* then decides to accredit, conditionally accredit or not to accredit the agency. Subsequently, the *Akkreditierungsrat* monitors the implementation of any conditions imposed and, if the agency was accredited, monitors the observance of the targets agreed with that agency. Each accreditation is issued for a limited time period (three to five years), which is then followed by a re-accreditation procedure.

The Actors in the Accreditation Scheme

In the course of its three-year pilot phase, the *Akkreditierungsrat* accredited four single-discipline agencies, and three cross-disciplinary agencies, i.e. agencies with

---

2   The *Akkreditierungsrat* considers 'participation by higher education institutions' to mean the academic and scientific community, including especially teachers and students, and by 'professional practice', representatives of economic life who will be proposed by both employer and employee organisations.

responsibility for degree courses across the whole spectrum of subjects. 'Single-discipline' and 'cross-disciplinary' agencies may accredit programmes in all geographical regions, with teaching being the main part of the respective schemes.

The cross-disciplinary agencies are:

- ACQUIN (Accreditation, Certification and Quality Assurance Institute): members are mainly the universities and universities of applied sciences in several *Länder* as well as in Austria.
- AQAS (Agency for Quality Assurance through Accreditation of Study Programmes): members are mainly the universities and universities of applied sciences in North-Rhine Westphalia and the Rhineland-Palatinate.
- ZEvA (Central Evaluation and Accreditation Agency): members originally were mainly the universities and universities of applied sciences in Lower Saxony; it is now open for membership from other *Länder* and from abroad.

The single-discipline agencies are:

- AHPGS (Agency for Study Courses in Medical Pedagogy, Care, Health and Social Work): members are mainly the conferences of faculties and deans, and professional associations in the respective fields.
- ASIIN (Agency for Study Courses in Engineering/Informatics and Chemistry, Biochemistry, Chemical Engineering): in 2002 ASII (Accreditation Agency for Study Programs in Engineering and Informatics) merged with A-CBC, the accreditation agency for chemistry, biochemistry, chemical engineering, to form ASIIN.
- FIBAA (Foundation for International Business Administration Accreditation): founded by the leading organisations of industry and commerce in Austria, Germany and Switzerland.

Other Actors

A crucial role in the accreditation procedure is played by the peers who should represent higher education institutions, professional practice and the student body. In view of the *KMK* resolution of 2002, the equivalence of corresponding study and examination achievements and academic degrees can be sufficiently ensured by subjecting the content of degree courses to peer review. Hence, it is assumed that the peers have reached disciplinary consensus regarding the essential standards and requirements for a degree course. However, when developing and assessing new, innovative degree courses, peers often have to make far-reaching and crucial decisions. The fact that they wish to see their respective disciplinary societies actively involved in the accreditation processes is only natural. The range of these societies extends from faculty and dean conferences via disciplinary work groups to the asso-

ciations and umbrella organisations – above all in the field of science and engineering – where science and research and business and industry work together in specialist fields (cf. Wissenschaftsrat, 1992).

There is no professional accreditation of graduates, but there is an accreditation
network – which co-operates with agencies – in which the chamber of architects in
its capacity as the association of the profession has been involved in the development of standards of accreditation, for example.

The Procedure for Degree Courses

The accreditation procedure aims to ensure equivalence, facilitate diversity, guarantee quality and create transparency. Allowing higher education institutions as much
freedom as possible in structuring their courses, without, however, jeopardising the
comparability of future study opportunities, resulted in the *Akkreditierungsrat* formulating relatively general criteria that should be applied to the accreditation of
degree courses. In contrast to the somewhat rigid standards and specifications contained in the framework examination regulations, the criteria now provide a flexible
content examination framework for the review of degree courses and thus clearly
demonstrate the quality dimension of accreditation.

The *Akkreditierungsrat* developed specifications on the accreditation application
process for degree courses which mainly cover:

- reasons for the degree course, such as mission statement, goals and aims;
- the planned degree course structure and requirements in terms of content and
  specialisation, such as organisation, structure and content of the programme,
  professional qualification of graduates, assessment of foreseeable developments
  in potential career fields;
- human, financial and infra-structural resources;
- quality assurance measures, such as data on completion rates, student satisfaction, etc. and
- study-related co-operation, especially concerning international programmes (cf.
  Akkreditierungsrat, 2002, p. 11).

In the course of processing the application for degree course(s) to be reviewed, a
review report is produced by the team of reviewers appointed on a case-by-case
basis by the agency. This report takes account of the institutional profile submitted
by the applicant, and includes an on-site inspection by the team of reviewers. It is
presented for a decision to the agency's Accreditation Commission, which must be
made up of representatives from higher education institutions, professional practice
and students. The Accreditation Commission comments on the review team's report
and decides to accredit, conditionally accredit or not to accredit the degree course(s)

in question. Accreditation can be awarded for a maximum of seven years. After that, a re-accreditation procedure must follow.

A summary of the results of the accreditation procedure is published on the website of the *Akkreditierungsrat* (www.akkreditierungsrat.de), as from 2003 also in English.

Implementation Problems and Shortcomings

The gradual concession of autonomy will only lead fully to the aspired quality increases if the education institutions receive support to achieve it. Accreditation can be used to avert the danger of education institutions developing in different directions in terms of quality. State supervision should concentrate less on cases of isolated crisis management and should be geared more towards system control and results responsibility (Arbeitsstab Forum Bildung, 2001). The accreditation process which is being developed in connection with the introduction of the new academic degrees redefines the accountability and responsibility of higher education and the state. State approval[3] now relates, in particular, to guaranteeing the availability of basic resources, the incorporation of degree courses into the higher education planning processes of the respective *Land* and the keeping of structural targets and standards.

There is no law on accreditation but recommendations and regulations by *KMK* and *HRK* serve as a basis for the accreditation system. The legal quality and stability of these foundations is made clear by the fact that they are based neither on an administrative agreement nor on any state treaty. While several agencies are registered associations, a status which provides them with a legal entity and makes them capable of acting, the status of the *Akkreditierungsrat* remains legally undefined. In contrast to the situation in other European countries, where accreditation was introduced and its key factors defined by act of law, the equivalent in the Federal Republic of Germany lacks a foundation which, for example, would allow the *Akkreditierungsrat* to impose sanctions when an agency has failed to observe the directives or standards set by it (see Erichsen, 2003, p. 102). Moreover, there is no appeals or objections procedure, although there is monitoring of the agencies' work by the *Akkreditierungsrat*.

The accreditation system plans to have a competitive relationship between the individual accreditation agencies. This means that one of the *Akkreditierungsrat's* responsibilities is to ensure fair conditions for competition between agencies. How-

---

3   Some *Länder* already dispensed with the approval procedure and now use service and performance
     agreements (*Leistungsvereinbarungen*) to steer the higher education institutions, including the range
     of studies and degree courses which they offer.

ever, the agencies carry out their accreditation work on the basis of process and quality criteria set by the *Akkreditierungsrat*, and so the quality seal awarded at the end of a successful accreditation is always the same. Hence, since the agencies all offer the same 'product' in the course of a comparable procedure, competition seems, at first glance, to be restricted solely to pricing and services. Recently, a kind of 'co-operation competition' between the agencies emerged which involves appropriate co-operation agreements with individual societies or networks in which recognition of the quality seal – for example by international professional associations – is linked to the name of the agency. Specifically, this could mean, for example, that a university is forced to use a specific agency if the graduates of a degree course to be accredited are to be accepted in the international job market. Since such a monopoly position would concern the whole structure of the accreditation system, the *Akkreditierungsrat* will also have to prove that it is a competition guardian.

From the outset, using accreditation to guarantee minimum standards triggered a controversial debate. On the one hand, critics saw a danger of 'downward' levelling. On the other hand, it was taken for granted that there was generally no need to worry about minimum standards, since, as a rule, these were ensured. The background to the concept of a definition of minimum standards that have to be met by individual programmes is the idea that institutions can develop profiles which extend beyond these minimum standards and can be steered and controlled by the principle of customers' power of demand. In order to allow this principle to unfold, it is necessary to make sure first that the potential customers have that power of demand. This calls for transparency, i.e., customers must be able to obtain information about the quality of the programmes, products and services on offer and compare these. A first step towards such transparency is the establishment of minimum qualities through accreditation.

Of the 1,500 or so bachelor's and master's degree courses currently on offer, more than 250 were accredited by April 2003. The great discrepancy that still exists between approved and accredited degree courses, and which critics like to cite as proof of the inadequacy of the accreditation system, comes primarily from the simultaneous introduction of the new graduation system and the accreditation scheme. There is, however, a discussion about the further development of the procedures of accreditation (e.g. leaner procedures for re-accreditation, combined procedure for related study programmes, etc.) to master the large and ever growing numbers of accreditation procedures.

8.2.2   Accreditation Scheme for Private Higher Education Institutions

Because most of the German higher education institutions are recognised and funded fully or partly by the state, institutional accreditation has not been discussed widely. However, with increasing globalisation and internationalisation and the growing autonomy of the higher education institutions, more and more private (corporate) higher education institutions have been established as foundations. While the minimum requirements for state approval of private higher education institutions are laid down in the *HRG*, the *Länder* use different models to recognise private institutions.[4]

The number of education providers in the field of higher education has increased recently. Recent private initiatives are to found universities that offer study programmes in various co-operative and organisational formats (e.g. domestic universities running programmes in co-operation with foreign educational institutions, foreign universities running their programmes in Germany). For example, such institutions are independent higher education institutions or institutions affiliated to existing state-maintained universities.

The *HRG* defines the requirements needed for state recognition. Recommendations adopted by the *Wissenschaftsrat* on the accreditation of private universities follow the approach taken by degree course accreditation and the system used to accept state-maintained universities for entry into the list of universities qualifying for the *HBFG*[5] university infrastructure-building system (Law on the Joint Task of 'Extending and building new universities') and relate to the establishment and organisation of an institutional accreditation procedure in order to make sure cross-*Länder* minimum quality standards apply to private universities. Any introduction of such a system needs the agreement of the *Land* in which the university is located (cf. Wissenschaftsrat, 2000, p. 4).

The following fundamental principles, procedures and institutional guidelines apply to the accreditation of private universities. An accreditation aims to check and determine that the defined minimum quality standards have been met. These minimum standards are based on those requirements contained in the *HRG* or in the respective *Land*'s higher education act and must take into consideration the particular profile of the university in question. The following general requirements need to be met:

- The university must have the status of a legal entity in Germany.
- It must present policy concepts on its structure and operations that must correspond to the quality level of a state university.
- The university must have its own controlling and quality assurance system to target performance areas that allow for continuous monitoring and improvement of internal processes and achievement of defined objectives.

---

4   There is a special case of accreditation of study programmes by accreditation agencies where the *Land* ministry takes this as precondition for the application of the private institution for full or partial university status. These are the same procedures as described above.

5   *HBFG = Hochschulbauförderungsgesetz* (University Construction Funding Act)

- Based on feasibility studies, the university must have adequate qualitative and quantitative resources at its disposal to put its concept into practice, in particular, sufficient human resources, material equipment and infrastructure.

The review of the universities' performance areas is based on the principle of the coherence of the set objectives and their achievability, of the envisaged processes and of the resources provided to this end.

8.2.3   Evaluation Schemes

Based on recommendations of the *HRK* and *Wissenschaftsrat,* evaluation procedures for teaching[6] were introduced in the mid-1990s to increase transparency, strengthen institutional responsibility, support higher education institutions in the introduction of systematic quality-promoting measures and promote the profile, image and competitiveness of German higher education institutions (see HRK Project Q, 2000; Wolf, 2002, for details). The evaluation procedures are expected to highlight the particular strengths and weaknesses of the evaluated institution and thus lead to more systematic strategies of quality assurance and quality improvement. Evaluation as a general task of higher education institutions has meanwhile been introduced by higher education laws in all the *Länder*.

The main elements of the evaluation procedures – a cycle of five to eight years is recommended – are internal self-evaluation, external peer review, and follow up.

Content and focus on self-evaluation are primarily in the following fields:

- structure and organisation of the respective department,
- teaching and learning objectives,
- programmes of study,
- academic staff and resources,
- students and course of study,
- teaching and learning,
- opinions of staff and students on teaching and learning,
- situation in the job market and graduate employment.

There is no national institution to co-ordinate evaluation activities. But there are initiatives at *Länder* (agencies), regional and cross-regional level (networks) between higher education institutions. Some other institutions carry out evaluations at

---

6   In some *Länder*, especially in Lower Saxony, there is also evaluation of research which is separate from the evaluation of teaching but with an attempt to link the two procedures. This is done by other institutions, cf. www.wk.niedersachsen.de.

the request of single universities or faculties. Their procedures differ to some extent from the recommendations made by the *HRK* and *Wissenschaftsrat* (cf. HRK Project Q, 2000). Agencies at *Länder* level are for example:[7]

- Central Evaluation and Accreditation Agency (ZEvA) in Lower Saxony,[8]
- Evaluation Office of the Universities in North Rhine-Westphalia,
- Evaluation Office of the Universities of Applied Sciences in North Rhine-Westphalia.

The networks are, for example:

- Association of Northern German Universities (*Nordverbund*),
- Evaluation Network of the Universities of Darmstadt, Kaiserslautern and Karlsruhe, with the ETH Zurich acting as an external moderator,
- Evaluation Network of the Universities of Halle, Jena, Leipzig.

The regional agencies are responsible for the preparation and administration of the entire evaluation procedure, including keeping of the time schedules and checking completeness of data provided by the departments under review, organisation of site visits, publication of final reports, etc. At first, the higher education institution must carry out a self-evaluation and write a corresponding self-report. The agency then distributes this report to the peer group members. The site visit by the peers that follows includes interviews with different status groups in the institution. The report written by the peers with support from the agency includes a critical review of the internal evaluation, a definition of problems and an outline of possible solutions. It is becoming increasingly common to find, after the final report, agreements between departments and the head of the institution about measures to be taken to improve teaching and learning, optimise the outcome or make sure that certain standards are met within a fixed period, as well as performance agreements (*Leistungsverein-barungen*) between the institution and the funding ministry.

Since 1998, the *HRK* has run a national programme – the Quality Assurance Project – to enhance the exchange of information and experience in the field of quality improvement measures in German higher education institutions across the Federal States. The key tasks for 'Project Q' are to ensure and develop common standards of evaluation at the national level, collect data on quality assurance, advise higher education institutions, disseminate best practice in the institutions and inform the public.

---

7   Information on all evaluation agencies and networks can be found at www.evanet.his.de.

8   ZEvA is an agency with two departments, the accreditation and the evaluation departments.

8.2.4 Other Assessment Activities

Besides the activities mentioned above, several departments in many higher education institutions have launched evaluation initiatives using different approaches and perspectives. Besides the cyclical evaluations of the disciplines, there are thematic evaluations. For example, the Association of Northern German Universities (*Nordverbund*) has carried out an evaluation on internationalisation (Fischer-Bluhm & Zemene, n.d.).

As another quality assurance procedure, a very limited number of institutions are employing benchmarking, the ISO-9000 certification or TQM/EFQM (cf. HRK Project Q, 2003). Moreover, a ranking procedure has been developed and is regularly carried out by the Centre for Higher Education Development (Centrum für Hochschulentwicklung (CHE), 2002) and special questionnaires on student satisfaction are used (cf. Evanet). So far, there has been no link between these activities and accreditation.

8.3 Relationships Between the Evaluation and Accreditation Schemes

8.3.1 Driving Forces for Decision-Making by Owners, Initiators and Controllers of the Schemes

Evaluation primarily serves as an analysis of strengths and weaknesses of an institution, department or faculty. Accreditation aims to contribute to improving and ensuring the quality of teaching and research by basing the review process on previously and externally defined standards and gives a study programme the right to exist. Because of these differing aims, the procedures are not closely linked since there are different owners of the procedures.

Experience has shown, however, that there is a whole range of overlapping areas. In the longer term, accreditation will need previous evaluation. This applies, in particular, to the future re-accreditations. Previous evaluation could additionally serve to reduce the accreditation load problem. Moreover, it will not be possible, from an economic perspective, to separate evaluation and accreditation in the long run, because the time and cost factors would be too high for institutions. The common features of the two processes, as well as a lower 'burden' for reviewers and higher education institutions justify tighter dovetailing of the processes. If the strict division of evaluation and accreditation were to be maintained, there would additionally be a danger that the quality assurance system could disintegrate into two parts: one for comparability and the other for quality improvement.

8.3.2 Political Framework

The most significant reforms observed in higher education in the last two decades (see Eurydice 2000) have been the greater autonomy given to higher education institutions in most European countries and the move away from the 'interventionary state' towards a more 'facilitatory state' (Neave & Van Vught, 1991). This often entailed releasing higher education institutions from control through legislation by giving them the right to establish their own statutes in the broadening area in which they are autonomous. The main focus was on reforms in institutional management, in financing institutions and the procedures for assessment and quality control of the educational provision. This has been strengthened with the introduction of accreditation procedures (cf. the reports in Bretschneider & Köhler, 2001).

As a response to the fundamentally different needs and conditions of a higher education system which had undergone transformations because of a long term expansion process and challenges of international competition as well as in the role of the higher education sector, quality assurance measures are of great importance. The expectation is that bachelor's/master's degree courses will be able to meet some new demands more flexibly (see the reports in Gützkow & Köhler, 1998). Accreditation is expected to play a role in solving quality problems and problems of international recognition of German degrees, while at the same time increasing student mobility and demand on the part of international students for study places in Germany.

8.3.3 Consequences for Institutions, Students and Other Stakeholders

As already stated, the discussion on accreditation is closely linked to that on bachelor's/master's degree courses. The introduction of these new degree courses – as research results show – is not without difficulties and obstacles for the institutions (see Schwarz, 2001). The development of new programmes based on the new scheme (modularisation, ECTS, etc.) has resulted in long discussions in the departments and has created additional work for the faculties and institutions. All the more so since the former system of Diplom/Magister degrees still exists.

The institutional differentiation between universities and universities of applied sciences has entered a new phase. Both are allowed to offer bachelor's and master's degree courses and the question of the blurring of the distinction between the two types is on the agenda. The introduction of the accreditation system is meant to solve problems raised in this debate. For example, there is a distinction between more research-oriented and more professionally-oriented degree programmes. In its accreditation application, the institution makes a claim to fit one or the other profile, and the accreditation procedure then has to lead to a final decision on whether the programme can be considered research-oriented or profession-oriented.

In the state-financed system, there are no tuition fees for students as yet.[9] There is, however, a discussion that tuition fees could be introduced for master's programmes: this is already the case for master's programmes which are not designed as consecutive programmes. Financial support for students for the whole bachelor's/master's programme is being discussed. Moreover, it is increasingly expected that the bachelor's should be the regular first professional degree.

The Federal Government and the Länder pointed out that the introduction of the new graduation system must be accompanied by measures that encourage the acceptance of these degrees by industry and society and open up new opportunities in the labour market for graduates (cf. KMK, HRK & BMBF, 2002). But as experience shows, labour market acceptance of different degrees is still not clear. This makes it difficult for students to decide whether to enrol in the new programmes. The expectation of more transparency has been met, however, since the *Akkreditierungsrat's* information on accredited programmes is increasingly used by 'customers' to make informed choices.

8.3.4   Projections for the Future

A strong network and close negotiations between all stakeholders and actors in the field of quality assurance are essential. And it makes sense to improve quality assessment activities in faculties and institutions and to encourage discussion on quality (see Berner & Richter, 2002). As Teichler (2003) pointed out, the multiple quality assessment in German higher education institutions shows that there is a danger that a new system of assessment could be developed for each occasion. This would lead to a 'super complex system of quality assessment'. Because of the challenge of continuing financial constraints and the overkill with procedures, an integrated system of quality assurance in higher education seems to be inevitable.

The strong participation of representatives of higher education institutions in the *Akkreditierungsrat* and the agencies is proof that accreditation stands for a system of quality standard development and assurance with science and education substantially sharing responsibility in this field, and participation by trade unions, etc. However, one must be wary of more state control and bureaucratisation (see Erichsen, 2002, p. 13).

---

9   Some *Länder*, e.g. North-Rhine Westphalia, are developing study accounts as an alternative to fees, cf. www.bildungsportal.nrw.de.

8.4   European and International Influences

The objectives of the Bologna Declaration correspond to the goals which the Federal Government and the *Länder* developed to modernise higher education in Germany and enhance the country's international attractiveness (cf. KMK, HRK & BMBF, 2002). With the Bologna Declaration another change was supported: institutional autonomy over the process (especially teaching and curriculum) of higher education was strengthened. There is a multilateral agreement that higher education institutions must play an important role in creating and structuring the European Higher Education Area through continuous efforts to remove barriers and develop a framework for teaching and learning which would enhance mobility and closer cooperation.

This trend towards greater institutional autonomy was accompanied by the establishment of new systems of quality assurance, not least in order to make institutions responsible and more accountable for the use of public funds. Evaluation schemes have been developed and used in nearly all Member States of the European Union over the last few years. At present, additional accreditation procedures are being discussed in many countries as a possible way of making quality assurance systems more effective (see Van Damme, 2001). This efficiency has yet to be proven.

Most of the German agencies, be they evaluation or accreditation agencies, as well as the 'Quality Project', are members of ENQA and other international networks, such as INQAAHE. These international perspectives influence national accreditation. With the advent of GATS, which bans any discrimination of foreign suppliers of services (see Yalçin & Scherrer, 2002), and the growing interest of higher education institutions in international accreditation, quality foreign assurance agencies may bring their services into the German market. This is already true of agencies from the USA.

Through the paradigm shift to neo-liberalism, which underlies GATS, the main philosophy of administration regulation and management moved away from direct control to indirect (market) control, deregulation and participation, but by no means does this shift mean the end of control and regulation as such. First, as we have experienced in Germany, a shift is not a complete replacement of one system by another. Second, there is also much resistance, and even in the organisations concerned with steering that process, various interpretations and changes are experienced over time (cf. von Kopp, 2002). Concerning accreditation, the *Akkreditierungsrat* will open up the system for agencies from other European countries, but as a controlling actor which opens the market for foreign applicants by forcing them to undergo the same procedure as the German agencies.

References

Akkreditierungsrat (2002). *Work Report 2000/2001*, Bonn: Akkreditierungsrat.

Arbeitsstab Forum Bildung (ed.) (2001). *Empfehlungen des Forum Bildung*. Bonn: Arbeitsstab Forum Bildung.

Berner, H. & R. Richter (2001). Accreditation of Degree Programmes in Germany. *Quality in Higher Education, 7(3)*, pp. 247-257.

Bretschneider, F. & G. Köhler (eds.) (2001). Autonomie oder Anpassung. *Frankfurt am Main, Paris.*

Bundesministerium für Bildung und Forschung (2002). *Zahlenbarometer 2001/2002.* Bonn: Bundesministerium für Bildung und Forschung.

CHE (2002). Das Hochschulranking, Arbeitspapier Nr. 36, Gütersloh: CHE.

Erichsen, H.-U. (2002). 3 Jahre Qualitätssicherung durch Akkreditierung – zur Emanzipation der Hochschulen im Bereich der Qualitätsverantwortung, *Gewerkschaftliche Bildungspolitik* (9/10 – 2002).

Erichsen, H.-U. (2003). Drei Jahre Qualitätssicherung durch Akkreditierung. Eine Zwischenbilanz, *die hochschule (1)*.

Eurydice (1999). *Europäisches Glossar zum Bildungswesen. Prüfungen, Abschlüsse und Titel, Vol. 1*, Brussels.

Eurydice (2000). *Two Decades of Reform in Higher Education in Europe: 1980 Onwards*, Brussels.

Eurydice: Eurybase (www.eurydice.org).

Evanet (www.evanet.his.de).

Fischer-Bluhm, K. & S. Zemene (n.d.). *Verbund Norddeutscher Universitäten: Von Programm-evaluationen zu thematischen Evaluationen – Erfahrungen des Verbunds Norddeutscher Universitäten aus der Evaluation der Internationalisierungsstrategien*, (www.evanet.his.de).

Gützkow, F. & G. Köhler (eds.) (1998). Als Bachelor fitter für den Arbeitsmarkt?, *GEW Materialien und Dokumente Hochschule und Forschung 92*, Frankfurt: GEW.

Higher Education Compass (www.higher-education-compass.de).

HIS-Ergebnisspiegel 2002 (www.his.de).

HRK Project Q (2000). *Quality Assessment and Quality Development in German Universities with Particular Reference to the Assessment of Teaching*, 1. Bonn: HRK.

HRK Project Q: *Wegweiser 2003* (in print).

Kehm, B.M. (1999). *Higher Education in Germany: Developments, Problems and Perspectives.* Wittenberg, Bucharest.

KMK, HRK & BMBF (2002). National Report Germany: Realizing the goals of the Bologna Declaration in Germany. Present situation and follow-up until the conference in Berlin 2003, (www.bologna-berlin2003.de).

Kopp, B. von (2003). GATS and National Education Systems – Changing Paradigms of Administration and Management, in: H. Döbert et al. (eds.), *Bildung vor neuen Herausforderungen*, Neuwied: Leuchterhand.

List, J. (2000). *Bachelor und Master – Sackgasse oder Königsweg?*, Cologne: Institut der deutschen Wirtschaft.

Neave, G. & F. van Vught (eds.) (1991). *Prometheus Bound. The Changing Relationship between Government and Higher Education in Western Europe*, Oxford: Pergamon Press.

Schwarz, S. (2001). 'The Point of Departure', in: Bretschneider, F. & G. Köhler (eds.). *Autonomie oder Anpassung*, Frankfurt am Main, Paris.

Teichler, U. (2003). Die Entstehung eines superkomplexen Systems der Qualitätsbewertung in Deutschland, in: E. Mayer, H.-D. Daniel & U. Teichler (eds.): *Die neue Verantwortung der Hochschulen*, Bonn: Lemmens.

Van Damme, Dirk (2001). *Policy Making in Europe: Convergence and Conflict*. Vienna.

Verbund Norddeutscher Universitäten (www.uni-nordverbund.de).

Wissenschaftsrat (1992). *Zur Förderung von Wissenschaft und Forschung durch wissenschaftliche Fachgesellschaften*, Bremen.

Wissenschaftsrat (2000). *Empfehlungen zur Akkreditierung privater Hochschulen*, Cologne: Wissenschaftsrat.

Wissenschaftsrat (2002). *Empfehlungen zur Reform der staatlichen Abschlüsse*, Cologne: Wissenschaftsrat.

Wolf, C. (2002). Evaluation von Studium und Lehre in Deutschland – eine Synopse, in: T. Studer (ed.): *Erfolgreiche Leitung von Forschungsinstituten, Hochschulen und Stiftungen*, Hamburg.

Yalçin, G. & C. Scherrer (2002). GATS-Verhandlungsrunde im Bildungsbereich. Report for the Max-Traeger-Stiftung. Kassel: University of Kassel.

9 The National System of Higher Education in Greece: Waiting for a Systematic Quality Assurance System

HARILAOS BILLIRIS

9.1 Preliminary Remark

Evaluation and accreditation procedures have not yet been formally established in Greece. Therefore, the presentation of the Greek case cannot fully follow the general guidelines of the other national chapters.

9.2 Higher Education in Greece

9.2.1 Higher Education Institutions

The higher education sector in Greece consists of 19 universities (including the School of Fine Arts) and the Hellenic Open University and 14 Technological Educational Institutions (TEIs) which belong to the technological (non-university) sector. They are all public.

There are 240 university departments and 170 departments at the technological educational institutions, a number that has increased by 43 % over the last ten years. For the academic year 2003/04, 21 new departments are going to open their doors to new students. Six are university departments. In Greece, each department corresponds to a specific subject or discipline leading to a degree. Approving a new department means approving a new degree. The Ministry of Education is responsible for the approval of new institutions and new departments. However, the development of the corresponding study programme is the responsibility of the institution.

9.2.2 Duration of Studies; General Degrees

There are three levels of study in Greek universities. The first is the undergraduate level, which leads to the basic degree, called 'diploma' or *ptychio*. The length of studies at this level varies from four to six years. Studies in medicine last for six years, whereas in engineering, agricultural studies, dentistry and pharmacy, fine arts and music they last for five years. In all other fields, they last for four years.

Postgraduate studies are divided into two levels. The lower level is of one year's duration in most cases and leads to the equivalent of a master's degree. This first

S. Schwarz and D.F. Westerheijden (eds.),
Accreditation and Evaluation in the European Higher Education Area, 197–205.
© 2004 *Kluwer Academic Publishers. Printed in the Netherlands.*

degree is called *metaptychiako diploma idikefsis*, the 'postgraduate specialisation diploma'. In 1993, there were 53 postgraduate programmes in universities, 111 in 1995 and 212 in 2000. The higher level is the doctorate level and it lasts for at least three years.

Studies in the technological educational institutions last for three and a half to four years. Graduates have access to postgraduate studies, which are offered exclusively by the universities.

9.2.3   Size of the Higher Education System

In the academic year 1999/2000, there were 276,902 enrolled undergraduate students (of which 141,942 were women) at the universities and 129,683 (of which 65,623 were women) at the technological educational institutions. In the same year, 40,641 (24,195 women) were new undergraduates students at the universities and 34,355 (17,953 women) were new entrants at the technological educational institutions. In the academic year 2000/01, there were 45,224 (28,085 women) new undergraduate students at universities and 34,574 new students at the technological educational institutions.

In the academic year 1999/2000, 128,976 were active university students. 38 % were under the age of 20. At the technological educational institutions, there were 79,102 active students and 47 % were under 20.

In the academic year 1999/2000, there were 8,170 postgraduate students (4,375 women) and 8,335 students on a doctorate course (3,392 women).

9.2.4   Lifelong Education

Lifelong education is considered a priority for the educational policy of Greece. In this context, the Hellenic Open University, which opened in 1999, is the main provider.

Table 1. Student numbers in the Hellenic Open University

	2000/01	2001/02	2002/03	2003/04
Undergraduate students	2,556 (women 53 %)	3,340	2,355	3,397
Postgraduate students	1,981 (women 57 %)	2,160	1,970	2,115

Students are charged annual tuition fees (€ 600 per thematic unit). The thematic unit covers a distinct subject in undergraduate or postgraduate studies. Every thematic unit includes three semester subjects. During one academic year, students can attend one to three thematic units in graduate programmes of study and up to two thematic units in the postgraduate programmes. Some students are granted partial or total scholarships for economic, social and academic reasons.

9.2.5   Scholarship Options

Scholarships, grants and financial support through various local bequests and donations by citizens and private legal entities are awarded to students at all levels of education. The State Scholarship Foundation (IKY) is the official institution that grants student scholarships. IKY scholarships are awarded both to undergraduate students who have excelled in the university entrance exams, and to those who wish to do a postgraduate degree in Greece or abroad and have succeeded in the corresponding exams.

Table 2. Number of scholarships awarded by IKY

	1999/2000	2000/01	2001/02
Graduate scholarships	2,415	2,654	2,796
Postgraduate and doctoral scholarships	279	138	222

Every year, the Ministry of Education awards a scholarship to the first three students who succeed in the National Examination System in each department of the universities and of the technological educational institutions. There are also scholarships awarded to a number of students by the research committees of certain universities.

9.2.6   Transition from Higher Education to Work

The following three tables present the number of graduates in the different levels of higher education in Greece, as well as unemployment statistics.

Table 3. Output figures by type of institution

	Universities		Rate	Technological educational institutions		Rate
	Total			Total		
Academic year	Enrolled	Graduates (Women)	Enrolled / Grad.	Enrolled	Graduates	Enrolled / Grad.
1999/2000	40,641	22,774 (13,623)	1.8/1	34,355	9,211	3.7/1
2000/01	45,224	22,495 (13,414)	2.0/1	34,574	10,071	3.4/1

Table 4. Output figures by level (total number and number of women)

Academic year	Postgraduate		Doctoral	
	Enrolled	Grad.	Enrolled	Grad.
1999/2000	1,908 (913)	1,972 (1,061)	890 (345)	779 (228)
2000/01	2,687 (1,475)	2,859 (1,590)	2,546 (1,276)	875 (321)

Table 5. Unemployment of higher education graduates

	TEI graduates	University graduates	Grad. (Post. + Doct.)
1990	7.6 %		5.5 %
1995	10.1 %		5.6 %
2000	13.2 % (M: 7.9 %, W: 18.6 %)	7.5 % (M: 4.9 %, W: 10.6 %)	5.7 % (M: 4.1 %, W: 8.5 %)

Some professions require a professional licence. 75 % of graduates could register with professional organisations (for example chemists), while 31 % of graduates should have a professional licence from their own Professional Associations or Chambers (Lawyers Association, Medical Association, Technical Chamber of Greece). According to a questionnaire to which 70 % of the departments replied, 60 % of the graduates find work that is related to their studies.

9.2.7   Teaching Staff

The main teaching staff at universities in Greece in the last seven years grew from 7,258 in the academic year 19961997 to 9,776 in the academic year 2002/03. In the academic year 1999/00, 128,976 students were active at the universities. This gives a ratio of main teaching staff to students of about 1/16. In the academic year 2000/01, 148,772 were active students at the universities, bringing the ratio down to 1/17.

At the technological educational institutions, the main teaching staff numbers grew slightly over the last seven years, from 2,201 (1996/97) to 2,302 in 2002/03. With 79,102 active students in the academic year 1999/2000, the ratio of main teaching staff to students was 1/34. In the academic year 2000/01, when 86,659 students were active, it dropped to 1/38. We must mention here that there is an extra number of teaching staff who are contractual and part-time teachers.

9.2.8   Governance and Steering of Higher Education

Higher education in Greece is governed by article 16 of the 1975 Greek Constitution, which states that higher education is public and free of charge. The Greek Constitution also refers to state control over the universities and the technological educational institutions, which is the responsibility of the Ministry of Education.

Universities and technological educational institutions in Greece are all funded by the state. They must allocate the government funding by establishing their own budget. The budget of each institution has to be approved by the Ministry of Education and the Ministry of Finance.

The existing legislation allows institutions to set fees only for postgraduate studies. 4 % apply annual tuition fees of up to € 1,500 and another 4 % apply tuition fees that range between € 900 and € 1,500.

Each academic unit has its own leadership and decision-making structure. There is a hierarchical relationship between the levels of these structures (Institution – School – Department – Sector). The rector and the two vice-rectors are elected for a three-year mandate by an electoral body. Undergraduate students make up part of the electoral body of 80 % of the part of the main teaching personnel of the institution. The dean of the school is elected for a three-year mandate by an electoral body consisting of the electoral bodies for the election of the presidents of all the departments that constitute the school. The president of the department is elected for two years by an electoral body in which undergraduate students again have 80 % of the votes of the main teaching personnel of the department.

The senate of the university consists of the rector, the two vice-rectors, the deans of all schools and the presidents of all departments, six to eight representatives of the main teaching staff, one representative of the undergraduate students of each department, two representatives of the postgraduate students, and four representatives of all other categories of personnel.

9.3   Evaluation of Higher Education in Greece

9.3.1   An Historical Review

In Greece, assessment or evaluation could not be discussed by the university community until the early 1990s, since all initiatives in the past were taken by the Ministry of Education. The evaluation concept mainly consisted in greater state control through financial cuts and institutional rankings, and there was no preliminary dialogue between the state and the universities. This inflexible and inefficient policy of the Ministry of Education led to a general opposition of the universities to the idea of evaluation. Evaluation thus became another field for the traditional opposition between universities and state in Greece. This opposition goes much further than the typical tension between university autonomy and state control, as it has its roots in a lack of mutual trust. It was in this context that the first attempts of the Ministry of Education to legislate the establishment of an evaluation procedure for universities emerged in 1992 and 1995. The opposition of the universities to the legislation was so great that it was never implemented.

To make better understand the climate in Greece, we can note another interesting and relevant phenomenon, which is the negative stance of Greek universities regarding the review process of the educational system carried out by an expert team of the OECD between 1995 and 1996 at the request of the Ministry of Education. It must be noted that the university students' and teachers' syndicates at all educational levels (primary, secondary and higher education) also adopted this stance. Strangely, the mass media, which are supposed to express but also to form common opinion, supported it. Notwithstanding, the OECD review was completed in 1996, and it included a section on evaluation of the Greek higher education system.

9.3.2   The Present Situation

The Ministry of Education in Greece is working on the establishment of new evaluation and quality assurance structures. The most positive and promising aspect is the gradual change in climate throughout the higher education system due to the combination of two significant factors.

The first has to do with the sensitisation of some Greek universities, as well as of some technological educational institutions, to the whole concept of quality and evaluation, which resulted in a number of initiatives that were taken by the institutions themselves and were simply supported by the Ministry of Education.

The second has to do with the change in the policy applied by the Ministry of Education. In fact, we can speak of a transition from a top-down process (where the Ministry of Education centrally plans and controls the evaluation procedures) to a bottom-up process (where the institutions are taking initiatives). In this bottom-up process, the role of the Ministry of Education is encouraging and supportive.

This change in the climate and in the stance on the concept of quality and evaluation led to a number of significant initiatives. First, two faculties (one in each higher education sector) participated in the pilot project to evaluate quality in higher education in the European Union that was carried out between 1994 and 1995. Then, two institutions (one in each higher education sector) participated in the project of the IMHE (Institutional Management in Higher Education) Programme of OECD on quality management, quality assessment and the decision-making process, which began in 1994. Moreover, five Greek universities participated in the institutional quality evaluation programme of the CRE.

In the same context, the Ministry of Education set up a huge quality assessment pilot programme for higher education institutions (both of the university and the non-university sector) for the two-year period 1998/99. This programme was financed by the European Union through the Second European Support Framework. The programme included both institutional and faculty (departmental) or programme assessments. The number of institutions or individual faculties that participated on a voluntary basis was quite impressive. In the university sector, seven institutional assessments were organised, as well as 42 faculty (departmental) or programme assessments. In the non-university sector, the corresponding numbers were five for institutional assessments and 31 for faculty (departmental) or programme assessments.

The main objectives of this programme were to help to develop a quality culture throughout the higher education system in Greece. The general methodological characteristics of the programme included a self-evaluation procedure and review by external reviewers (including a site visit and preparation of an evaluation report). The publication and the wide dissemination of the results of each evaluation procedure are prerequisites for the participation of an institution or a faculty in the programme. The completion of the programme must be followed by the publication of a final report, under the responsibility of the Ministry of Education, that summarises the results of the exercises and analyses examples of good practice.

This vast exercise obviously had many weaknesses, especially as it was not supported by expertise. Among these we can note the lack of concrete and clear directives as regards the methodological aspects, as well as the lack of an effective centralised monitoring and steering mechanism. However, these weaknesses are considered of minor importance, given the objectives of the overall process.

The involvement of a large number of Greek higher education institutions in several international or national quality evaluation processes on a voluntary basis, has already established a positive climate, which is quite different from the negative one that existed only a few years ago. It is worth noting that after the completion of these programmes, eleven out of the 19 Greek universities participated at least once in a national or international institutional evaluation procedure and similarly 45 out of the 240 university departments participated at least once in a faculty or programme evaluation procedure. Similar numbers can be given for the non-university sector of higher education. The change in the overall climate is evident, and therefore the prospects for future developments must be considered quite promising.

9.3.3   The Immediate Future

On March 15, 2003, the Minister of Education notified the Rectors' Conference of the draft law for the National Council of Quality Assurance and Assessment

(NCQAA) of Higher Education. In his letter, the Minister underlines that the draft law emerged from:

- An analysis of all the European quality assurance systems and discussions with specialists in Europe, which were adjusted to our national characteristics, needs and goals.
- The experience gained by the evaluations of the Greek higher education institutions.
- The exchange of opinions and suggestions between the higher education institutions.

The NCQAA will be an independent advisory body which will help the institutions to reach their goals and advise the state and government on higher education. It will not engage in any kind of marking, grading, ranking or accrediting the higher education institutions or impose penalties and give awards.

The draft law proposes one National Council for both sectors of higher education as an independent authority, which will consist of eleven members (nine academics and two students from both sectors). The members of the Council will be appointed by the Council of Ministers on the proposal of the Minister of Education, from a list of candidates made up by the Rectors' Conference, followed by the opinion of a relevant Committee of the Greek Parliament and the students from their own national bodies.

The Council will have the following competences:

- It will design the four-year operational programme of quality assessment in higher education in Greece.
- It will provide every support to the higher education institutions from the perspective of knowledge and experience.
- It will be responsible for analysing and developing the results of the quality assessment.
- It will keep and update a database on the progress in the quality assessment system and the development in an international context.
- It will be responsible for assigning external evaluators.
- It will elaborate and organise research concerning the methodology of the quality assessment system.
- It will organise special courses for members of the institutions to acquire experience in quality assurance and assessment systems.
- It will co-operate with international organisations and research centres dealing with evaluation in higher education procedures.
- It will organise the statistics and documentation of the Greek higher education institutions.

The higher education institutions had until the end of May 2003 to express their reactions to the Minister of Education and the law was expected to be passed by the Greek Parliament at the end of June 2003.

10 Quality Assurance in Motion. Higher Education in Hungary after the Change of Regime and the First Cycle of Accreditation

CHRISTINA ROZSNYAI

10.1 Introduction

10.1.1 Higher Education Statistics

Before the 'regime change', i.e. the fall of Soviet-dominated socialism, in 1989/90, roughly 12 % of 18- to 22-year-old Hungarians were enrolled in college or university education. Currently some 35 % of the age cohort participate in some form of tertiary education,[1] though selection now includes not only college and university studies but also two-year vocational and other programmes (see section 10.1.3). The distribution of students among all forms of tertiary education is 34 % (117,947 persons) in university-level programmes, 56 % (195,291 persons) in college-level schemes, 7 % (24,558 persons) in specialised post-graduate programmes, 2 % (7,030 persons) in doctoral programmes, and 1 % (4,475 persons) in vocational higher education programmes (Central Bureau of Statistics, 2002, http://www.ksh.hu). The declared intent is to raise the overall ratio to 50 % by 2010.

Hungary has 18 state universities, twelve colleges, five church-maintained universities and 21 church-maintained colleges, and eleven private colleges. In addition there are eight state-recognised foreign higher education institutions, with a licence to operate granted by the minister of education (see Törvény a felsőoktatásról, 1993). Only one of them opened after 1996, when an amendment to the 1993 higher education act specified that foreign higher education institutions can only be established if their application has been evaluated by the Hungarian Accreditation Committee. These institutions do not receive state funding. Church institutions receive similar normative funding as state institutions and are accredited by the Hungarian Accreditation Committee, whose mandate, however, pertains only to secular programmes. Private institutions that wish to be recognised by the state must also be accredited and may receive state financing if they sign an agreement with the government, but here tuition covers a major part of their costs. Tuition at state and

---

1   Web site of the Hungarian Ministry of Education at http://www.om.hu, 'Hungarian Higher Education System: an Overview' and 'The Future University: A Great Choice in Education'.

S. Schwarz and D.F. Westerheijden (eds.),
Accreditation and Evaluation in the European Higher Education Area, 207–232.
© 2004 *Kluwer Academic Publishers. Printed in the Netherlands.*

church institutions has been introduced and revoked by consecutive governments, but was minimal when it existed. A viable and popular student loan system was introduced in 2001 (see A Kormány 119, 2001).

10.1.2   Types of Higher Education Institutions

Hungary has a binary higher education system. The higher education act differentiates between universities and colleges (Act Sections 3 and 4). Education at universities is research-oriented, which means that the approach to teaching is more theoretical and that the academic staff is more involved in theoretical research than at colleges. They, in turn, aim to provide more applied knowledge and skills. According to the law, the difference between the two categories of institutions is in the length of studies required for a first degree (minimum four years for universities, three for colleges); the minimum areas of knowledge or science and different programmes taught ('several' areas each with 'several' programmes, and one area with 'several' programmes respectively); and the level of the degrees of their academic staff (doctorates already for 'docents' at universities, only for professors at colleges). Additionally, universities must have the material and intellectual resources for conducting scientific research, for training for and granting doctorates and for conducting habilitation procedures. Colleges must provide the conditions for conducting research and development. Both types of institutions may be state, private and/or church establishments.

10.1.3   Main Types of Degrees

It follows from the binary system that Hungarian higher education offers college and university degrees. The law allows either type of institution to offer both types of study programmes, provided that their resources meet the requirements. There have been discussions and agreements relating to the transition from one type to the other. Very often institutions require an additional one year of study to make up for the lack of research-oriented or practical-oriented courses, as the case may be, for students switching from one type of establishment to another. As a credit system is not yet in place at the national level by the time this report has been written (the government has postponed the deadline for the introduction from 2002 to September 2003), there may be additional requirements for students changing institutions even within the same type.

The higher education act declares that for use abroad college degree holders may refer to their degrees as 'bachelor's' and university degree holders may refer to their degrees as 'master's' (Act Section 24 § 97.6.a and b). The legislators' intention was to define the level of the two degrees, without considering the two-tier character of 'real' bachelor's/master's studies. However, discussions are currently accelerating to work out a system of studies where one level builds on the other, as foreseen in the 'Bologna Declaration' for the 'European higher education area' in 2010. Only universities grant Ph.D. degrees.

In the 1996 amendment to the higher education act, Hungary instituted two-year vocational higher education programmes, one third of which may count towards college or university studies. These may be offered at higher education institutions or other establishments. Also stipulated in the act are 'complementary undergraduate' programmes, which are either university programmes for college graduates or teacher training programmes for graduates with a first degree (Act Section 124/E.f). 'Specialised post-graduate education' stipulated in the act (Section 124/E.k) does not lead to an additional degree, rather it provides in-depth training in an area, which leads to a certificate.

Figure 1. Types and levels of higher education provision in Hungary

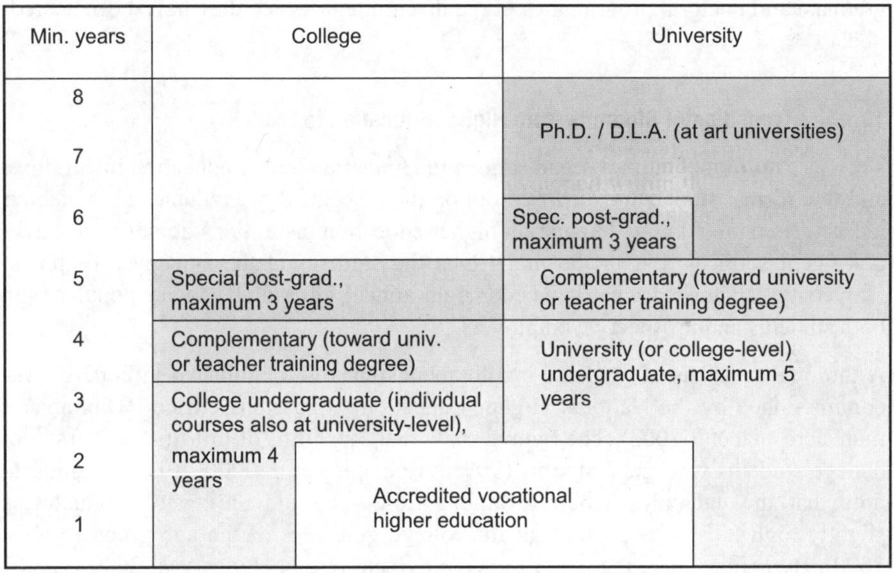

Min. years	College		University
8			Ph.D. / D.L.A. (at art universities)
7			
6			Spec. post-grad., maximum 3 years
5	Special post-grad., maximum 3 years		Complementary (toward university or teacher training degree)
4	Complementary (toward univ. or teacher training degree)		University (or college-level) undergraduate, maximum 5 years
3	College undergraduate (individual courses also at university-level),		
2	maximum 4 years	Accredited vocational higher education	
1			

10.1.4   Main Types of Programmes

The previous section dealt with programme types from the perspective of the degrees they lead to. With regard to the levels of education the higher education act specifically lists them as being accredited vocational higher education; college undergraduate education and college postgraduate education; university undergraduate education; university postgraduate education; and doctoral education (Act Section 84 § 1 and 2). Undergraduate, specialised postgraduate and vocational higher education programmes may be offered in full-time, correspondence, evening or distance education programmes.

As far as subject areas are concerned, a Government Decree (A Kormány 169, 2000) lists 56 disciplines within eight areas of knowledge to which study programmes must be assigned. As of February 2003, the Hungarian Accreditation Committee (HAC) registered over 430 different accredited first-degree programmes, which make up 1,640 programmes taught in the 67 accredited institutions.

Another set of government decrees concerns the national qualification requirements for all degree programmes. They describe the required content and outcomes of all undergraduate and postgraduate (but not Ph.D.) programmes offered in the country. Higher education institutions are free to set up vocational higher education programmes, undergraduate programmes and their specialisations, specialised postgraduate and doctoral programmes in the discipline in which they have been accredited.

10.1.5   Transition of Students from Higher Education to Work

There are no formal alumni organisations in Hungarian higher education institutions, and few formal studies were carried out on the placement of graduates in the labour market. As far as I know, Hungarian higher education institutions do not have career placement services, but in the mid-1990s the students at the Budapest Technical University established what has become an annual job fair. It is very popular with both students and prospective employers.

A thorough analysis of graduate employment trends was published in 2002. It was commissioned by the National Higher Education Admissions Office ('Diplomák a munkaerő-piacon', 2002). The figures show that four fifths of full-time university or college students who graduated in 1999 were employed in 2000. It is interesting to note that the unemployment rate among 20-24-year-old university graduates is slightly higher (7 % in 2000) than for college graduates of the age group (5 % in 2000). By coincidence, the overall unemployment rate in Hungary in 2000 was the same as that of university graduates (7 %). That general unemployment ratio is down from almost 13 % in 1993, when the unemployment rate for university and college graduates was 3.4 % and 3.2 % respectively, but, as noted, with a higher education attendance rate within the age cohort of roughly one third of present figures.

10.1.6   Governance and Steering of Higher Education

The higher education act describes the positions and levels of institutional govern-ance. Section 12 outlines the structure of institutions, which may be divided into faculties, departments, institutes, etc. Higher education institutions are established by parliament and are listed in the higher education act. Faculties are established by government and legislated by government decrees. All other units are established by the institution. That means that higher education institutions have the autonomy to establish their own divisions only below the faculty level. To establish a new higher education institution or faculty, an institution has to submit an application to the minister of education, who, in turn, has to ask the Hungarian Accreditation Commit-tee to evaluate the application. The application is also analysed by the Higher Education and Research Council, an advisory body to the minister (see below, sec-tion 10.2.3), which checks the feasibility of the new institution or faculty within the whole higher education context.

Section 13 of the act deals with the operation and management of higher education institutions, which are based on their by-laws passed by their senate. Universities are headed by rectors, multi-faculty colleges by college rectors, single-faculty colleges by directors elected by the senate and university rectors are confirmed by the presi-dent of the republic, while college rectors or directors are confirmed by the prime minister. Section 14 deals with the operation of faculties and units of instruction.

10.2   Accreditation and Approval Schemes

10.2.1   Accreditation

According to Hungary's first higher education act of 1993, all higher education institutions must be accredited to be state-recognised. The act requires all Hungarian higher education institutions and their programmes to be accredited every eight years. In addition to institutional accreditation, the HAC also conducts separate programme accreditation under a variety of schemes required by law.

Accreditation is carried out *ex post*, via institutional accreditation, which involves all the degree programmes of the institution, and *ex ante*, via preliminary accreditation for institutions applying for licence to operate; via the approval of degree pro-grammes to be launched for the first time in the country (in the form of qualification requirements); and via the approval of new degree programmes at an institution (which have to meet the standards set down in the qualification requirements).

Institutional Accreditation

The first cycle of institutional accreditation was completed in 2001, while the second round began in autumn 2003.

Institutions and Their Units Involved in the Scheme. The law calls for all higher education institutions in Hungary and their study programmes to be accredited every eight years. Under this mandate the HAC worked out its specific standards and procedures. The premise was that the products of higher education institutions are the diplomas or degrees they issue and that therefore all elements contributing to that degree should be evaluated to arrive at a quality assessment.[2] 'All elements' was defined primarily by input factors. With this approach the three 'units' asked to prepare separate self-evaluation reports encompassed (1) the institution as a whole, (2) the faculty and (3) the study programme leading to the degree. The department, and any other unit contributing to a study programme (e.g. institutes, laboratories, clinics, practice farms, etc.), were assessed and included in the team visits from the perspective of how they contributed to the degree as the ultimate output. At the institutional level, the institution's mission statement and strategic plan, management and governance, regional role, approach to research, and basic statistics regarding infrastructure were inspected, but none was of primary importance. The same items were evaluated at the faculty level.

For study programmes one set of general questions involved everything from its broad aims, including curriculum development policies, to admission requirements, the make-up of the curriculum (including type of work involved, work-load, examination schedule). Another set studied in depth the courses and subjects (including the academic staff qualifications and subject content, teaching materials and related research). The HAC's *Accreditation Guidebook* (1995-1998) contained a detailed description of the accreditation procedure, the HAC's standards for evaluation, and an elaborate set of chapters and tables of facts and figures to be supplied in the institution's self-evaluation. Separate sections were added to accommodate the special considerations for evaluating church-run institutions and distance education programmes. A separate set of criteria exists for the preliminary accreditation for new institutions. Applications should supply some data on the foreseen purpose and role of the institution, the professional background of its contracted academic and non-academic staff, the institution's available infrastructure and its foreseen development, and detailed curricula for the degree programmes to be offered. Preliminary accreditation, as opposed to institutional accreditation of already existing establishments, usually did not involve site visits.

---

2   I use the term 'quality assessment' in the general sense, i.e. any approaches of checking quality without wanting to indicate one particular form of it in this particular context.

Before working out the next round of institutional accreditation the HAC elaborated a Strategic Plan.[3] It encompasses all aspects of the HAC's mission and purpose, an interpretation of its legal mandate and its tasks, as well as its operation. The Strategic Plan stakes out the basic premises within the legislative requirements under which institutional accreditation should proceed.

Programmes, Subjects and Disciplines Involved in the Scheme. In addition to degree programmes evaluated in the eight-yearly institutional accreditation process, the HAC accredits national qualification requirements and all new programmes launched at an institution.

As noted before, national qualification requirements, issued in the form of government decrees, set the framework for all degree programmes taught in Hungary. The requirements describe the requisite content and outcomes, including the main examinations, the knowledge and skills to be attained, and the credit points of all undergraduate degree programmes (divided into university and college sections), and specialised postgraduate study programmes offered in the country. New qualification requirements are initiated by institutions. An application for launching a degree programme in which there already are accredited national qualification requirements focuses on the local context in which the proposed programme will run, i.e. the teaching staff and infrastructure, as well as the curriculum. All undergraduate programmes must be accredited. These include full-time, evening, correspondence and distance education tracks, as well as off-site provision.

There is also a government decree that lists the disciplines under which degree programmes in Hungary are grouped. The list must also be approved by the HAC. Institutions which have accredited undergraduate programmes in a given discipline may launch postgraduate programmes (and doctoral schools for universities) in the discipline without further accreditation.

In parallel to launching the second round of institutional accreditation in fall 2003, the HAC began to conduct programme accreditation for selected disciplines in the whole country within a short time-span. History and psychology were selected for the initial review.

Geographic Range Involved in the Scheme. All institutions and their programmes in the country must be accredited. Additionally, off-site campuses of Hungarian higher education institutions in neighbouring countries must also be accredited by the HAC.

---

3   The Hungarian Accreditation Committee Strategic Plan, drafted by senior staff member Tibor Szántó, was written with input from an internal committee, and accepted by the HAC plenary pursuant to resolution 2002/1/II/2.1 in February 2002.

Research and Teaching. The higher education act stipulates that the HAC assesses the quality of education and 'scientific activity' in higher education institutions. The HAC has not evaluated research per se, but has focused on the research qualifications and activities of the academic staff as the background for the education they provide. In both colleges and universities, the scientific achievements of the teaching staff constitute an important factor in judging the quality of educational provision.

Programme Accreditation

The HAC conducts programme accreditation within and separately from institutional accreditation. The types of programmes are listed in the higher education act (Section 81 § 1.a and 2.c, d, f), as are doctoral schools; national qualification requirements; new programmes to be launched at institutions; specialised postgraduate programmes (whereby the HAC only examines if the institution meets quality standards, based on its undergraduate provision, in the discipline in which such a programme is to be launched); vocational higher education programmes (only the discipline as above).

As noted, the Hungarian government issues decrees on national qualification requirements, as well as on a set list of disciplines. The list of disciplines is grouped into eight areas of science: natural sciences; engineering; medicine; agriculture; social sciences; humanities; arts; and theology. Each, except for the last with only one discipline, has listed between five and eleven disciplines grouped into one of the areas.

Institutions, Programmes, Subjects and Disciplines Involved in the Scheme. The units involved in teaching the programme are listed in the application and include the faculty (if there is one), as well as the department(s) and, if applicable, laboratories, institutes, practice farms, clinics, etc. In addition to a description of the basic requirements for an institution, new higher education institutions seeking licence to operate must submit the programmes they wish to launch. For colleges these have to be at least two undergraduate programmes, and for universities at least four undergraduate programmes with two each in at least two areas of science.

An institution granted accreditation in a discipline may run vocational or specialised postgraduate programmes in its accredited discipline. Once an institution is accredited for a discipline, only new undergraduate programmes have to be accredited. Doctoral schools at universities must be accredited and have to belong to one of the listed disciplines. That means that an institution must meet quality standards in a given undergraduate programme before it can run any higher-level programme.

Geographic Range Involved in the Scheme. Any programme at any level may be offered outside the institution's main campus. In this case the HAC reviews whether the infrastructure and academic staff involved in the programme meet the necessary requirements. The degree issued for an off-site programme should be equal in content and quality to the one offered at the institution's main campus, and is technically a degree issued by the main institution.

10.2.2 Supra- and Intra-Institutional Evaluation Schemes

Supra-Institutional Evaluation Schemes

Two Hungarian higher education institutions (Attila József University of Arts and Sciences, Szeged, 1995, and Lajos Kossuth University, Debrecen, 1997) have undergone evaluation by the CRE (now European University Association, EUA). The focus of institutional evaluation by the CRE was the institution's management and quality assurance, as compared to the programme-centred approach of the HAC.

Intra-Institutional Evaluation Schemes

Higher education institutions are free to devise their own internal evaluation schemes to meet their particular circumstances. Both the ministry of education and the HAC have extended their assistance and provided guidelines for institutions. In the new round of institutional accreditation it is foreseen to assess the annual reports for progress in the institutions' quality management and educational provision.

An amendment to the higher education act, which went into effect in September 2000, introduced a clause that authorises the government to 'determine the system of requirements for higher education quality policy' (Section 72.o). Accordingly, the minister of education set up a team to elaborate guidelines to assist higher education institutions in developing their internal quality assurance mechanisms. Nóra Halmay, a member of the HAC staff and author of its *Accreditation Guidebook*, was invited to join the team and has contributed to the document. The guide, issued in October 2001, is based on the EFQM (European Foundation for Quality Management) model and on the TQM (Total Quality Management) philosophy, and can be downloaded from the ministry web site at http://www.om.hu.

10.2.3 The Actors

The higher education act regulates quality assurance in Hungary. It authorises the HAC to carry out external evaluation for accreditation, the higher education institutions to take responsibility for their internal quality assurance, and the minister of education to oversee the quality of higher education institutions with respect to their compliance to legislation.

At a broader policy level, the Hungarian parliament and government (which in Hungary is understood to mean the prime minister and all the ministers) also influence the process to varying degrees. Parliament passes laws whereby it determines higher education development and its annual budget, establishes or closes state higher education institutions and endorses non-state institutions (following HAC preliminary accreditation or accreditation), and determines fundamental policy. It also determines the budget of the HAC. The government passes government decrees whereby it establishes or closes faculties (or recognises these as non-state institutions, following HAC preliminary accreditation or accreditation in each case), appoints HAC members, and issues other decrees on higher education, such as on the national qualification requirements for degree programmes or the list of disciplines (the latter two after having received the HAC's opinion), or the decree on the 'fundamental regulations concerning the organisation, operation, and accreditation procedure of the Hungarian Accreditation Committee' (A Kormány 66, 1997). Furthermore, the government fixes the number of students who may enrol into state-financed higher education institutions each year. With the 2000 amendment to the higher education act, the government also determines the 'system of requirements for the quality policy of higher education.' The minister of education authorises the establishment of undergraduate study programmes (following HAC preliminary accreditation), determines the national qualification requirements for specialised postgraduate programmes (after receiving the HAC's opinion), and appoints the HAC's secretary-general in agreement with the committee's president.

An additional body, the National Higher Education and Research Council (FTT), acts as an advisory body to the minister of education in matters of financial support, feasibility and strategy for higher education institutions and programmes, including state-financed student numbers (Act Sections 76-79). The council works with its own pool of evaluators.

The Hungarian Accreditation Committee (HAC)

The HAC consists of 30 members, in addition to non-voting members brought in to cover major disciplines which are not represented by the full members. One representative from the national student union is, by law, a permanently invited, non-voting member. In addition, the HAC invites one representative from the national union of doctoral students, one from the FTT, and one from the National Doctoral and Habilitation Council. The HAC also has an International Advisory Board, currently with ten members from Western and Central Europe and the U.S.A., to review the HAC's work and make recommendations for improvement as well as to propose foreign reviewers.

Half the members are delegated by higher education institutions (as agreed upon by the Hungarian Rectors' Conference, the Conference of College Directors, and the

Chair of Art University Rectors). Ten members come from scientific research institutions (the Hungarian Academy of Sciences and the National Committee for Technical Development). The remaining five members are delegated by professional organisations and chambers, who must consult with each other to chose the delegates. The one area where the HAC has decision-making powers is the establishment of doctoral schools. The HAC's basic authority is to 'express opinions' on various issues, i.e., it has an advisory function and the final decision is made by the minister of education, government or parliament, as the case may be.

For institutional as well as all types of programme accreditation procedures, the HAC involves external evaluators. For institutional accreditation the evaluators make up the visiting team. Separate visiting teams are set up for the different faculties of an institution. They consist of academics and professional experts in the main disciplines taught at the evaluated faculty.

Programmes are evaluated by means of a written application package. The evaluation is carried out by two expert reviewers, with a third one stepping in if the first two were inconclusive. The reviewers' reports are discussed by the HAC's expert committee which is most closely related to the discipline of the programme applied, and the expert committee's report, in turn, is discussed by one of three expert committees for the main areas of science (medicine and agricultural sciences; technical and natural sciences; social sciences, humanities, theology and arts) before going up for vote by the plenary. With the 2000 amendment to the higher education act the HAC was given the additional task of evaluating applications for professorial appointments, announced in open tenders by higher education institutions. The idea was to curb the proliferation of professorships institutions in order to ensure a higher salary on the public pay scale for their teaching staff and to receive additional public financing.

The HAC was evaluated by an international panel co-ordinated by the CRE (now EUA). The report, together with the HAC's reply, was published in 2000 (see http://www.mab.hu/english/a_links.html).

The Higher Education Institution and the Minister of Education

All levels of an institution are involved in the accreditation process, because they contribute to the institutional self-evaluation report. With the exception of doctoral schools, on which the HAC has decision-making powers, the minister of education makes the final decision, or passes on the HAC's opinion on issues that are under the authority of the government or parliament. The minister may overturn the HAC's decisions, but must provide a reason which must be published (Government Decree § 20.6, pursuant to Act Section 74 § 2).

General Formal Rules and Legal Regulations

An intricate set of regulations is related to accreditation by the HAC. The highest level is the higher education act, first passed in 1993 and amended several times. (A new law is currently under discussion). The HAC as an organisation is legislated in the act, a related government decree, and its own by-laws. It establishes its own by-laws, which encompass its procedures for all levels and types of accreditation. According to the government decree, the by-laws must be published in the official gazette of the ministry and hence endorsed by the minister. The membership of the HAC must also be published in the ministry gazette, but here the minister does not even have indirect endorsing powers, since the members are appointed by the prime minister. In addition, the HAC draws up its accreditation requirements and standards, which must also be published in the ministry gazette. The HAC also issues the above regulations, from the by-laws down to any of its lesser regulations which are not promulgated in the ministry gazette, in its own *Accreditation Newsletter* and its website, http://www.mab.hu.

Formal Financing

Section 80 § 6 of the higher education act states that 'The HAC is a legal entity, an independent professional body in the service of Hungarian higher education, its secretariat is an organisation with full authority and a public budget. The money for its operation shall be ensured by Parliament separately within the annual budget.' The government decree on the HAC states in § 27 that 'The HAC president and members shall receive a fee. The amount and conditions for payment shall be set down in the HAC by-laws.' In § 18.7 the decree states that 'The members of ad hoc committees and experts shall receive a fee for their work. The fee and the conditions for payment shall be set down in the by-laws.' With respect to financial administration § 31.4 stipulates, 'The chief financial officer of the secretariat shall be appointed and dismissed by the minister on recommendation of the Secretary General.' Further, § 32 sets down that the budget must be approved by the HAC plenary, as well as other details of procedure.

The HAC by-laws contain a separate annex on financial and budgetary procedures, which regulate the amounts and modes of payment of specific items derived from the act, government decree and by-laws.

Formal Stages of the Procedure

Two documents regulate the formal procedures for the tasks set down for HAC in Section 81 of the higher education act. These are the HAC's by-laws and its accreditation requirements (see http://www.mab.hu/english/a_regulations.html). The procedures and criteria for institutional accreditation are additionally described in the HAC's *Accreditation Guidebook*. The new edition was published late 2003.

a) Institutional Accreditation. The procedure is set down in the HAC by-laws, the accreditation requirements, and the *Accreditation Guidebook.* For institutional accreditation, the by-laws contain appendices that regulate the requirements and procedures for the preliminary accreditation of new institutions (Appendix 5) and faculties (Appendix 6) as well as foreign higher education institutions to be established in Hungary (Appendix 7) and the accreditation of institutions (Appendix 8). These procedures set down very briefly what the evaluation will cover and describe the steps of the procedure.

A second set of regulations governing the accreditation of institutions (and programmes) is the accreditation requirements. In terms of the accreditation of institutions the requirements set down the minimum conditions for teaching staff, facilities and equipment, and programme provision which must be met for university and college faculties, for universities, for colleges, and for foreign higher education institutions applying for permission to operate in Hungary. The accreditation requirements concerning the accreditation of institutions are very general, leaving the detailed criteria and procedures to the *Accreditation Guidebook.*

The following round will retain many of the procedural elements, and will continue to focus on the educational provision, with more emphasis on the institutional dimension. Key elements that will be different are as follows. The HAC will no longer assign a grade (on a scale of four) to the evaluated degree programme but will instead provide a detailed analysis; it will examine the institution's quality assurance system; accredit disciplines instead of individual programmes by spot-checking a few programmes and, if the evaluation is positive, will consider all programmes within the discipline accredited (but if the evaluation is negative, all programmes will be evaluated); select the programme for evaluation based on the annual quality audit reports of the institution; and concentrate more on process and output factors of a programme. The institution will have more leeway to focus its self-evaluation report on its own perceived strengths and weaknesses. Concerning its own role and responsibility in the accreditation process, the HAC wants to increase the proficiency of its members and experts in accreditation.[4]

b) Programme Accreditation. For programme accreditation, the by-laws contain appendices that regulate the requirements and procedures for the preliminary accreditation of new undergraduate and specialised postgraduate programmes, i.e. national qualification requirements (Appendix 1), for vocational higher education programmes (Appendix 2), for launching an undergraduate programme at a higher education institution (Appendix 3), and for doctoral schools (Appendix 4). The procedures for the first three types of programmes set down very briefly what the

---

4   The information is taken from a draft document on the planned approach to institutional accreditation
     presented to the HAC plenary for discussion on February 1, 2003.

evaluation will cover and describe the steps of the procedure. The appendix concerning doctoral schools contains the full procedures and criteria (which for other types of programmes are regulated in multiple regulations), since doctoral schools, which run doctoral programmes within a broad disciplinary area, were only introduced with the 1999 amendment to the higher education act to supersede the accreditation of individual doctoral programmes. Technically, all programme accreditation that is not conducted within the eight-yearly institutional accreditation procedure is preliminary accreditation, since it concerns future programmes.

The accreditation requirements constitute the second set of procedures governing the accreditation of programmes. They apply to both preliminary accreditation and to the accreditation conducted within the institutional accreditation process. The requirements set down what each type of programme must contain in terms of minimum content (teaching staff number and qualifications, curriculum, facilities and equipment) in order to be accredited. The types of programmes are vocational higher education programmes, national qualification requirements, undergraduate programmes, specialised postgraduate programmes, distance education programmes, programmes taught in a foreign language.

Added to the general requirements are the additional criteria for programmes in particular disciplines established by the expert committees of the HAC.

Formal Duration of the Stages of the Process

a) Institutional Accreditation. The entire institutional accreditation procedure lasts for eight to twelve months.

b) Programme Accreditation. The deadline for the preliminary accreditation of doctoral schools, for national qualification requirements, for new programmes to be launched at institutions, for specialised post-graduate programmes, and for vocational higher education programmes is six months.

Formal Rules for Objection Regarding the Procedures. The HAC's decisions regarding its assessment of Ph.D. programmes are binding to the minister of education. All other decisions are 'opinions', but the minister can require the HAC to repeat a procedure if s/he believes that the HAC did not observe the regulations. The minister has rejected no more than 1 % of the HAC's decisions, mainly in the last two years. The increase is probably due both to a maturing critical attitude towards external assessment (and demand for more substantiated explanations backing up decisions) that goes along with a growing quality consciousness on the part of higher education institutions, and to a particular government's greater propensity to exert its leverage.

Formal Rules for Information; Distribution of Outcomes

The HAC issues decisions concerning applications to establish doctoral schools, and 'opinions' on all other issues. Its decisions and opinions, in the form of resolutions, are published by HAC in its *Accreditation Newsletter* and website. Resolutions on institutional accreditation, with an explanation of one to several pages (depending on the number of programmes accredited at the same time), were published in the first cycle. The HAC's strategic plan foresees that an exhaustive evaluation report be published in the upcoming round. As regards programme accreditation, decisions or 'opinions' are published in the *Accreditation Newsletter* and web site along with a brief explanation of two to three sentences. With both institutional and programme accreditation, the decisions passed by parliament, government or the minister of education subsequent to the HAC's 'opinion' are also published in the *Hungarian Gazette* and/or the *Gazette of the Ministry of Education.*

Following a decision in 2001 by the ombudsman for the protection of information, the HAC must publish its reasons for issuing specific decisions more extensively. The HAC conducted a survey of higher education institutions on whether they wished to make the accreditation reports public, and 76 % of those that replied were in favour.

10.2.4   Implementation of Formal Rules

Practical Application of Procedures

The principal concerns regarding the application of procedure in the Hungarian accreditation system stem from the dichotomy between the profuse regulations, which establish one set of expectations (namely towards their adherence), and the engagement of acknowledged scientists and scholars, whose predominantly scientific or scholarly expertise (rather than in accreditation methodology) raises another set of expectations. The acknowledgement of the importance of some formal training in accreditation methodology is difficult to obtain. The report of the panel which evaluated the HAC, organised by the then CRE, recommended 'that the HAC reconsider its requirement that everyone involved in its work hold a scientific degree' (CRE, 2000, p. 173). Since then, the HAC has engaged practising professionals in its expert committees and as external evaluators. It remains to be seen to what degree some sort of formal training for evaluators, set down in the draft document on the future round of institutional accreditation, can be realised. The consequence of the former practice was inconsistency, lack of transparency and insufficient justification in the HAC's judgements.

Practical Application of Legal Regulations

The HAC membership is nominated by higher education institutions, research institutions, and professional organisations (see 10.2.3). The nominating procedure, as set down in the government decree on the HAC, calls for the delegating organisations to each send the name of their nominee to the outgoing HAC president, who forwards the full 30-member list to the ministry. That means that while the ministry technically proposes the HAC members to the prime minister for appointment, the committee is in fact independently selected by the delegating bodies. The negative implication is, however, that the delegating mechanism does not guarantee the body's continuity nor sure that all major disciplines are represented. Another practical consequence of the legislation regulating the HAC is that the ministry of education is mandated by law to supervise the HAC's observance of legality in its procedures. Furthermore, all HAC's regulations are checked by the ministry before being made public. Thirdly, all HAC's decisions are in the form of 'positions' and 'opinions' (with the exception of decisions on doctoral schools, where the HAC has decision-making powers), with the final decision being taken by the minister. The minister has the right to reject the HAC's resolutions, but in this case he must publish the reasons for doing so. In the last few years this has occurred more frequently (as I mentioned above).

Handling of Financial Matters

The HAC's budget is allocated by parliament through the annual budget law (Act Section 80 § 6). The annual amount, however, is controlled by the ministry of education to which the HAC's budget plan must be submitted and which then submits it within its own plan to parliament. As far as payment is concerned, here too, the money is paid out via the ministry on a monthly basis. In effect this means that the ministry exerts direct control over the overall funds and specific components available to the HAC for its operation.

Time Frames for the Procedures

The HAC generally adheres to the time frames set down in the by-laws and procedures, which in their current form reflect years of experience. The last tally conducted in 2000 shows that between 1994 and 1999 the HAC exceeded the time frames in 15 % of institutions and 20 % of programmes. The reasons for the lags were mainly because of the request for additional information from the applicants and the slow return of evaluations by external reviewers.

Handling of Rejection Procedures

If the required information is missing in the application, the HAC requests it. Concerning the content of an application, the HAC requires that institutions or programmes meet the criteria set down in its quality requirements. Expert committees do have room for individual judgements, however. In institutional accreditation, no institution was closed because of a HAC decision. In a number of cases, however, institutions were asked to elaborate action plans to alleviate their problems, which were reviewed regularly before final accreditation was granted. In programme accreditation, some programmes were discontinued, but the great majority of rejections concerned applications for new programmes. A number of professorial appointment applications have been rejected. The HAC sends its reports to the applicants, including the detailed decisions for approval or rejection.

10.3 The Driving Forces Behind, and the Consequences of Accreditation

10.3.1 Other Schemes

As I have noted, the higher education act recognises only one official form of external quality assurance for higher education institutions in Hungary, namely accreditation, as carried out by the HAC, with the final decision (with the exception of doctoral schools) being taken by the minister of education. Any other quality evaluation is carried out by individual institutions or units as they see fit.

10.3.2 The Driving Forces behind Accreditation, and Ongoing Qualitative Changes in Hungarian Higher Education

Since the higher education act makes accreditation in Hungary mandatory, the owners, initiators and controllers of the process carry it out in compliance with the law. Exploring the underlying reasons why accreditation was introduced in Hungary is another question, and to my knowledge there has not been any systematic research on this topic. Studies carried out by foreign scholars have tried to summarise the reasons for accreditation versus other schemes in Central and Eastern Europe. Of course there are several common denominators (see below), but these essays examine the common trends and do not consider the substantial differences between these countries (e.g., Tomusk, 1997; Westerheijden, 2001). The handful of Hungarian studies I am aware of are mainly descriptive and not very analytical (e.g., Rébay, 2001).

Accreditation as the approach to quality assurance[5] in Central and Eastern Europe is in many ways more rigid than the quality assurance approaches in Western Europe. The choice of accreditation, as opposed to quality evaluation or review of quality

---

5   I use 'quality assurance' as a collective term, i.e. without wanting to indicate one particular form of quality assurance, such as accreditation or evaluation, in this particular context.

without a pass/fail judgement, has its roots in the historical and cultural context of the countries in the region, and therefore varies from one country to the next not only in the details, but also in the degree of rigidity. When developing its accreditation model, the HAC's intention, beyond passing a yes/no decision on the institutions or programmes it evaluated, was to act as a quality consultant and bring constructive criticism into its evaluation procedure and reports. How far it has succeeded in this may be open to debate. The introduction of new mechanisms of social and political interaction is far from linear and affects the higher education sector.

Accreditation was the preferred method of quality assurance in Central and Eastern Europe because:

> ... the need with the emergence of democracy to establish comparability with Western higher education; the necessity to re-evaluate the curricula to rid them of politically distorted content; the urgency to modernise programme content and approach as well as to introduce more flexible programme structures. (Tomusk, 2000, pp. 175-185.)

> Answers such as a steep rise in private institutions in some countries, and in pressure to allow access for a large number of students to a previously elite sector may also be part of the explanation, although these trends were experienced in Western Europe as well, albeit more gradually. There has been the blunt postulation that accreditation is the approach most suited to a region accustomed to an autocratic mentality. (Campbell & Rozsnyai, 2002, pp. 60-61.)

I surmise that the introduction of accreditation in Hungary was a trade-off for the state relinquishing the total control over higher education institutions that existed before the regime change, and granting them a certain degree of autonomy. Accreditation was to ensure that the quality of higher education, which enjoyed international recognition – at least until the early 1990s – should not be lost. I also surmise, however, that over the years state control has grown as compared to the launching phase of the new national higher education system in the early 1990s, just as the legal structure has become increasingly intricate with the multiplication of amendments to the higher education act and the ongoing consolidation of the political environment. A new higher education act is currently on the drawing board and it is hoped that it will grant institutions more autonomy. A number of factors point in this direction. Whereas Hungarian rectors and college directors had practically no experience in institutional management in the business sense of the word, a decade of immersion in international trends and practices and increasing responsibility to keep their institutions afloat under considerable financial pressure is beginning to change this tendency.

Moreover, the ministry of education has launched a broad programme to develop higher education, which includes a finance reform. Part of the programme focuses on restructuring the entire financing system. A preliminary study analysed the current weaknesses of higher education institution budgetary allocation and financing, and the higher education system as a whole (Matolcsy, 2001, pp. 19-20). The aim of the reform, if and when it becomes reality, is to ensure more rational, transparent and efficient expenditure of public money by higher education institutions in a budgetary system which can better adapt to social changes and to give institutions more flexibility in the use of the money they receive from the state budget, while ensuring greater co-ordination of the projects on which the money is spent. Growing financial responsibility must be accompanied by greater liberty in management, including less over-regulation, and covering everything from enrolment quotas to study schemes.

In September 2002, the pay-scales for college and university teaching staff were raised by 54 % (see Stark, 2003), and it can be hoped that the practice of teaching staff having several jobs in various parts of the country will give way to the conviction that the quality of higher education must be safeguarded by all players involved. This topic also comes up in discussions concerning the quality of education, and in preparation of the new higher education act it is to be hoped that a balance will be found to regulate multiple positions without infringing on the teaching staff's personal rights.

The introduction of the ECTS-compatible credit system in September 2003, and the variety of study schemes that will gradually follow, will loose up the educational structure and its regulations in favour of broader guidelines.

Finally, as the 'European higher education area' is increasingly becoming a reality and Hungary continues to establish its niche in it, the global forces will have many positive consequences for the country's educational system.

10.3.3   The Consequences of Accreditation for Higher Education Institutions, Departments and Scholars

In the first round of accreditation, Hungarian higher education institutions learned the implications of quality assessment. By conducting self-evaluation from the institutional to the department level, the notion of 'quality culture' has become a reality. Beyond saying that an accreditation decision has the potential to threaten the very existence of a higher education institution, the HAC has functioned as much as a consultancy as a bureaucratic authority. This, together with the institutions' own self-evaluations, have helped institutions to recognise their strengths and weaknesses and to act on them. I realise that my statement may not meet with the unanimous agreement of those who work in higher education institutions. Yet a survey the HAC conducted among all higher education institutions in Hungary for its external evaluation by the CRE panel (see section 10.2.3) shows that about 80 % were satisfied with the HAC's work up until 1999 (CRE, 2000, p. 55).

How far the next cycle can improve on the first, in particular by shifting its focus on input to output data and tailoring the procedure to the individual institution, remains to be seen. Perhaps a more important question is to what degree accreditation has contributed to the improvement of the quality of higher education in Hungary. One must look at the complexity of problems facing Hungarian higher education before trying to answer the question. The study for the financial reform project mentioned above pinpoints the weaknesses of the Hungarian higher education system.

- 'Characteristic of the system is the low efficiency of its operations, marked by acute shortages and visible squandering,
- Elected institution heads with limited authority and with accountability to their own institutional senate find it difficult to tackle even those problems which could still be solved, as this would involve conflicts of interest,
- The structure of provision is determined more by tradition, the teaching staff's preferences, and by what changes additional state financing might promise,
- The minimum income institutions earn points to their low integration in the economy and society, due in part to the lack of any institutional framework for setting up such relationships, and in part to private companies' distrust of state-financed institutions,
- The effort of university staff to obtain a higher income manifests itself in the form of private businesses that use the university facilities and equipment and its name, and which are tolerated by the institutional leadership,
- The frequent changes in the framework for institutional operation determined by the state (which stem from the state's dilemma as to whether it should play a direct or indirect role in higher education) make it difficult for institutions to see their long-term incentives and to make long-term plans,
- Institutions are dissatisfied with the many regulations on financial management (earmarked budgetary estimates, the required spending of surpluses within a limited time period and fixed in form, etc.) stemming from the law on the state budget, which they perceive as a strait-jacket but which, in the present system with no practical structure for the flow of information and no ownership rights, provide necessary but not apparently sufficient guarantees for the state to supervise the autonomous institutions,
- Recurring cases of bankruptcies or near-bankruptcies of institutions, which come as a surprise to the administration, stem not just from the lack of sufficient financing but also from the status of the institutions and the internal leadership structure, i.e. the system of responsibilities.' (Matolcsy, 2002, p. 22. Translation by C.R.)

Faced with such formidable problems, which may be explained by the legacy of a dictatorial regime and the lack of a model for transforming higher education into an educational service sector of the kind required by a new democratic society, the remit of the HAC to 'accredit the educational and scientific activities in higher education and to carry out quality assessment' (Act Section 80 § 1) is not broad enough to safeguard the quality of the sector. Beyond the political power plays that Hungary, like most new democracies in Central and Eastern Europe, continues to witness, it may have been the feeling that the HAC alone could not deal with the complex problem of safeguarding the quality of higher education that led the policy makers in the 2000 amendment of the higher education act to authorise the government to oversee higher education quality (Section 72.o), while taking away the remit of the HAC to function 'for the ongoing supervision of the standard of education and scientific activity in higher education, … and for the supporting of quality assurance' (Act prior to 2000 amendment, Section 80 § 1).

Let us now answer the question: to what degree has accreditation contributed to the improvement of the quality of higher education in Hungary? Though not quantifiable, higher education quality is generally perceived to have deteriorated in the past decade. The reality alone that attendance has tripled would have required enormous flexibility in the sector, while many players in all parts of the sector put great efforts into conserving the status quo, even if that could only be an uphill struggle. Another consideration is that competition for students in Hungarian colleges and universities is just beginning (and only in a few financially profitable fields as economics and law). The government sets the number of students who may enrol and institutions receive normative financing according to student numbers.

However, several studies have investigated the comparative market value of diplomas from particular institutions (e.g., a study that was supported by the Ministry of Education: Galasi, Timár, & Varga, 2001, pp. 46-48, or the earlier mentioned study, 'Diplomák a munkaerő-piacon', 2002). And from the study cited above, as well as from the many discussions brought about by the Bologna process (e.g., as seen in the Hungarian Rectors' Conference statement from its December 17, 2002 meeting) concerning the plans to restructure educational programmes to accommodate the credit system and the two-cycle structure, it appears that both the government and the sector's leadership are taking action to tackle the problems.

As far as the HAC is concerned, it has formulated the implications of the committee's role within Hungarian higher education together with the complex of tasks derived from it in its Strategic Plan. The plan sees the HAC as a service organisation within higher education and within society, and stakes out the HAC's challenges for the future in the light of the changes higher education must undergo to accommodate the Bologna process. The plan has also set down the principles along which the second round of institutional accreditation should proceed. It should be less formalistic than before and focus more on substance than on indicators, should develop the improvement of the accreditation process and the HAC's advisory role rather than call on institutions to account for their quality. The staff and the committee's members should receive more methodological training. The HAC's activities and decisions should become more transparent and public. Listing these aspirations means that these features were not sufficiently present before and that they are necessary to fulfil the HAC's stated role.

10.3.4   The Consequences of Accreditation for Students and the General Public

While accreditation reports issued by the HAC could inform prospective students, their parents and the public at large, of the quality of provision at a given institution or programme, this was not the case. One reason was that the report and the reasons behind the decisions were not published, only the accreditation decision and a short explanation. With the publication of the full report, it is hoped that this requirement to serve the public will be fulfilled.

The HAC and accreditation have not been able to balance the threat to the quality of higher education posed by the rise of mass education. Higher enrolments were actively promoted by government until recently. Even though the demographic decline Hungary is experiencing is reaching the age cohort, the structural demands the numerical increase brings to higher education are evident. A new tendency seems to be arising to curb the expansion of higher education until the financial and system changes that can ensure its quality are in place.

10.4   International Influences

10.4.1   The Effects of the Bologna Process and Globalisation

The Bologna process affects two aspects of Hungarian higher education: the restructuring of the traditional binary system into a two-cycle system of studies, and the introduction of the credit system.

The recalculation of programmes and curricula to make up credit units is probably the easier of the two tasks. Yet this too requires a change of mentality, which is not unanimously accepted by all the actors involved. The fact that students are offered a variety of curriculum structures is perceived by some as a loss of the well-established fundamentals on which traditional curricula were built. But both the credit system and the loss of traditional structures are a consequence of mass education and hence an unavoidable development. The Credit Decree (A Kormány 200, 2000) requires all higher education institutions in Hungary to have the credit system, as defined in the law, in place by the academic year 2003/04. The national qualification requirements for degree programmes (see above) already assign credit points to all programmes.

A much more difficult problem is the conversion of the traditional binary higher education system into a two-cycle, bachelor-master structure. The ministry of education has set up a working group to define the core issues and to integrate the input of professional groups. At the time of writing it can be said that every participant in Hungarian higher education is aware of the momentum of the Bologna process that will ultimately result in the introduction of the two-cycle structure in many, if not all, degree programmes. It appears now that medicine, law and some humanities programmes will continue to be offered only at the master's level (though, of course, there will also be shorter health care and legal studies).

Student mobility is relatively low compared to many Western European countries. Hungary has been involved in TEMPUS programmes since 1990. In the academic year 2000/01, 2001 Hungarian students studied abroad under Socrates–Erasmus. More than a quarter (536) went to Germany, with 275 going to France, 205 to Italy, 199 to Finland, and 135 to Great Britain. Under CEEPUS, the Central and Eastern European Higher Education Exchange Programme, there were 184 undergraduate and master's students from Hungary in 2000/01 (see TEMPUS Hungary, http://www.tpf.iif.hu/newsite/tka/sajtoszob.htm, Statisztikák [Statistics]). In addition, there are some government and international scholarships. An estimated 3 % of full-time students study abroad on a private basis. The recognition of studies abroad is proceeding smoothly at the national level, as the Hungarian Equivalence and Information Centre, a department of the ministry of education, is an active member of the ENIC/NARIC network. Information is much less unequivocal concerning the acceptance of foreign studies of returning students at specific higher education institutions. It seems to be dependent both on the flexibility of the institutional department and, to some degree, the subjects studied.

Concerning the effects of the Bologna process on the 'quality assurance' (cf. Bologna declaration) of higher education in Hungary, the HAC is a participant in many international organisations and events and is an active actor in the Bologna process in the area of accreditation at the European level. HAC members are aware of the many projects on multilateral and international accreditation schemes. Discussions have been held within the HAC on the transformation from the binary to the linear, two-cycle study structure. The HAC has guidelines (as part of its by-laws) to deal with the evaluation of foreign institutions and has set up an ad hoc committee to deal with special problems arising in this regard. Moreover, the committee has discussed the evaluation of transnational distance education programmes as an issue to be dealt with in the near future. But these programmes have not yet made their mark on Hungarian higher education.

All in all it can be said that higher education and the HAC are reacting with some delay to the Bologna Declaration, to which Hungary was a signatory, but that discussions at many levels have taken off in the last year or so. The rigidity of the Hungarian structure of higher education poses an enormous challenge to the whole system and to all players concerned. While the Bologna process is providing the momentum to rethink the structure and purpose of higher education, I am not sure that a flexible, market- and consumer-oriented, financially feasible higher education system that is open to change, ready to promote mobility, to accept a variety of compatible educational patterns and is service oriented and sensitive to the needs of all levels of society, is imminent.

A complete reconsideration of the existing value system is necessary and a frame of mind that revolves around elite education must adapt to a new reality. While the transformation that took place in higher education after 1989/90 was a step towards a more flexible system than the congealed structure of the previous decades, the Bologna process is providing the impetus for a truly qualitative change. The HAC has recognised the need for change, as can be seen in its Strategic Plan and the actions it has taken and is planning to take. I can only hope that it will not lose the capability and authority to be a proactive player in the quality assurance of Hungarian higher education.

10.4.2   International and Local Models of the Hungarian Accreditation Scheme

In the three years leading up to Hungary's first higher education act in 1993, many players contributed to the discussion about the future architecture of Hungarian higher education. These were the Rectors' Conference, the College Directors' Conference and the Chair of Art University Rectors, as well as policy makers following the change of regime in 1989/90. The methodology for accreditation was taken from the U.S.A. and evaluation models from Western Europe. In this regard, the first president of the Hungarian Accreditation Committee, András Róna-Tas, deserves credit for exploring a number of systems and adapting the main components to a feasible scheme for Hungary.

The first accreditation scheme was developed by the HAC after consultation with higher education institution academics and staff, and was tested in a pilot phase in 1994, in which two universities and four colleges were accredited. Subsequently, the HAC contracted a consultant, Ágnes Kaposi of Kaposi Associates in London, who worked out the principles and procedural guidelines for a new guidebook. Dr. Kaposi was already involved in evaluating a college in Hungary and had some insight into the local conditions. The second and subsequent editions of the *Accreditation Guidebook*, written by staff member Nóra Halmay, have remained fundamentally the same.

The new accreditation guidelines for the second round will be based on a number of sources. First, the HAC has been actively involved in international quality assurance organisations and meetings in the last ten years and has gained considerable experience. The basic concept is set down in the HAC's Strategic Plan. The HAC has set up an internal committee, which has discussed this aspect of the Strategic Plan and the future accreditation scheme in great detail. Finally, Nóra Halmay, who is contributing to the new guidebook, has actively participated in a team created the Hungarian ministry of education, which has produced guidelines to set up internal quality evaluation schemes that are intended to assist higher education institutions.

10.5 Other Quality Assessment Activities in Institutions or Units

Higher education institutions have their own teaching and research requirements which form part of their by-laws which set down the obligations regarding teaching load, publications, etc. for positions of all levels. In addition to these requirements, individual merit is recognised when renewing contracts and including staff in external research projects. This can supplement the staff member's income. Teaching staff in Hungarian higher education institutions are public employees. Their remuneration follows a pay-scale set by government, although it has recently raised professors' salaries to what is considered an acceptable level. The salaries of lower-level teaching staff continue to be far below earnings in industry.

There is no tenure *per se*, and permanent status is linked to the level of a position. The higher education act (Section 6 § 14.2) states that lecturers and readers can be appointed for a term of four years, which is not renewable for lecturers but renewable once for readers. Full and assistant professors may hold their positions until they reach the retirement age of 70. One important quality control mechanism is the introduction in the 2000 amendment to the act (pursuant Section 81 § 2.j) of the requirement that the HAC evaluate applications to positions of full professor. Here, the HAC checks the educational and scholarly or scientific background of applicants. This is, in fact, a form of peer review.

Promotion is decided at the appropriate levels of the institution, depending on the level of the position. (Section 6 of the act describes the achievements, such as teaching and research experience and scientific degrees, that applicants to the various positions must possess.) No doubt, merit, and hence quality, does play a role in the promotion of teaching staff. Once the senior level has been attained there is little quality control. It follows from the above that there are no financial bonuses for special achievements in Hungary. External research contracts in fields where these exist may bring additional income to departments and individuals, but they are *ad hoc* and are by no means a systematic way of rewarding quality.

References

A Kormány 66/1997 (IV.18.) Korm. rendelete A Magyar Akkreditációs Bizottság szervezetéről, működéséről és az akkreditációs eljárás alapvető szabályairól [Government Decree 66/1997 of April 18 on the fundamental regulations concerning the organisation, operation, and accreditation procedure of the Hungarian Accreditation Committee]. In: *Magyar Közlöny* 1997/33. pp. 2073-2080.

A Kormány 169/2000 (IX.29.) Korm. rendelete az egyes tudományterületekhez tartozó tudományágak, valamint a művészeti ágak felsorolásáról [Government Decree 169/2000 of November 29, Listing the Disciplines Within the Different Areas of Science, and the Areas of Art]. In: *Magyar Közlöny* 10/10/2000, pp. 6095-6096.

A Kormány 200/2000 (XI.29.) Korm. rendelete a felsőoktatási tanulmányi pontrendszer (kreditrendszer) bevezetéséről és az intézményi kreditrendszerek egységes nyilvántartásáról [Government Decree 200/2000 of November 29 On Introducing the Credit System in Higher Education and Unified Registration of Institutional Credit Systems. *Magyar Közlöny* 2000/116. pp. 7260-7265.

A Kormány 119/2001 (VI.30.) Korm. rendelete a hallgatói hitelrendszerről és a Diákhitel Központról [Government Decree 119/2001 of June 30 2001, On the System of Student Loans and the Student Loan Center]. In: *Magyar Közlöny* 2001/74. pp. 5452-5458.

Campbell, Carolyn, & Rozsnyai, Christina (2002). *Quality Assurance and the Development of Course Programmes*. Papers on Higher Education. UNESCO.

CRE (2000). *The External Evaluation of the Hungarian Accreditation Committee*. Budapest. http://www.mab.hu/english/a_links.html.

Diplomák a munkaerő-piacon [Diplomas On the Employment Market] (2002). Study headed by Péter Galasi. In: *Mit kínál a magyar felsőoktatás? Felvételi Tanácsadó 2002* [What Does Hungarian Higher Education Offer? Advice for Admission 2002]. Budapest: Országos Felsőoktatási Felvételi Iroda [National Higher Education Admissions Office], pp. 649-674.

Galasi, Péter, Timár, János, & Varga, Júlia (2001). Pályakezdő diplomások a munkaerőpiacon I [Fresh College and University Graduates in the Labor Market I]. *Magyar Felsőoktatás* 2001/1-2.

Hungarian Accreditation Committee (1995-1998). *Accreditation Guidebook for Higher Education Institutions*, by Nóra Halmay, based on guidelines by Agnes Kaposi. 7 eds., 2 English eds.

Matolcsy, János (2001). A magyar felsőoktatás finanszírozási rendszerének reformja [The Reform of the Financial Structure of Hungarian Higher Education]. *Magyar Felsőoktatás* 2001/9.

Matolcsy, János (2002). Megkezdődött a finanszírozási rendszer reformja projekt [The Reform Project on the Financial Structure Has Started]. *Magyar Felsőoktatás* 2002/1-2.

Rébay, Magdolna (2001). Felsőoktatási akkreditáció, európai trendek [Higher Education Accreditation, European Trends]. *Educatio* 2001/4. pp. 719-723.

Stark, Antal (2003). A felsőoktatás 2003. évi költségvetése [The Higher Education Budget for 2003]. *Magyar Felsőoktatás* 2003/1-2 http://www.magyarfelsooktatas.hu.

The European Higher Education Area. Joint declaration of the European Ministers of Education, Convened in Bologna on the 18th of June 1999. http://www.mab.hu/a_linkek.html.

Tomusk, Voldemar (1997). External Quality Assurance in Estonian Higher Education: Its Glory, Take-off and Crash. *Quality in Higher Education*, 3, No. 2, pp. 173-181.

Tomusk, Voldemar (2000). When East Meets West: Decontextualising the Quality of East European Higher Education. *Quality in Higher Education*, 6, No. 3.

Törvény a felsőoktatásról (1993) évi LXXX. [Law on Higher Education LXXX/1993]. In: *Akadémiai értesítő*. Sept 15, 2000, pp. 72-105. Main amendments 1996, 1999, 2000. See English version (1996) at http://www.om.hu/english.

Westerheijden, Don F. (2001). Ex Oriente Lux? National and Multiple Accreditation in Europe After the Fall of the Wall and After Bologna. *Quality in Higher Education*, 7, No. 1. pp. 65-75.

11 Practice and Procedures Regarding Accreditation and Evaluation in the Irish Republic

MAUREEN KILLEAVY

11.1 Introduction

Third level education in the Republic of Ireland has undergone considerable expansion in recent years both in terms of the numbers of student registered in the various institutions, and the extent of institutional provision and the range of courses of study available to students. During the ten year period between the academic years 1989/90 and 1999/2000 the numbers of students registered at third level rose from 62,137 to 115,696 representing an overall increase of over 80 %. The marked rate of increase in the numbers of students taking part in third level education was consistent throughout the period although some small variations occurred from year to year. At an institutional level also, there has been substantial expansion of the system both in the enlargement of existing institutions and in the establishment of new universities and institutes.

The structure of the Irish third level education system is binary or two-tier comprising the university sector and the institutes of technology. Traditionally, the universities have institutional autonomy, a right that has been underwritten in the legislation of 1997 (i.e. the Universities Act, 1997). The universities are, however, funded by the state and are not independent of external control in that their duties and responsibilities have been laid down in the new legislation. They are also monitored by a statutory body, the Higher Education Authority (HEA), which allocates state funding to the universities. The other major sector of the two tier or binary third level education system is made up largely of the institutes of technology (ITs) which operate under the monitoring agency, the Higher Education and Training Awards Council (HETAC).

It is necessary to point out that the term *accreditation* as it is used in Ireland does not refer to the same process as it does in other European countries. In this state it is customary for universities to award or confer degrees while it is usual for most of the non-university institutions, to have their qualifications awarded by the Higher Education and Training Awards Council, the statutory body instituted by government for this purpose. In some higher education institutions outside the university sector however, degrees are validated and awarded by one of the universities with which the institution has an association. Accreditation as it is used in Ireland refers to the process by which relevant degrees are accredited by professional bodies as

S. Schwarz and D.F. Westerheijden (eds.),
Accreditation and Evaluation in the European Higher Education Area, 233–250.
© 2004 *Kluwer Academic Publishers. Printed in the Netherlands.*

appropriate qualifications for membership of the profession in question. Some of these professional bodies which grant accreditation are national bodies while others are organised at an international level. Throughout this study the meta-terminology devised by the editors of this volume is used as far as possible to facilitate the comparative focus of the project.

11.2   The National System of Higher Education in Ireland

11.2.1   Size of the Irish Higher Education System

The third level education system in Ireland is broad in scope and encompasses the university sector, the technological sector, the colleges of education and private independent colleges. The first three groupings comprise 34 institutions including eight universities that are largely autonomous and self-governing while being substantially state funded. Because of this it would be incorrect to categorise them as either solely public or private as they have, in varying degrees, characteristics or attributes of both types of institution.

The 14 institutes of technology that are located throughout the country provide a range of courses from craft to academic level. While there is a difference in the degree of state control across the Irish higher education area this difference is not directly attributable to the private vs. public nature of the institutions. Both the universities and other third level institutions receive their funding in varying amounts from the state to defray part or all of their costs. As a consequence, they are publicly accountable and they are also subject to legislation. There are a number of private third level institutions in Ireland, some of which operate under HETAC regulations while others operate independently on a commercial basis.

The number of students participating in higher education in Ireland has increased substantially in recent years with an estimated 55 % of students now going on to higher education on completion of post primary school. Unlike a number of countries that experienced a decline in the numbers of students entering third level education, the participation rate in Ireland has continued to increase each year. At present it is among the highest in the world. The Higher Education Authority suggests that these rapidly growing numbers reflect growing retention rates within post primary schools, demographic trends and increasing transfer rates into higher education.

Entry to third level education for Irish students is based upon performance in the final post primary state examination, the Leaving Certificate. This form of selection was introduced in 1968 when students entering the medical faculty in University College Dublin were selected on the basis of their results in the Leaving Certificate Examination. The system was gradually developed and extended during the following ten years to become a common, centralised selection system for entrance to all the Irish universities and most of the third level higher education institutions. Currently, the vast majority of students entering higher education in Ireland are selected on the basis of points attained in the Leaving Certificate. The minimum points requirement for various courses of study at university are laid down by the institutions and places are then allocated to students on the basis of merit.

11.2.2   Sectors in the Higher Education System

Traditionally, the higher education system in Ireland has comprised two sectors, the university sector including the recognised colleges and the colleges of education, and the technological sector, reflecting the binary structure of the system. All of these institutions are substantially funded by the State. In recent years, however, a number of independent private colleges have been established. These offer a range of courses, some of which are accredited by the relevant statutory body, while other private institutions offer degree courses that are validated by universities outside Ireland.

There are eight universities in Ireland. Four of these are now separate but linked institutions reflecting their former federal organisation within the National University of Ireland following the reconstitution of the sector by the Universities Act 1997. These four include:

- University College Dublin (UCD), the National University of Ireland, Dublin;
- University College Cork (UCC), the National University of Ireland, Cork;
- The National University of Ireland Maynooth (NUIM); and,
- University College Galway (UCG), the National University of Ireland, Galway.

The remaining four institutions comprise:

- The University of Dublin (Trinity College);
- Dublin City University (DCU);
- University of Limerick (UL); and,
- St. Patrick's College Maynooth (The Pontifical University).

The National University of Ireland also includes five separate recognised institutions:

- The Royal College of Surgeons in Ireland, (RCSI);
- National College of Art and Design, (NCAD);
- The Institute of Public Administration, (IPA);
- The Shannon College of Hotel Management; and,
- St. Angela's College of Education for Home Economics in Sligo.

These five institutions are designated recognised colleges. Courses and academic staff in these colleges are recognised by the NUI, which awards degrees to students who successfully complete recognised courses.

Trinity College Dublin (TCD), the first and only constituent college of the University of Dublin was founded in 1592 by Queen Elizabeth I. Three colleges for the education of primary school teachers and one college specialising in the education of teachers of home economics are associated with Trinity College. The University of Limerick was established in 1972 as the National Institute for Higher Education Limerick and Dublin City University was established in 1980 as the National Institute for Higher Education Dublin. Both institutions became universities in 1989 following the passing of amendments to the relevant legislation. There are two colleges of education; St Patrick's College, Drumcondra, and the Mater Dei Institute of Education associated with Dublin City University. Mary Immaculate College, Limerick, is similarly associated with the University of Limerick. St. Patrick's College Maynooth, which was founded in 1795, incorporated the national seminary for the education of Roman Catholic priests and the Pontifical University founded in 1896.

The third level institutions are associated with the National University of Ireland including the Royal College of Surgeons in Ireland, (RCSI); the National College of Art and Design, (NCAD) are designated recognised university colleges. The RCSI that was established in 1784 became a recognised college of the National University of Ireland in 1977. This College provides a full-time undergraduate degree course in Medicine together with specialist postgraduate training in the medical area. Institutionally, and in a similar manner to Trinity College Dublin, it has certain characteristics of a private institution.

Three of the eight colleges of education located throughout Ireland: Mater Dei Institute of Education, St. Angela's College of Education, and St. Catherine's College of Education for Home Economics, offer programmes leading to a teaching qualification for specialised subject areas at post primary school level. The five remaining Colleges of Education provide approved degree courses that lead to a BEd degree qualifying the successful candidate as a primary teacher. The Church of Ireland College of Education, Froebel College of Education, and Coláiste Mhuire, Marino, are associated with Trinity College Dublin. Mary Immaculate College of Education and St. Patrick's College of Education are associated with the University of Limerick and Dublin City University respectively. The undergraduate programmes in these colleges entitle successful candidates to the award of a BEd degree.

The National College of Art and Design (NCAD) which is a recognised college of NUI can trace its origins back to 1746. It provides a wide range of certificate, diploma, primary degree and graduate programmes including teacher education courses. The Institute of Public Administration (IPA) in its capacity as a recognised college of NUI offered degree and diploma courses some by distance education

The other major sector within the Irish third level education system involves the 14 institutes of technology which are located throughout Ireland and provide higher education to large numbers of students. These developed from the earlier Regional Technical Colleges (RTCs) which were established nation wide as part of the major expansion in third level education provision which occurred in the 1970s. (HEA, 2003). The largest IT, the Dublin Institute of Technology, (formally established under the Dublin Institute of Technology Act, 1992), has been granted the right to award degrees. This new institution incorporated seven existing institutions, covering a wide range of courses in such areas as Architecture, Technology, Marketing, Catering, Commerce and Music. In the past a considerable number of these courses had been offered at degree or professional qualification level.

As part of 1970s expansion in third level education provision the National Council for Education Awards (NCEA) was set up in 1971 with academic responsibility for the non-university third level sector. The Higher Education and Training Awards Council (HETAC) was established in 2001 as a national body under the Qualifications (Education and Training Act) 1999 to take on the role formerly the task of the NCEA. The HETAC is the validating body for most of the courses run by the Institutes of Technology and this body confers national certificates, diplomas and undergraduate and postgraduate degrees up to doctorate level.

11.2.3 Types of Degrees

The Irish universities and the Dublin Institute of Technology confer academic awards on successful students in their own colleges. Most non-university colleges receive academic qualifications at degree level from the Higher Education and Training Awards Council which also sets and monitors standards at all levels of higher education and training up to PhD level. Typically teaching at undergraduate level is by way of a programme of lectures supplemented by tutorials and, where appropriate, practical demonstration and laboratory work. Masters degrees are usually taken by course work, research work or some combination of both. Doctoral degrees are awarded on the basis of research.

Trinity College Dublin and the NUI Universities, UCD, UCC and NUIG offer undergraduate and postgraduate degree courses in Arts, Human Sciences, Commerce/ Business Studies, Science, Engineering and Medicine. In addition UCC offers courses in Dentistry, UCD offers courses in Veterinary Medicine and Architecture while NUI Maynooth provides programmes in Arts and Science. DCU offers courses in Business, Computing and Mathematical Sciences, Engineering and Design, Science and Health, Education and Humanities. The University of Limerick provides courses in Business, Education, Engineering, Humanities, Informatics and Electronics and Science. In general the provision of professional studies, particularly in the medical and associated areas is centred in Trinity College Dublin and the former university colleges of the NUI. The programmes of two new universities that were formerly National Institutes of Higher Education (DCU and UL) are concentrated (although not exclusively) in the sciences and technological areas. A number of courses leading to non-degree qualifications are available, usually confined to graduate students, in the universities.

The institutes of technology provide a comprehensive range of courses ranging from second-level craft apprenticeship programmes right through to two year National Certificate, three year National Diploma and four year degree programmes in the applied fields of Engineering, Science (including Computer Science), Business Studies and Humanities and postgraduate studies. In addition, these Institutes play an important role at regional level in providing for recurrent educational needs by way of part-time day and evening programmes. The DIT offers a broad range of courses covering Apprentice, Certificate, Diploma, Degree and Professional awards and is the validating body for its own awards. The provision of third-level part-time evening courses is a very important function of the DIT.

Table 1. Level and duration of qualifications in the non-university sector of the Irish third level education system

Type of award or degree	Duration of programme
One year certificate	One year full-time course
National certificate	Two year full time course
National diploma	One year post National Certificate. Three years in total
Graduate diploma	Usually a one year course. Designed for graduates seeking a vocational reorientation
Bachelor's degree	One year post National Certificate. Three years in total
Master's degree	One-two year(s) duration. Either by research or through a taught programme
Doctorate PhD	Three years or more of original research

Table 1 presents a broad outline of the courses of study at certificate, diploma, undergraduate and postgraduate degree level offered in institutions in the non-university sector of the Irish third level education system. The awards in question are most usually granted by bodies outside the institutions attended by the students; however, it should be noted that the Dublin Institute of Technology grants its own awards. While some of the courses offered are of pre-degree level they may, in certain circumstances entitle successful candidates to transfer with credit to one of the universities to complete a relevant course for a higher qualification. A similar initiative was announced by the National University of Ireland in its qualifications framework policy document relating to student access, progression and transfer.

These innovations, although not relating to degree level courses, are a significant development in that they anticipate a more widespread introduction of a credit system within higher level courses.

11.3   Accreditation and its Evaluation Framework

As has been pointed out, Irish universities award or confer degrees which are validated by these institutions themselves while the term accreditation refers to the recognition of academic qualifications by professional bodies as appropriate for membership of various professions. Most of the non-university third level institutions have their qualifications awarded by the Higher Education and Training Awards Council, the statutory body instituted by government for this purpose. One institution outside the university sector, the Dublin Institute of Technology has been granted the right by government to confer degrees and in some cases third level institutions outside the university sector have their degrees validated and awarded by one of the universities with which the institution in question has an association. No formal system for the accreditation or quality assessment of degrees at a national level is in place in Ireland, However, quality assessment does take place within various rubrics and both quality assurance and accountability are mandatory within the third level education system. In Ireland, Quality Assurance (QA) and the assessment of quality within QA is not focused on the degrees conferred by the university but rather on fostering a quality culture in all the activities of the institution.

The accreditation of degrees in the Irish universities is a matter for the institutions themselves as is the assurance of quality within the various departments of each university. Over the years serious attention has been paid to issues of quality and procedures, and structures have been developed in relation to these matters. Since the Report of the Commission on Higher Education (1967) which was followed by the establishment of the Higher Education Authority (in 1971) the importance of quality in higher education has grown. In some countries this trend followed a model involving direct state intervention and the institution of special quality assurance bodies. In Ireland, however, a 'more devolved model of self-regulation within a clear legislative framework' has been devised for the purpose. This was in accordance with the partnership model that has continued to typify policy development within the public sector in Ireland over recent years. The Conference of Heads of Irish Universities has been the body that has shaped policy and developed the area of quality improvement and quality assurance with the close collaboration of all the universities across the sector. The development of the self regulatory type of procedures that are now in place has been made possible by the provisions of the Universities Act, 1997, which guaranteed 'the autonomy of each university to determine its own quality assurance procedures free of the bureaucracy which has become associated with quality assurance procedures in other countries.'

While the regulation and formalisation of accreditation is in certain respects a novel development within the Irish universities, the assurance of the quality of degrees has always been undertaken in a serious and organised manner. The sector has traditionally utilised the services of international experts within the external examination system to ensure the quality of both the degrees and research activities of the institutions. This system involves an annual external quality review of primary and higher degrees by international experts who act as assessors. In 2002, over 90 experts from 16 different countries examined and reported on all aspects of degree programmes including assessment procedures in each department within the Irish university system. In addition external agencies and professional bodies grant recognition to a number of university degrees through a process of continuous monitoring and review. At a less formal but nonetheless important level the system of peer review of research publication and the peer assessment of applications for research funding are important elements of the Irish university system. The fact that a major criterion of suitability for academic appointment, tenure and promotion is a candidate's research record is indicative of the importance of peer evaluation. This is established on the basis of scholarly publications in refereed academic journals that have achieved a creditable standing in the Citation index.

11.3.1   Quality Assurance in Irish Third Level Education: Current Developments and Procedures

Section 35 of the Universities Act (1997), requires the Chief Officer of the university to establish procedures for quality assurance aimed at improving the quality of education and related services provided by the university. This section of the Act with its emphasis on quality improvement and on university autonomy provides the framework for the achievement of this goal. While the Higher Education Authority has a monitoring function in relation to quality assurance and quality improvement (QA/QI), the duty of operationalising the scheme in each university lies with Chief Officer and the Governing Authority of the university itself. University College Dublin was one of the first universities to develop new Quality Assurance/Quality Improvement procedures under the recent Irish legislation and its lead has been followed by the other institutions. The procedures developed by UCD include the establishment of a QA Office and the appointment of a Director and a Standing Committee on Quality by the Academic Council of the university. The mission statement of the Quality Assurance Office outlines the rationale and values that underpin the operation that is documented fully.

> The Quality Assurance Office is dedicated to enhancing the quality of all aspects of the work of the University through co-operation with staff and students as they interact with one another for the advancement of teaching, learning and research. Our activities are based on respect for the individual, on fair and equal treatment of all col-

leagues and on gaining the respect of the University community through the quality of our own work.

The evaluation process for academic departments in University College Dublin is based on EU methodology and refined by the experience gained during the three-year pilot project involving ten departments that had volunteered to participate. The evaluation included a self assessment report prepared, in consultation with all staff in the department; and included an evaluation by students as required by the Universities Act 1997, 35(2). Follow-up was an integral part of the process and each reviewed department is provided with a Quality Improvement Plan (QIP) based on the self-assessment report and the peer review report. The QIP includes proposals for implementing improvements relating to the following organisational and administrative matters, shortcomings in services, procedures and facilities, inadequate staffing facilities and other resources. The original five-year plan for the review of academic departments has been extended to ten years by which time, in 2008, the academic departments will have been reviewed.

The aim of the QA/QI process in UCD is to provide a framework within the university that can work toward achieving the goal of a quality culture. The other universities have adopted similar procedures and structures. University College Cork (UCC, NUI,C) has appointed the Quality Promotion Unit to operate QA/QI in the institution and similar developments have been put in place throughout the sector. The growing approval of the way QA/QI has been developed within the sector is due the democratic nature of the model that reflects the idea of partnership advocated in the National Development Plan 2000–2006. While the universities have institutional autonomy they are subject both to the Higher Education Authority which has responsibility for monitoring policy matters, accountability quality assurance and budgetary allocation, and to the Universities Act (1997) and other relevant legislation such as the Freedom of Information Act (2000).

Accreditation within the institutes of technology and issues related to QA are subject to the conditions laid down in the Qualifications (Education and Training) Act, 1999. This Act provided for the setting up of the National Qualifications Authority of Ireland to establish and maintain a framework of qualifications, to act as the overall guarantor of the quality of awards and to facilitate and promote access, transfer and progression. As a result the Further Education and Training Awards Council and the Higher Education and Training Awards Council was set up to provide certification within the framework of qualifications. The latter is the validating body for most of the courses run by the ITs and confers National Certificates, Diplomas and Degrees up to doctorate level. HETAC/DIT Diploma or Certificate holders may, in certain circumstances, be able to transfer to the Universities to complete courses for a higher qualification.

The 1999 Act heralded an important difference in the assessment of degree and diploma courses in the non-university sector of Irish higher education. The HETAC and formerly its predecessor the NCEA were responsible for the appointment of external examiners for their courses for which they were the validating body. That arrangement is no longer in place from the beginning of the academic year 2004 in accordance with section 23 and section 28 of the Qualifications (Education and Training) Act 1999. From 2004 the responsibility to establish procedures for both the assessment of learners and quality assurance is to be devolved to the providers in question. This is similar to the protocols in operation in the Higher Education Authority institutions.

The development of a national framework of qualifications setting out arrangements for access, transfer and progression for learners is a key feature of the Act. Thus each learner will be able to determine her or his own educational goals and see how they can be fulfilled. This will make achieving educational and training goals a continuing and lifelong ambition. All Irish awards are included in the national framework of qualifications maintained by the National Qualifications Authority of Ireland. In 1999 a similar initiative by the National University of Ireland relating to its diploma and certificate courses was announced. This innovation was undertaken in response to the 'need for the greater integration of all the University's awards and for the promotion of the concept of a ladder of qualifications that would be compatible with developing structures outside the University and specifically with the National Framework'.

The National Framework of Qualifications was designed to be a single, nationally and internationally accepted certification structure covering all extra-university third level courses. It also includes all further and continuing education, and training programmes must be strategically placed between the second level and university qualifications systems. The purpose of this holistic approach is to ensure that access and progression into higher education are made flexible and amenable to those who had heretofore found such access or progression difficult if not impossible.

The Qualifications (Education and Training) Act, 1999, stipulates that the standards set for awards are informed by internationally accepted best practice and brings the operation of the National Academic Recognition Information Centre (NARIC) under the umbrella of the National Qualifications Authority (NQA). Founded 20 years ago, NARIC is the official body for the regulation and recognition of higher education diplomas that are awarded on completion of professional education courses of at least three years. In this way it is envisaged that NARIC, in co-operation with similar bodies in other countries, will also facilitate the integration the education systems throughout Europe.

11.3.2 Time Span and Scope of Procedures

The time-span and scope of procedures related to accreditation and quality assessment varies throughout the third level education system although certain features, most notably those related to frequency and transparency, are common throughout third level education. The system of external examination of degrees operates annually and involves the inspection and assessment of course work, the examination procedures and the standards achieved by candidates for degrees. Typically, an oral assessment (including practical tests where appropriate) of a representative selection of degree candidates by the external assessor form part of the external examination system.

Proposals to institute a new degree or qualification within the university sector involve lengthy procedures. The academic standards and the need for the new course must be examined at departmental, faculty and academic council level within the university. With individual departments in competition for scarce resources and funding, the proposals for establishment of new courses must be accompanied by a certified impact statement detailing the costing implications. Currently, proposals that are not self-funding are not considered except in the exceptional circumstance in which an outside body guarantees to provide the financial resources necessary.

Apart from these considerations a number of features that derive from recent legislation have implications for the maintenance of standards and accountability within the higher education system. The Freedom of Information Act (1999), which applies to the education system, provides for a measure of public accountability. At an individual level this legislation also gives students the right to view the papers they presented for examination and the institutions have appeals procedures in place to deal with any alleged injustice in assessment. The most powerful role related to rewards and sanctions in the university sector lies with the Higher Education Authority which has the responsibility for reviewing the strategic development and the quality assurance procedures of the institutions. When viewed in conjunction with its monitoring responsibility and its annual role in allocating governmental funding its power is of major significance.

11.4 Accreditation in Higher Education: Main Actors and Procedures

11.4.1 The State

State involvement in accreditation and evaluation within the Irish higher education system is not based on direct intervention. Proximate and immediate matters concerning the operation of the third level education system are delegated to the statutory bodies instituted for the purpose. More broadly based policy matters are developed following extensive consultations with the relevant stakeholders in the system.

This practice is in accordance with the partnership model that has been the basis for policy development within the public sector in Ireland. Widespread discussions such as those during the National Convention on Education, 1994, and the Commission on the Points System, 1998, are typical of the consultative process in the partnership model.

The state is the main provider of funding and resources for the Irish higher education system and this provision is made through the Higher Education Authority to the university sector and similarly through the Higher Education and Training Awards Council to the institutes of technology. The functions of these statutory bodies include the monitoring of the system in terms of both quality assurance and standards.

11.4.2 The Higher Education Authority

The Higher Education Authority is the planning and development body for higher education in Ireland. It was set up on an ad hoc basis in 1968, and was given statutory powers in the Higher Education Authority Act 1971. The Authority has wide advisory powers throughout the whole of the third level education sector. In addition it is the funding authority for the universities and a number of designated institutions. Its principal functions are:

- to further the development of higher education;
- to maintain a continuous review of the demand and need for higher education;
- to assist in the co-ordination of state investment in higher education and to prepare proposals for such investment;
- to allocate among universities and designated institutions the grants voted by the *Oireachtas*;
- to promote the attainment of equality of opportunity in higher education and democratisation of higher education.

The Authority was given additional responsibilities under the Universities' Act, 1997. These include reviewing the following:

- University strategic development plans;
- University quality assurance procedures;
- University equal opportunity policies and their implementation.

The legislation also charged the Higher Education Authority with the tasks of 'advising the Minister for Education on the establishment of new institutions of higher education; continually reviewing the demand for higher education; and making recommendations on the provision and distribution of places for students throughout the national system of higher education.' A major function of the HEA is the overseeing of the financial operation of universities and colleges and the seeing of the financial operation of universities and colleges and the distribution of government funding within the sector.

The extension of the remit of the Higher Education Authority, initially suggested in the Government White Paper of 1995 and contained in the Universities Act of 1997 include:

> advising the Minister in relation to higher education policy generally across the whole sector, and on specific issues; overall responsibility for the operational decisions arising from the implementation of agreed policies, including budgetary allocations to the colleges; ensuring that all higher education institutions put into effect policies which promote equality of access, participation and benefit ...; ensuring ... a balance of level, type and variety of programmes among the various institutions ...; ensuring that systems and processes are in place which will facilitate the necessary public accountability and provide for the evaluation of cost-effectiveness ...; ensuring that quality assurance procedures are in place in all institutions and ... are monitored; promoting links between institutions, society and the economy.

This extension of the functions of the HEA, in particular the linking of the responsibility for policy matters, budgetary allocations, accountability, the evaluation of cost effectiveness and the monitoring of quality assurance procedures in one body gives that body a very powerful role within the third level sector.

11.4.3 The Higher Education and Training Awards Council

The Higher Education and Training Awards Council is the statutory body responsible for the co-ordination, development and promotion of higher education outside the universities. It approves courses and confers degrees, diplomas, certificates and other educational awards. It sets and monitors standards in the colleges and, through it, a transfer network operates whereby students can move from Certificate to Diploma to Degree level depending on examination performance. Qualifications awarded by this body are internationally recognised by academic, professional, trade and craft bodies. Apart from the Institutes of Technology, HETAC has a range of designated institutions including national institutions such as the National College of Ireland (NCI) and a wide range of religious and other private colleges.

11.4.4 Professional Bodies

A number of the professional areas of study in third level education are regulated by professional bodies, some of which have a legal charter. While some of these bodies provide courses of study which they assess themselves, others validate or accredit the degrees awarded to students by one of the universities or institutes of technology as suitable for entry to the profession in question. Legal studies leading to an academic award are provided by the universities. Such courses, however, are academic and while they may be the first steps in a legal career, they do not entitle the recipient to professional accreditation. Legal studies leading to a professional qualification in Ireland are provided by two bodies, The Honorable Society of King's Inns, and the Law Society of Ireland. These bodies are responsible for professional training in one of the branches of the two-tier legal system. The courses run by the Honorable Society of King's Inns lead to the professional qualification of barrister-at-law, while the courses run by the Law Society of Ireland lead to qualifications enabling the holder to practise as a solicitor.

The more usual practice for entry to the professions is for professional bodies to give recognition or validation to a degree awarded by an academic body. This applies in a number of areas including architecture, engineering, nursing, psychology, teaching, and social work. The usual practice is for the professional body in question to set up an accreditation committee for a degree for which recognition is requested by the awarding institution. If the degree is assessed as a suitable entry qualification for the profession, accreditation is given and the course in question is monitored annually by the professional body to ensure the maintenance of standards. Some of the professional bodies involved in this process are nationally based while others are European or international bodies.

11.4.5   International Actors

International and EU involvement in the accreditation process is customary rather than subject to regulation or legislation. The practice of external examination of degrees by international experts is a time-honoured practice in Irish universities. Further, student and staff exchanges under the various EU programmes such as Erasmus and Comenius have necessitated the provision of courses of a comparable standard to that in other EU countries. Apart from these institutionally based considerations the fact that many Irish graduates find appointments in other countries means that their qualifications are accepted internationally. However, as in other countries, further progress is required in developing equivalencies between programmes to facilitate inter institutional developments.

11.5   Developments and Current Trends in the Area of Evaluation During the Last Two Decades

During the last two decades in Ireland there has been a growing impetus to codify and regulate the provision of higher education both in the university sector and in the institutes of technology and other institutions. The changes that have been introduced involve legislative provision and the setting up of new and the strengthening of existing statutory bodies. These changes have occurred, in part, as a result of the growing numbers of students taking part in third level studies and the consequent funding requirement on the exchequer to fund the system. Alongside the gradual massification of Irish third level education the growing closer association between countries in the European Union and the effects of globalisation generally have signalled a need for a process of standardisation. Such a system would facilitate the establishment of equivalencies, similar to those existing between qualifications at post primary or second level education. The Irish government and the universities and other institutions have indicated their acceptance of such developments in their co-operation with the initiatives associated with the Bologna Declaration.

Within the university sector significant developments in the area of evaluation involve the recent legislation codifying the role and functions of the university and the establishment and strengthening of the HEA as the body with the remit reviewing the demand and need for higher education together with the allocation of the monies voted by government among universities and designated institutions. This conjunction of the functions of the monitoring of the universities; the allocation of funding; the review of each university's strategic development plan; and the co-ordination of state investment in higher education in one statutory Authority gives that body a pivotal role in relation to evaluation (Higher Education Act, Universities Act 1997).

Within the non-university sector the major development in the area of evaluation has been the passing into law of the Qualifications (Education and Training) Act 1999. This act provides for the setting up of the National Qualification Authority of Ireland (NQAI) for the purpose of establishing and maintaining a framework of qualifications, acting as the overall guarantor of the quality of awards and facilitating and promoting access, transfer and progression. This Act also provided for the setting up in the following year of the Higher Education and Training Awards Council (HETAC) and the Further Education and Training Awards Council (FETAC) to provide certification within the framework of qualifications.

While FETAC is concerned with the non-higher education provision within the post second level sector, its linkage with HETAC under the NQAI is a significant development in relation to higher education. The qualifications provided by the institutions accredited by FETAC will, as part of the national framework of qualification, provide students with access, transfer and progression routes to both further qualifications and higher education as appropriate. This ensures that the national framework of qualifications will function as the accepted certification structure covering all extra-university third level, and all further and continuing education and training programme at post second level education.

11.6   Accreditation and the Internationalisation of Higher Education: Range of Activities, Level of Involvement

The Bologna Declaration has sign-posted an era of increased emphasis on both quality assurance and standards so as to facilitate the comparability of qualifications throughout Europe. The 1999 declaration gave a commitment to the promotion of European co-operation in quality assurance as a basis for developing 'comparable criteria and methodologies.' The authorities of universities throughout Europe, including the European University Association (EUA) and 32 rectors' conferences have supported the development of quality benchmarks for their institutions. To meet the challenges for Irish universities the Conference of Heads of Irish Universities has proposed a Framework for Quality in Irish Universities and issued guidelines for implementing quality assurance and quality improvement. This has been supplemented by the establishment of the Irish Universities Quality Board (IUQB).

One of the most urgent of the Bologna Declaration provisions for Irish third level institutions is student mobility. Governments and institutions are required to remove obstacles to student mobility, according to the Declaration. This means that the European Credit Transfer System which is now widespread in Ireland must be extended to allow for credit transfer as well as credit accumulation.

Issues relating to accreditation cannot be viewed in isolation but rather must be examined within the changing landscape of the sector as an entity with interlocking and interdependent parts. In Ireland both the government and the stakeholders in the system have been concerned that while the last decade was marked by a continuous growth in student numbers, current projections suggest that the number of students leaving post primary schools will decrease by 35 % in the coming decade. Further, concern has been expressed that the attrition rate among students, which can exceed 30 %, is an indication that colleges are not meeting the needs of students. This is likely to result in surplus capacity across a sector that may have difficulty in responding to changing demand. To combat this, and to deal with other problematic factors recent policy initiatives in Irish third level education have focused on integrating planning and on making the system more responsive to regulation and control by governmental agencies and statutory bodies which operate within the system.

The climate of opinion among policy makers in Ireland has been changing in recent years; this is evident from the nature and type of policy documents not only from official sources including the Department of Education and Science and the statutory bodies but from the institutions themselves. The emphasis is no longer on third level education as being of value in itself and as the right of all students. Rather, it is viewed as an important, if indirect, input into the future economic growth and prosperity of society and as a right that carries duties and responsibilities. These and other indicators of change are highlighted in the Skilbeck Report, which was commissioned by the Higher Education Authority and published in the first years of the 21st century. Professor Skilbeck formerly was the Deputy Director for Education, OECD. This report does not advocate a pre-eminent cultural role for the university in Ireland but rather applies the language of commercial activity to the sector. The report argues that universities should attract funds from a variety of sources while focusing on improving quality and 'value for money'. It also identifies the need for greater flexibility in the system to facilitate responsiveness to changing demands and needs.

The development of a transparent system of assessment and marking, cross-disciplinary courses and cross-institutional arrangements are recommended by the Skilbeck Report. Such developments at local level would serve to facilitate co-operative endeavours between universities in different countries and pave the way for some of the aspirations noted in the Bologna Declaration. However, although some of the Skilbeck proposals are not without merit, they are embedded in procedures and structures with slight reference to cultural and socio-political values. Facing University Challenges: An IFUT View asserts that the arguments presented by the report overemphasise the short-term economic challenges and are based on a narrow view of the university – that of an educational business responsive to the marketplace.

The future focus of higher education in Ireland may well be largely determined by economic considerations and by the forces of globalisation. Perhaps the most far-reaching proposal suggested in the Skilbeck Report, and the one most pertinent to the future role of Irish universities is the recommendation that the institutions recreate themselves. It is suggested that they should do this by broadening their horizons, enhancing their power and capabilities and becoming global players. This suggests that not all universities are sufficiently well placed to enter the highly competitive global market and consequently, some institutions may be more suitably placed within a local and regional context. The focus of such regional institutions should be the building of partnerships with local industry and community and they should have as their primary target the growth and development of the region. The other universities with the capability of following the global course as a competitive force should focus on 'selling such services as undergraduate and post graduate places and consultancies on the global market as Australia, Japan, Switzerland and the UK among others no do so successfully'. This recommendation seems to suggest that the future for Irish third level education depends on the ability of the system to exploit the world market for services as envisioned in the General Agreement on Trade and Services.

This suggestion that the Irish university sector should subdivide into two strands with two markedly different functions would, if put into practice, have major policy implications. While this suggestion is not emanating from governmental sources *per se* it is very significant in that it comes from a report published by the Higher Education Authority, the statutory body whose functions include the monitoring and funding arrangements for the sector and the Conference of Heads of Irish Universities. The division of the university sector in terms of function and focus and the need for all institutions 'to demonstrate maximum efficiency, ability to generate resources and a readiness to reform' is proposed as a response to the challenges of modernisation and more particularly to globalisation. The emphasis on this aspect of developments within the sector would seem to indicate that the major stakeholders in the university sector not only favour globalisation but also are ready to recommend strategies for dealing with it.

The climate of opinion among the policy makers and stakeholders regarding the role and functions of the university is currently undergoing major change. The emphasis is no longer on education as of value in itself and the vision of the university as advanced by Newman in the nineteenth century seems to have faded. The representatives of government and the university authorities are in agreement on the need for change and the direction in which change should occur. The Skilbeck Report stresses the responsibility of the university to contribute to the future economic growth and prosperity of society. Skilbeck proposes that third level institutions continually appraise the quality of their teaching, research and service roles and set standards based on international benchmarking for their future development within an increasingly global environment. These views were echoed by Dr Roger Downer, President of the University of Limerick, who emphasised the vital role that universities must play in shaping tomorrow's world in his speech on behalf of Conference of Heads of Irish Universities. These views were also echoed by Dr Don Thornhill, Director of the Higher Education Authority, who stressed that universities must accept that new strategies are inevitable if universities are to remain competitive and relevant to Ireland of the 21st century. The intended result of such policy proposals would seem to be the standardisation, integration of structures and procedures and the systemisation of accountability measures within an increasingly globalised third level education system.

12   Italy: Accreditation in Progress. Autonomy, Minimum Standards, Quality Assurance

CARLO FINOCCHIETTI & SILVIA CAPUCCI

12.1   The National System of Higher Education in Italy

12.1.1   Size of the System

Italian higher education is organised in a binary system: university education, and non-university education. The university sector consists of 77 institutions subdivided into two main categories: state universities (63 institutions) and non-state universities legally recognised by the competent State authority (14 institutions). The university population currently is 1,800,000 students.

The non-university sector covers, first, higher education institutions for music, dance, figurative and applied arts (fine art academies, national academies for dance and drama, national school for cinema, music conservatories, higher institutes for applied arts). Next, there is higher integrated technical education and training (IFTS programmes). The sector also comprises second level professional programmes under the responsibility of the Regions. Finally, there is higher education for languages (interpreters and translators).

12.1.2   Outcomes of the Bologna Declaration: Reforms of Higher Education Cycles and Qualifications

The main purpose of the 1999 reform was to endow all higher education institutions – and above all universities – with greater teaching autonomy, which was unprecedented in the Italian educational tradition. With reference to the university sector, the 1999 reform has now been fully implemented. Universities autonomously define the teaching rules of their degree programmes in their institutional teaching regulations *(Regolamento Didattico di Ateneo*, RDA); in particular, the RDA determines the name and the educational objectives of each degree programme, the general framework of the teaching activities to be included in the curriculum, the number of credits to be attributed to each teaching activity, and the modality of the final degree examination.

S. Schwarz and D.F. Westerheijden (eds.),
Accreditation and Evaluation in the European Higher Education Area, 251–274.
© 2004 *Kluwer Academic Publishers. Printed in the Netherlands.*

In conformity with the objectives of the Bologna Declaration, the 1999 university reform has also defined the new architecture of the system. Italian university studies are now organised in three cycles.

The *first cycle* (undergraduate studies) consists of one type of degree programme, called *Corsi di Laurea* (CL), which aims at providing undergraduate students with an adequate command of general scientific methods and contents as well as specific professional skills. Access is based on the Italian school leaving qualification, which is awarded after passing the relevant state examinations, following completion of 13 years of schooling; equivalent foreign qualifications may also be accepted. Admission to individual degree programmes may be subject to specific course requirements. First degree programmes last for three years. The first degree *(Laurea,* L) is awarded to undergraduates who have earned 180 credits.

The *second cycle* (graduate studies) includes three types of degree programmes: *Corsi di Laurea Specialistica*, CLS; *Corsi di Specializzazione di 1° livello*, CS1, and *Corsi di Master Universitario di 1° livello*, CMU1.

CLS are aimed at providing graduates with an advanced level of education for the exercise of a highly qualified professional activity in specific areas. Access to CLS is based on the Italian first degree (L) or an equivalent foreign qualification; its length is two years. The degree, *Laurea Specialistica*, LS (second degree), is awarded to graduates who have earned a global amount of 300 credits, including those of the first degree that have been recognised for access to the CLS (maximum 180); it is also compulsory to write an original dissertation. A limited number of CLS regulated by specific EU directives (dentistry, medicine, veterinary medicine) share the following features: the educational requirement for access is the Italian school leaving diploma or an equivalent foreign qualification; admission is always subject to entrance exams; courses last for five years, except medicine which takes six years.

CS1 are devised to provide the knowledge and abilities needed for the practice of a few specialised or highly qualifying professions (e.g. teaching, legal professions); they may be established exclusively in application of specific Italian laws or EU directives. Access is by a *Laurea* (first degree) or an equivalent foreign degree; admission is subject to the passing of a competitive examination; the course length varies between two and three years. The *Diploma di Specializzazione di 1° livello*, DS1 (first level specialisation degree) is conferred to graduates who have earned 300 to 360 credits, including those of the first degree that have been recognised for access to the CS1.

CMU1 are advanced scientific programmes or continuing education courses open to the holders of a *Laurea*, L, or an equivalent foreign degree; admission may be subject to additional conditions. The course lasts for a minimum of one year. The *Mas-*

ter Universitario di 1° livello, MU1 (first level university master), is awarded to graduates who have earned at least 60 credits.

Third cycle degree courses (postgraduate studies) consist of *Corsi di Dottorato di Ricerca*, CDR (research doctorate programmes); *Corsi di Specializzazione di 2° livello*, CS2 (second level specialisation programmes); *Corsi di Master Universitario di 2° livello*, CMU2 (second level university master programmes).

CDR aim at training postgraduates for very advanced scientific research or for very high professional appointments; they envisage the use of suitable teaching methodologies such as updated technologies, study periods abroad, internships in specialised research centres. Access is based on an Italian second degree (LS) or an equivalent foreign degree; admission is subject to passing very competitive exams; the official length of studies is at least three years; the writing of an original dissertation is necessary to obtain the third degree called *Dottorato di Ricerca*, DR (research doctorate).

CS2s provide postgraduates with the knowledge and skills required to exercise highly specialised professions (e.g. medical specialities); they may be established exclusively in application of specific Italian laws or EU directives. Access is through an LS (second degree) or an equivalent foreign degree; admission is subject to a competitive examination; the course normally lasts for one year, except for all the CS2s of the health sector which may take up to five years.

CMU2s are advanced scientific programmes or continuing education courses that are open to holders of an LS or of an equivalent foreign degree; admission may be subject to additional conditions. Studies take at least one year. The degree *(Master Universitario di 2° livello*, MU2) is awarded to postgraduates who have earned a minimum of 60 credits.

Finally, the reform included the adoption of the Diploma Supplement (DS) and of a national credit system based on the ECTS. Therefore, Italian degree programmes are now structured in credits (CFU = *crediti formativi universitari)*; a university credit corresponds to 25 hours of work, including personal study. The average annual workload of a fulltime student is fixed at 60 credits.

12.1.3 Governance of the University System: From Centralisation to Autonomy

In the last decade, there have been substantial developments in terms of distribution of power in the management of university education. The first important step towards decentralisation was made in 1989, when the Ministry for Universities and Scientific and Technological Research (MURST) was established as a separate entity from the Ministry of Education with a view to further promote the two sectors of university education and scientific research by attributing their co-ordination to the same authority. One of the purposes of this reform was to separate the responsibility for decisions in matters of university policy, entrusted to MURST, from their actual management, a task attributed to individual universities and research bodies. Another objective was the implementation of university autonomy. At the end of this reform process, MURST merged once again with the Ministry of Education to form the present Ministry of Education, University and Research (MIUR).

A second significant development was the transfer of power from the central government to individual universities. Full institutional autonomy was gradually achieved through a series of legislative acts: statutory and operational autonomy was sanctioned by Law 168 of 1989, financial autonomy by Law 537 of 1993, autonomy for the recruitment of the teaching staff by Law 210 of 1998, and finally teaching autonomy by ministerial decree 509 of 1999.

A third important change consisted in the transfer of normative and regulative powers from Parliament to the Government by means of provisions leading to deregulation, power delegation, the decentralisation of functions, and administrative simplification.

The fourth important modification took place in the organs representing the different components of the academic community as well as in the advisory bodies assisting the Minister in matters of university policy. Most were reformed or newly established (e.g. National University Council, Italian University Rectors' Conference, National Council of University Students, National Committee for the Evaluation of the University System).

Concerning the management of the system, the most significant innovation was undoubtedly the gradual decentralisation of competences from the central government to individual institutions. This has resulted in a shift from a type of management based on strong ministerial authority to a new model in which the central government has yielded all operational powers to universities, even though it retains some financial and policy responsibilities. Universities have increased their power over the management of operational processes and achieved full autonomy (statutory, financial, didactic, staff recruiting).

12.2   Accreditation, Approval and Evaluation

12.2.1   Why Programme Accreditation?

In Italy, the system of accreditation of university degree programmes was launched in 2001. On the one hand, universities had just designed the new degree programmes and were applying to the state for funding. On the other, in order to allocate funds efficiently, the Ministry of Education (MIUR) asked the National Committee for the

Evaluation of the University System (CNVSU) in order to elaborate a scheme of programme accreditation. Only accredited programmes would obtain ministerial financial support.

As a consequence, two distinct but correlated procedures came simultaneously into being: one for formal approval of new university curricula (see section 12.2.3), and one for the accreditation of the programmes themselves, after checking if they met the minimum quality standards (see below).

12.2.2 Accreditation of Degree Programmes: CNVSU's Proposal

In its proposal, CNVSU adopted the definition of accreditation proposed in the 2001 CRE report: 'Accreditation is a formal, published statement regarding the quality of an institution or a programme, following a cyclical evaluation based on agreed standards'. If we analyse that definition, the essential feature of accreditation is evidently the need to pre-determine the requirements that are unanimously regarded as indispensable ('agreed standards') to guarantee the desirable quality levels. It is useful, therefore, to adopt a system of 'cyclical evaluation' based on quantifiable, verifiable and representative indicators. Eventually, the publication of the evaluation outcomes ('published statement') aims to provide an explicit, substantial – and not purely formal – acknowledgement of the qualitative levels ascertained.

The objectives of the Italian system of programme accreditation have been determined as follows:

• reduce auto-referential elements as well as the merely bureaucratic respect of the formal requirements typical of the Italian system centred on the legal validity of study qualifications;

• create a system of clear information and transparent, verifiable guarantees on the qualitative standards of individual study programmes; this objective leads to greater rationality in the choices made by those subjects that apply to the university system from the outside as interested actors: the students and their families who have to decide how and where to invest in education, as well as companies, industries and bodies, both private and public, that need graduates.

• contribute to a competitive system that can operate fairly within a university context that is characterised by a wide and diversified educational offer; actually, this could cause the risk of the distribution of misleading information on very different programmes bearing the same denomination or on very similar courses with different names;

• promote within individual institutions a constant process for quality improvement by sensitising all actors involved to the necessity to verify regularly the consistency of pre-determined objectives, allocated resources, organisational commitment, educational outcomes.

CNVSU's working plan provided for two subsequent implementation phases. First, a starting phase – pre-accreditation – in which the minimum standards were determined in terms of resources for an institution to offer sound education in the different classes of degree programmes, and, within individual classes, in each programme (number of teachers, their qualification, number and sizes of classrooms, libraries, laboratories, etc.). The second phase of accreditation also had to consider the minimum standards in terms of the qualitative characteristics of the education process and of its outcome in terms of graduates.

12.2.3   The Approval of Degree Programmes

The procedure for the approval of university degree programmes is articulated in the four phases outlined below.

Phase 1 – Drawing up of University Teaching Regulations (RDA)

Individual institutions codify the rules for the organisation of the teaching of their degree courses in the *Regolamenti Didattici di Ateneo* (RDAs). University teaching regulations and their amendments are issued by rectoral decree. Each RDA determines:

- the names and objectives of the degree programmes and the numbers and definitions of the respective classes;
- the general framework of the educational activities to be included in the curricula;
- the number of credits to be attributed to each educational activity;
- the main features of the final examinations for the different degrees.

In conformity with the University's statutes, RDAs also regulate the organisational aspects of the teaching work that is common to all degree programmes. In particular they define:

- objectives, times and modalities for the competent authorities to jointly provide for planning, co-ordination and control of the outcomes of the different educational activities;
- the procedures concerning university teachers' and researchers' annual teaching duties, including integrative activities, guidance and tutoring;
- the procedures concerning the organisation of tests, subject examinations, and the final degree examination;
- modalities for the assessment of students' performance; the grading scales are 18-30 (subject exams) and 66-110 (degree examination); the highest grades (30 and 110 respectively) may be followed by a special distinction *(lode)*;

- the evaluation of the initial education of the students to be admitted to first and second cycle degree programmes (CL and CLS respectively);
- the organisation of educational activities for the evaluation of the initial education of students to be admitted to CL as well as those related to additional educational obligations;
- the setting up of a university service for the co-ordination of all guidance activities to be carried out in co-operation with upper secondary schools, and of a tutorial service for all students in each degree programme;
- the introduction of specific organisational modalities for teaching part-time students;
- the procedures to determine the university structure or person responsible for each educational activity;
- the evaluation of the quality of all activities;
- the ways to make both procedures and decisions public;
- the rules for the awarding of joint degrees.

The RDAs also determine the modalities according to which individual institutions must issue the Diploma Supplement. In conformity with the Lisbon Convention of 1997, it registers the main information on the specific curriculum completed by students to obtain that degree.

Phase 2 – Teaching Regulations of Degree Programmes (RDC)

The teaching regulations of each degree programme *(Regolamento Didattico di Corso di studio,* RDC) are determined by the competent teaching structure in compliance with the RDA, taking into account the respect of freedom of teaching and of teachers' and students' rights and duties. Individual RDCs define the organisation of the respective degree programmes. In particular, each RDC determines:

- the list of curricular subjects with the subject areas of reference; it also specifies all other educational activities and, if necessary, the modular structure of certain subjects;
- specific educational objectives, credits, and those subjects or other educational activities that may be propaedeutic;
- curricula offered to students; the rules are also laid for students to submit their individual study plans, if necessary;
- the typology of available teaching/learning activities, distance education included, exams, and other ways of assessing students' performance;
- provisions regulating attendance, when compulsory.

Phase 3 – Consultations and Approvals

The proposal a new programme must be accompanied by the opinions and supporting motivations of advisory bodies. First, the *University Evaluation Unit* gives its opinion on available resources and their congruence with the objectives of the programme.

The *Regional Co-ordinating Committee* (CRC) then advises on proposals for new programmes. The CRC is made up of the rectors of the universities in the same Region, the president of the Regional Council and a student representative. The CRC also co-ordinates initiatives in such matters as the planning of access to university studies, student guidance and welfare services, advanced professional education, lifelong and recurrent education, and the use of university facilities. Moreover, the CRC co-ordinates relations between the university system and the school system, the education institutions of the Region and the economic and social representatives of that territory.

The *employers'* advice is also compulsory. Universities must consult local organisations representing industries, services and the professions to check the congruency of the educational proposals with the economic needs of the regional territory and the occupational opportunities that may be realistically offered to future graduates.

The *National University Council* (CUN) must check the proposals to determine whether they correspond to the compulsory curricular content according to the decrees approving the various degree classes and the teaching activities provided for by the RDA (university teaching regulations). The CUN may either approve the proposal or ask the university authorities to reconsider their proposal.

Finally, the office for university autonomy and students' affairs of the Ministry of Education (MIUR) examines the proposals, checks their procedural correctness, the compulsory advisory opinions, and issues the decrees approving the respective university teaching regulations.

Phase 4 – Approval of RDAs

Once this process of consultations and control has been completed, the rectors of individual institutions approve the university teaching regulations. The RDAs are the internal legal basis to launch new degree programmes.

12.2.4   Minimum Standards for Accreditation

These are the aims that are agreed upon and the criteria that are adopted in the evaluation of the resources which are regarded as indispensable for the accreditation of new study programmes.

Objectives of the control of minimum standards:

- Ensure all students (and their families) that each university has the resources necessary to support its educational offer.
- Through the dissemination of information to those concerned, guarantee that the educational offer of each institution is transparent and can be compared with that of other universities.
- Check the congruence between the supply, the demand for education, and available resources.
- Allow both MIUR and universities to allocate available resources efficiently through specific incentives and disincentives.

General evaluation criteria:

- One credit (CFU) must include approximately eight hours of 'front' teaching.
- Different reference dimensions have been identified with respect to students who enrol in the degree programmes of the various classes.
- Each permanent teacher normally covers 120 teaching hours in the classroom. It is assumed that such a teaching engagement is mainly (50 %) for the *Laurea* programmes (first cycle) – E.g.: 60 hours x CL + 40 hours x CLS + 20 x CDR, master courses, etc.
- The subjects in which available teachers are competent must be consistent with the profiles offered in terms of number of credits assigned to 'basic', 'qualifying', 'similar/integrative' educational activities.
- University facilities (classrooms, labs, etc.) must be adequate for all enrolled students (full-time, part-time).

Variables used:

- Programmes offered by the Faculties (due to the transformation of already existing programmes and to the setting up of new ones).
- Enrolled students.
- Permanent teachers available in the different subject areas.
- Usable facilities (classrooms, laboratories, libraries).

Calculation of adequate student numbers:

- Full-time students are usually expected to have an average workload of 60 credits per year, corresponding to at least 1,500 hours. The institution must guarantee teaching services at least to the amount determined in the decrees that approved the degree classes (generally corresponding to 650-750 hours per year).

- Part-time students are required to engage in an average workload that corresponds to the number of credits for which they enrolled (less than 60). The teaching load for the educational activities reserved for such students (whose proportion will remain limited) is determined accordingly as the proportion of the 60 credits required from full-time students.

Diversified dimensions of degree programmes of the different classes: On the basis of preliminary analyses of the data concerning students who matriculated in 1999/2000, four groups of degree programmes have been identified with reference to the different classes; a referential quantity (maximum student number) and a variability interval have been attributed to each group. This type of evaluation was considered necessary to ensure minimum quality standards of the educational offer. It allows for timely adjustments of overcrowded courses through their diversification or subdivision, and avoiding courses with very few students, which could cause inefficient use of resources (excess educational offer). A higher number of matriculated students than the maximum value of the interval shows the need to adjust the resources and/or to provide for the subdivision or diversification of the offer. A lower number of matriculated students than the minimum shows a probably inefficient use of resources.

Number of permanent teachers: The minimum number of permanent teachers for a *Laurea* programmes is determined to cover at least 80 % of the subjects related to the main types of educational activities (basic, qualifying, similar and integrative).

- one-cycle CLS: 15;
- teachers engaged both in the CL and CLS in the first study programme of the class: 16; in the subsequent programmes: twelve;
- teachers engaged in one programme typology in the first study programme of the class: nine (CL) and seven (CLS); in the subsequent programmes: seven (CL) and five (CLS).

Facilities:

- *Classrooms* must be able to host all students enrolled in each course year for 15-20 hours per week at least (60 CFU x eight teaching hours in the classroom = 480 seat-hours per student). If we calculate teaching periods of 28 (24) weeks a year, it amounts to 17.1 (20) seat-hours per week. Hence, a classroom that can adequately host a full class for 30-40 hours per week during the teaching periods may meet the needs of the students of two classes.
- *Laboratories* must be suitable to give all students the opportunity to use them. Availability of work places must be compatible with the requirements fixed in the teaching regulations of the different programmes or in specific regulations (e.g. in the case of *numerus clausus* programmes such as dentistry, medicine, or veterinary medicine).

Application of Minimum Standards

Minimum standards have first been applied to first-degree programmes (CL). The total number of teachers needed for the programmes of a Faculty has been determined by the sum of a + b + c:

- a = minimum number of teachers for new and transformed CL = number of classes x 9 + (number of programmes – number of classes) x 7;
- b = minimum number of teachers for one-cycle programmes = number of classes x 15 + (number of classes – number of programmes) x 15;
- c = number of teachers employed in interfaculty programmes.

The number of teachers calculated according to the formula above must be subtracted from the number of teachers available in the Faculty. A result below zero shows a lack of minimum standards, whilst a result above zero shows the presence of teachers who are employable in CLS (second cycle programmes).

Criteria for Special Funding (Innovation)

The following criteria must be checked in the new CL for the allocation of special funds reserved for teaching innovation:

- Timeliness and completeness of procedures for the establishment and launch of the CL;
- Permanent group of teachers mainly engaged in the CL (minimum standards in terms of 'stable' teaching);
- Attractiveness: the number of students enrolled in the first year must be higher than the minimum planned;
- Evaluation of CL quality must be regular, and refer both to organisation and outcomes, according to both national and international criteria;
- Employability and connection with the context: clear definitions of the professional profiles and labour market; consultation with local representatives of the various socio-economic components (industries, services, the professions).
- Setting up of a 'trend committee' for each CL (which includes representatives of the labour market);
- Percentage of contract teachers who, hired from outside the academic world, are competent in specific professional fields;
- Inter-university and international co-ordination; regional planning of educational supply in conformity with the educational needs of the territory; international agreements for the co-ordination and exchanges.

Evaluation Effects

New CLs (i.e. not originating from previous *Laurea* programmes) must meet minimum quality standards to be included in the programmes that serve the objectives of the 2001-2003 planning and the related funding. If individual universities do not allocate the resources for teaching innovation in conformity with the pre-determined criteria, their quota of ordinary funding may be reduced.

Programmes that lack minimum quality standards are not funded nationally. Universities may decide to abandon them or to run them all the same using their own financial resources. In particular cases, it is also possible to submit an adjustment plan to the CNVSU to reach the minimum quality standards.

Agenda for the Development of CNVSU's Analyses

- 2001-02: check of compatibility of total number of teachers per faculty with the educational programmes offered.
- 2002-03: check the number of teachers available to ensure the CFU required (basic, qualifying, similar or integrative). Details on the availability of adequate facilities (classrooms and labs).
- 2003-04: check teachers' specialisations in relation to the areas of the subjects offered. Map of available classroom places, of the need for laboratories, and facilities to support students. Advertise the programmes.

12.2.5 Other Accreditation Systems

Degree Programmes in Engineering

The Council of the Presidents of the Italian Faculties of Engineering has elaborated SINAI (the national system of evaluation and accreditation of degree programmes in engineering). The Council had two main motivations: a) the on-going process for the implementation of university teaching autonomy; b) the academic and professional recognition of qualifications within the European Union.

Regarding the former, as a consequence of curriculum liberalisation, automatic validation of academic and professional qualifications will no longer be possible. Degree programmes belonging to the same 'class' may lead to professional profiles with diverse competences, not only in different institutions, but also within the same university. This may occur even if the degrees bear the same name. Besides, a further consequence of the institutional autonomy process will be greater competition among universities. Hence, the problem of quality assurance becomes extremely important: competition in educational goals of a high standard will be necessary. The implementation of institutional teaching autonomy must therefore be accompanied by a rigorous application of quality control of educational objectives as well as of the structuring process and final product of individual degree programmes.

The second reason why it is urgent to start a national scheme of programme accreditation is the academic and professional recognition of qualifications within the European Union. At the European level the emerging trends in quality assurance and mutual recognition of qualifications in engineering all point to the need for trans-European co-ordination to facilitate recognition and mobility.

The accreditation system of programmes in engineering is based on their evaluation. It is now an internationally shared opinion that a system of accreditation of degree programmes (CdS) must be based on an evaluation of the CdS. We note that evaluation of a CdS may concern either teaching (from the educational objectives of the CdS to the resources and methodologies which allow for their achievement) or organisation (the evaluation must make the application of the procedures devised for the observation and control of teaching and its outcomes credible). Some accreditation systems prefer to evaluate teaching rather than organisation (e.g. ABET); others (in particular those inspired by ISO-9000) prefer to evaluate organisation.

To achieve the highest objectivity and efficiency, the SINAI method integrates evaluation of teaching and of organisation in a single procedure, thus adopting an approach that is original at the international level. Its designers were conscious that the introduction of an evaluation culture in CdS must take place gradually. The procedure would consist in six fundamental steps: production of data, indicators, and parameters; their analysis; drawing up of an annual self-evaluation report; regular control and external evaluation by an independent body; quality improvement measures; observation of effects.

Master Programmes in Business Administration

Accreditation of MBA programmes has been consolidated over the years. The accrediting agency is an independent association, ASFOR (Association for business management training). Established in 1971 to promote a management culture and develop the educational offer in that field, ASFOR now has more than 50 members (higher schools, universities, and other institutions). It participates in the main European projects on the development of management and quality control.

The main objective of its accrediting process and of the granting of the label 'accredited by ASFOR' is to make a clear distinction between those Master programmes which meet a significant set of requirements – to be evaluated globally – and the thousands of programmes offered as 'Master's'. At present, there are some 20 programmes which are accredited by ASFOR. The decision on the significance and solidity of individual programmes is based on:

- check of existence of objective and explicit criteria that the organising institution sends in beforehand (objective and comparable basis for evaluation);
- partial evaluations expressed by each of the bodies involved in the accrediting process.

Through its accrediting operations, ASFOR intends to provide a useful service to the potential clients of master programmes: they may avail themselves of a guidance tool. It is also a service for companies: thanks to the existence of minimum quality standards, they may rely on a more homogeneous product. Finally, ASFOR aims to support the higher education institutions: when applying for accreditation, they accept to engage in the constant upgrading of their respective programmes.

The minimum compulsory standards for ASFOR accreditation are:

- applicants' selection: applicants' personnel data (age, academic qualifications, previous professional experience at managerial level) and admission procedures;
- teaching: minimum length in hours, study plan (compulsory subject areas), on-the-job projects, academic staff, teaching direction;
- evaluation of participants' performance: expected outcomes must be determined at the beginning of the programme, checked at regular intervals, formally assessed at the end;
- placement procedures: percentage of master's degree holders who are employed at their level within six months;
- programme funding.

Accreditation of Non-State Institutions of Higher Education

Italy has 14 non-State universities, almost one fifth of the present total number of Italian universities. Most have been established recently. In particular, the *Università Carlo Cattaneo, 'LIUC'*, at Castellanza, the *Università Campus Bio-Medico* in Rome (1991), the *libera Università degli Studi 'San Pio V'* in Rome, the *Università Vita-Salute San Raffaele* in Milan (1996), the *libera Università di Bolzano* (1997), the *Libera Univerrsità Europea 'Jean Monnet'* at Casamassima and the *Università della Valle d'Aosta* (2000).

In the history of Italian universities, institutional accreditation has taken different forms in relation to the main transformations affecting the university system. In the system in force in the post-war period up to the 1980s, institutional accreditation took place through a process which resulted in the legal establishment of a university or the transformation into State universities of private institutions *(libere università)* or of separate branches of State universities. It is possible to trace in all these procedures some implicit measures of quality assurance: certain minimum standards are required, together with the favourable opinion of the advisory bodies made up of representatives of the academic staff. Those involved in the process included the institution applying for accreditation and the Government, Parliament, the Ministry of Education and the National University Council.

Institutional accreditation changed when university planning on a national basis was introduced with the first four-year Plan of university development (1986-1990). The establishment of new universities lost its former element of spontaneity and became subject to criteria of rational planning and specific provisions to be included in pluri-annual plans for the development of the university system. This new phase involved the Regional Co-ordination Committee, made up of the Rectors of the universities located in the same Region, and CRUI (Conference of the Rectors of Italian universities): they both had to give their opinions on the individual proposals and the university development plan as a whole.

More recently (as from 1996), the legal process of formal approval has been supported by an external evaluation carried out independently of the Ministry of Education by the Observatory for the Evaluation of the University System, which later became the National Committee for the evaluation of the university system (CNVSU). CNSVU examines teaching, research and buildings; the availability of adequate human resources for teaching and administration; and the availability of necessary financial resources and the articulation of the budget. If CNVSU gives a favourable opinion, the next step is the formal establishment of the non-State university. The juridical instrument that is used is a ministerial decree which simultaneously approves the Statute and the RDA (university teaching regulations), legally recognises the institution, and authorises it to award legal degrees. The process for the accreditation of non-State universities does not only consist in an *ex ante* evaluation. CNVSU also periodically checks the situation *ex post* – that is after the formal approval of the institution and the publication of the related decree – to ascertain consistency of the subsequent development phases of the university with the development plan submitted for approval. Therefore, at later stages, CNVSU checks the existence of the minimum standards in relation to teaching, instrumental equipment, building structures, financial resources, and personnel in order to verify that there is an adequate number of permanent teachers, researchers and technicians, depending on the university, as well as adequate infrastructures and services for all students.

This is CNVSU's way of interpreting its role as the 'guide' of Italian universities towards the evaluation culture. Its methodology of *ex post* evaluation aims to control how far the newly recognised institutions carry out their initial development plan; how consistent a plan they have elaborated for the adjustment of their facilities during the first years of their newly-acquired legal status; time and modalities in which the new institutions succeed in obtaining all the resources needed to carry out a regular teaching and research work at university level; the availability of teachers in the transition phase in relation to those required for their future permanent status.

12.3   Analysis of the Processes: Actors and Regulations

Following the publication in the Official Journal of the Italian Republic of the legal tool introducing university teaching autonomy (DM 509 of 3 November 1999), universities actively engaged in designing new degree programmes. This took about one year (2000/01). As soon as the institutions officially presented their educational offer for the academic year 2001/02, the procedures for the approval and accreditation of the new programmes started in early 2001. The Ministry of Education (MIUR) decided to set in motion a monitoring process to check if individual universities, when designing the new curricula, complied with all features and requirements they had submitted for approval, and if the degree programmes really met the minimum quality standards agreed upon.

MIUR began by requesting the co-operation of CNVSU, the national committee for the evaluation of the university system (i.e. the Italian Agency for Quality Assurance in university education), but other actors were also rapidly involved in the approval and accreditation procedures.

It seems relevant to point out that, in the present phase of the process, a discrepancy has been observed between the accrediting actors on the one hand and a large component of the academic world on the other. While at the national level the complex legal provisions of programme approval and accreditation have been implemented, at the institutional level there is very limited awareness of what is going on among academics and administrative officers who are not directly involved. Action should therefore be taken to inform the academic and university staff about accreditation and to sensitise them to the need for regular quality evaluation in every day university life.

12.3.1   The Italian System of Programme Approval and Accreditation: The Actors

The procedures for the accreditation of degree programmes have been agreed upon by a technical team made up of CNVSU, MIUR, CRUI and CNSU.

CNVSU

The National Committee for the Evaluation of the University System (CNVSU) determines the criteria for the evaluation of all universities; draws up an annual report on the evaluation of the university system; promotes the experimentation and implementation of quality assessment procedures, methodologies, and practices. It also carries out technical evaluations of the proposals to establish new State or non-

State universities in order to authorise them to award legal degrees. Furthermore, CNVSU defines the data that universities must transmit periodically to the Committee itself. It elaborates and executes an annual plan of external assessment sessions concerning individual institutions or single teaching units. It reports on university planning (level of accomplishment and results), carries out research on the state of university education and student welfare services with a view to implement social justice and democracy in education, and on policies regulating access to university programmes. It carries out studies to define criteria for the redistribution to universities of the balance quota from the total funds for their ordinary financing. At the Minister's request, the CNVSU also carries out preliminary investigations and advisory sessions, defines standards and parameters and elaborates technical legal texts with reference to the different activities of individual universities and to the projects and proposals they submit to the Ministry.

CNVSU is an independent body that interacts autonomously with individual universities and the Ministry of Education, University and Research; it has a technical and administrative secretariat and has a specific place in the national budget.

MIUR

The Ministry of Education, University and Research (MIUR) was established in 1999. It merged the facilities, financial resources, staff and functions of the former Ministry of Education (MPI) and Ministry for universities and scientific and technological research (MURST). Concerning university education, MIUR plans the development of the university and research systems; is responsible for legislation on general education matters and financing of universities and public research bodies; monitors and evaluates the education system; transposes the EU and international legislation into the Italian education system; deals with European harmonisation and international integration; implements university autonomy; supervises non-university institutions of university level; regulates university access; participates in the activities related to the access to the civil service and regulated professions; ensures a connection between university and school education as well as between vocational and professional training.

CRUI

The Conference of the Italian University Rectors (CRUI) is an association of the rectors of all Italian universities, both State and non-State but legally recognised. CRUI pursues the following goals: a) present the needs of the university system to government and parliament, based on an in-depth analysis of issues; b) express its views on the university development plan and on the state of university education; c) promote and support university initiatives at national and international level by developing close relations with similar associations within and outside the European Union.

CNSU

The National Council of University Students (CNSU) was conceived as an advisory body of student representatives. It elaborates proposals for the Minister on: a) projects to restructure the university system; b) ministerial decrees on general guidelines for the organisation of degree courses, and providing means and methods to promote student guidance and mobility; c) criteria for the use of the balance quota, i.e. the amount of the total fund for the ordinary university funding which is determined through the re-equilibrium formula. In addition, CNSU: d) elects its representatives at CUN (National University Council); e) may submit proposals on other university matters of general interest; f) draws up for the Minister a national report on student conditions in the university system; g) may interrogate the Minister about facts of national consequence concerning teaching and student life.

CUN

University proposals for new degree programmes are also subject to the advice of the National University Council. CUN is an elective body representative of university autonomy. It formulates proposals and advice on: a) university planning; b) criteria for the use of the balance quota from the fund for the ordinary financing of universities; c) decrees regulating the structure of degree programmes; d) the definition of subject sectors; e) recruitment of university teachers and researchers.

Other Relevant Actors

Italian universities have set up a system for the internal evaluation of their operational management, teaching and research activities, and student welfare services. Availing themselves of comparative analyses of costs and results, all institutions verify the correct use of public resources, research and teaching productivity, the regular development and the fairness of their management. At each institution, evaluation is in the hands of a collegial body, the *university evaluation unit*. Its composition, objectives and functions are regulated by the university statutes: it is made up of five to nine appointed members, at least two of whom are chosen among scholars and researchers who have experience in the field of quality assessment, even if they do not belong to the academic community. University evaluation units are granted the following rights: operational autonomy, access to all necessary information, and dissemination of their proceedings within the legal limits of the respect for privacy. Evaluation units periodically collect anonymous students' opinions on the teaching activities of the respective institutions.

With respect to the new degree programmes, the approval and accreditation process made use of the database on the educational offer of all Italian universities (http://offertaformativa.miur.it), which was constituted to:

- provide telematic support for the elaboration of the new degree programmes, from their planning to ministerial approval and the control of minimum quality standards;
- provide full information on the educational offer of individual universities and on the teaching content of all their programmes (these are described by means of a common standardised grid) in order to guide students in their choice of studies.

12.3.2 Degree Programmes: From National Definition of Curricula to Institutional Teaching Autonomy

As with higher education systems in some other continental European countries, the Italian university model was based on academic programmes and degrees whose content was rigidly defined by national regulations under the supervision of the State. Because of such centralised control in addition to their academic significance, university degrees also had 'legal validity' and produced juridical effects (e.g. in relation to public competitions for functions in the civil service or for access to regulated professions).

Over the years, national university regulations have evolved considerably; the most interesting phases of their evolution are summarised in the following paragraphs.

In a first phase, the national teaching regulations consisted in a series of detailed rules and tables which fixed the names of the different programmes, their legal length, the number and names of compulsory subjects, the modalities of final degree examinations, and the names of the degrees to be conferred. The most obvious consequence was national homogeneity of degree programmes in the same field and of the same type. The laws that produced these regulations date back to the early 1930s; the act most commonly quoted as the main legislative reference is the decree No. 1652 of 1938.

A partial liberalisation was introduced in 1969 to satisfy the pressing requests from university student associations. Students were allowed to submit individual study plans, which were different from those defined by the teaching regulations, provided they respected the pre-determined number of subjects and chose from the list of subjects actually offered by the respective Faculties. These 'personal' study plans were subject to the approval of the competent Faculty Councils whose members, when making their decisions, had to take into account the educational level and the professional competence to be achieved by those students through the degree programmes concerned.

The national regulations underwent a substantial revision in 1990 with the *riforma degli ordinamenti didattici universitari* (reform of university teaching rules; Law No. 341 of 1990). Its main objective was to restructure all degree programmes on the basis of the greater university autonomy, and promote greater flexibility of the system. In this respect, the 1990 reform:

*   sanctioned revision of curricula of all degree programmes, defined criteria for their regular updating, and modified administrative revision procedures;
*   introduced the principle that the educational content of a programme is partly optional, meaning that national regulations must determine only general subject areas to be covered; hence, once the minimum standard of homogeneity necessary to preserve the legal validity of individual degrees was granted, much leeway was given to individual institutions;
*   pursued the re-composition of knowledge by opposing fragmentation in ever more specialised fields and in ever more subject courses, through the definition of subject areas.

The DM 509/1999 reform had to reconcile two conflicting factors: the institutional autonomy in the definition of university curricula and the need for legal validity of degrees through their reference to national regulations. The *'classe'* was introduced as a solution. The degree programmes of the same cycle and typology which share the same qualifying educational objectives and the related indispensable teaching/learning activities, independently of the names they are given in individual universities, were organised in groups called *'classi di appartenenza'*. In relation to each class of degree programmes, at national level the qualifying educational objectives were identified along with the teaching/learning activities necessary to achieve them; these activities have been grouped in six main types:

a)   basic education;
b)   subject fields characterising each class;
c)   subject fields connected with or integrative in relation to those characterising the class, with special reference to cultural contexts and interdisciplinarity;
d)   educational activities chosen by students;
e)   educational activities aimed to check students' competences in foreign languages, and to train them for the final degree examination;
f)   other educational activities devised for the students to acquire further competences in foreign languages, information technology and telecommunications skills, abilities to create relations, or any additional skill or competence that can help their transition to the labour market; these activities are also meant to fa-

cilitate students' choice of a future profession through direct contact with the labour market (e.g. professional guidance and training periods).

The central authority determines a minimum number of credits that are compulsory at national level for each of the above. Individual institutions autonomously define the content and development of the curricula in a national context.

12.4   Accreditation and Evaluation Schemes in Relation to Europe and Globalisation: The Italian Debate

12.4.1   The Debate on the Legal Validity of Study Qualifications

The internationalisation of Italian higher education opened a lively debate on the legal validity of both academic degrees and professional titles. Three main positions have emerged recently in this debate, ranging from the will to abolish legal validity definitively to the belief that it is still necessary and even useful.

Abolitionists

Associations in favour of free education are inclined to repeal the idea of legal validity by doing away with the national teaching regulations and the state examinations that entitle one to exercise a profession. The abolitionist position is based on the belief that educational initiatives arising from the social context need to be carried out freely. This opinion is shared by the representatives of the Italian liberal culture, large groups of the industrial world and some Catholic associations that are active in the educational sector.

Abolitionists generally take the USA as their model, focusing on the lack of state curricular control and on the qualitative competition among educational institutions at different levels. The issue of the value of degrees is left to the evaluation of the labour market rather than of the state.

Realists

The opposite position, although in favour of institutional autonomy, recognises the utility of the legal validity of qualifications and the need to retain it in a large number of sectors. The supporters of this opinion believe that global deregulation is promoted as a mythical device that is capable of eliminating the limitations of the Italian educational system, whereas in reality it would cause more problems than it would solve. The system of legal validity of qualifications has a function in many sectors, for example in the case of programmes for the health-related professions, as well as those for other regulated professions. More generally, it protects consumers. Besides, with respect to university education, the 'realists' maintain that the recent reform of the system has already considerably modified the concept of the legal validity of qualifications.

The realists' position has a wider cultural background. They fear that a generalised and drastic abolition of the legal validity may cause a transfer of powers in educational matters from the state to professional corporations rather than to the labour market. They also see the risk that deregulation may incur high social costs. It would offer greater opportunities to the economically powerful to obtain the most valuable qualifications (or simply the most advertised ones), thus countering values of equality and solidarity. Therefore, in the realists' opinion, a solution which provides for some public control over study programmes and qualifications is more democratic.

Accreditationalists

The third, more recent, position aims at gradually replacing the national teaching regulations by the new practice of programme accreditation for quality assurance. The supporters of the accreditation model associate its adoption with the processes of increasing teaching autonomy and stress its importance to ensure the quality of the educational offer of higher education institutions.

12.4.2 Italy and the Bologna Process

Italy immediately transposed the principles and criteria of the Bologna Declaration into national legislation. The ministerial decree 509/1999, while defining a number of detailed provisions concerning the university system, also determined the complete reform of its overall framework by dividing it into cycles, establishing first degrees which granted their holders an initial effective transition to the labour market, introducing a credit system based on the ECTS, and adopting the Diploma Supplement. This was in conformity with the two international agreements signed by the European Higher Education Ministers at the Sorbonne and in Bologna in 1998 and 1999, respectively.

In order to promote the Bologna Process further, Italy has modified its national legislation to allow Italian universities to design integrated curricula leading to joint degrees, in collaboration with foreign institutions.[1] Moreover, Italy has considerably developed the internationalisation of its university system thanks to two specific projects launched in 1999 and 2001 respectively.[2] Both are supported financially by the Ministry of Education through a co-financing plan.

---

1   See paragraph 9 of art. 3 of DM 509/99.
2   See art. 7 of Ministerial Decree 313/99, and art. 10 of Ministerial Decree 115/01, respectively.

These two projects undoubtedly encouraged the internationalisation of universities. They facilitated international programmes for mobility of students, teachers and researchers, which created a cultural climate in the universities that initiated and sustained international and intercultural initiatives. This stimulated the process of university self-assessment, as it gave greater opportunities for comparison with university systems of partner countries, the integration of curricula or the introduction of an international and intercultural dimension in teaching and learning activities, in research and in services.

The first internationalisation project resulted in the financing of 178 degree programmes (out of 477 proposals submitted by 68 institutions); the overall financial commitment amounted to ITL 52 billion (almost € 27 million), of which ITL 20 billion (ca. € 10 million) came from the Ministry and 32 billion (ca. € 16.5 million) from the universities concerned.

As the first project met with widespread approval (witness the number of submitted proposals), the Ministry decided to open a second round for the period 2001-2003. The new proposals, again based on the principle of co-financing, were to meet some more specific requirements. For example, the Ministry favoured inter-university cooperation proposals that aimed at the study of themes related to the Bologna Declaration's common European Area of Higher Education. Examples are accreditation, credits, diploma supplement, assessment, quality assurance, and academic recognition of qualifications. Besides, the proposed initiatives were to be devised to improve the quality of university organisation and its administrative structures from an international perspective and to produce positive effects on the university system. The overall financial commitment of the proposals submitted amounted to over € 22 million, € 15.5 million of which came from the universities concerned.

12.4.3 Italy and GATS

The principle of the free movement of professional services, which is one of the main GATS objectives, recently found a concrete application in Italy. In the legal process that led to the latest national legislation on immigration of citizens from non-EU countries, some regulations have been approved concerning the recognition of professional qualifications awarded to non-EU citizens by non-EU education institutions and professional bodies (cf. articles 49 and 50 of the Presidential Decree 394 of 3 November 1999). Italy has applied to these professional qualifications the same recognition mechanisms provided for by the EEC General Systems. In so doing, Italy has taken an innovative course aimed at facilitating the free movement of all professionals, independent of their nationality.

12.5   Other Quality Assessment Activities in Higher Education

Among the various actions for quality assessment in the Italian university sector, two initiatives should be mentioned in particular. They concern student evaluation of both university administrative structures and of teaching methodology.

The 'Good Practice' Project – financed by the National Committee for the Evaluation of the University System (CNVSU) – aimed at improving university management by analysing the effectiveness and efficiency of the administrative activities at different universities. Some specific objectives of the project were to:

- make adequate provisions for management effectiveness in relation to different types of 'clients', both inside each institution (teachers and researchers in particular) and outside each institution (mainly students).
- check the possibility of adopting the same testing model not only to compare the performance of different universities at the same moment, but also to analyse the development of a single university over a certain period.
- carry out the benchmarking not only of performance, but also of processes, to increase the number of available instruments to better understand the reasons for variations in results at various institutions;
- facilitate the dissemination of the project data and conclusions to all university administrative officers by creating a managerial panel for consultation.

The second is the 'Euro-Student' Project – currently run by the *Fondazione Rui*, which also started it in 1995 – consists of a national survey of the study and living conditions of Italian university students. The inquiry, which is updated every three years, is now in its third round. Data are collected by means of a questionnaire which the students fill in anonymously. Students' assessment of university teaching is examined with great care. In this respect, the final report offers interesting information at national level on the evaluation of different teaching modalities (in particular, university lectures), of university teachers' performance with reference to their professional competence, knowledge of their specialisation, teaching aptitude and method, ability to arouse their students' interest, etc.; and about the teaching facilities of individual faculties.

13 Latvia: Completion of the First Accreditation Round – What Next?

ANDREJS RAUHVARGERS

13.1 The Higher Education System in Latvia

13.1.1 Size of the Higher Education System

The stagnation – and even drop – in student numbers between 1990 and 1994 is usually explained by the economic situation of the transition years. On the one hand, young people needed to work and earn a living, and on the other, they felt it was not very clear if and which higher education qualifications were worth investing in, given the great changes in the national economy. A sharp increase in student numbers has, however, been observed since 1994. Out of a population of 2,450,000 inhabitants, the 110,500 students represented 32 % of the 19-24-year-old cohort in the year 2001/02.

The most popular fields are social sciences, accounting for 51 % of the students (including 28 % for business administration and economics); teacher training accounting for 16 %; and engineering accounting for 10 %. Humanities and natural sciences each attracted 7 %, services 3 %, health care 4 %, and agriculture 2 %.

There were 66,577 (60 %) full-time students in the year 2001/02 and 43,923 (40 %) part-time students. That year, 59 % of all students were enrolled in professional programmes, the remaining 41 % in academic ones. 12,395 students (11.2 %) studied towards the Master degree and 1,301 (1.2 %) were enrolled in doctoral programmes.

The five state universities and six other state higher education institutions (usually specialised university-level institutions, e.g. in arts) grant doctoral degrees. In the academic year 2001/02, they hosted 74,952 students (68 % of the student population). The nine state institutions which grant degrees below the doctoral level accounted for 13,901 or 13 % of the students, whilst the share of the 13 private institutions was 19,410 or 17 %.

13.1.2 Types of Institutions

The types of higher education institutions in Latvia must be interpreted with care. Although the law provides for a division into university and non-university type, it

275

S. Schwarz and D.F. Westerheijden (eds.),
Accreditation and Evaluation in the European Higher Education Area, 275–297.
© 2004 *Kluwer Academic Publishers. Printed in the Netherlands.*

only sets higher requirements for research and staff qualification in university-type institutions. At the same time, the features of non-university institutions do not differ substantially. Hence, a non-university higher education institution can strengthen its research activities and thus 'grow' into a university type institution. Accordingly, the formal division does not coincide with a division into academic and professional higher education institutions. At the same time, the law allows any institution to offer both academic and professional programmes, if it can obtain accreditation for the particular kind of programme. For these reasons, we shall avoid using the university or non-university division in this chapter, rather grouping institutions according to degrees or diplomas they are entitled to confer.

13.1.3 Main Types of Degrees

Inspired by the Bologna Declaration and aimed at a transparent and easily understandable degree system in Latvia, the Law of Higher Educational Establishments was amended in the year 2000. The system of degrees and qualifications was modified, mainly through the introduction of a two-tier bachelor–master structure in professional higher education. However, the transition is not yet complete. Hence, both programmes leading to the 'old' and 'new' degrees and qualifications coexist.

Before the Amendments of the Year 2000

In *academic higher education,* the two-tier bachelor-master structure began in 1991. However, the bachelor and master degrees were interpreted as purely academic qualifications, mainly aimed at preparing graduates for further research activities. Hence, the degrees could only be awarded 'in a branch of science', i.e. according to a list of branches of science approved by the Research Council. This implies that no interdisciplinary or professionally oriented bachelor or master degrees could legally be awarded. The duration of studies for the bachelor degree was three to four years and for the master degree no less than five years, including the bachelor stage.

In *professional higher education,* there were two main types of programmes: the 2- to 3 year programmes leading to 'first-level professional higher education diploma' which can be used as a labour market qualification or, alternatively, credit transfer towards the longer professional programmes. The mainstream was the longer programmes that lasted for a minimum of four years. Studies in some disciplines could last for up to five (dentistry, pharmacy, some other disciplines) or six years (medicine). They lead to diplomas certifying a 'Second level professional higher education qualification'. With the exception of the programmes in medicine, dentistry and pharmacy, holders of the level II professional higher education diplomas were not eligible for further studies towards doctoral degrees. If the programme comprised standards for a bachelor degree, the holders could be admitted to master studies, even though a bachelor degree was not awarded.

Figure 1. Current degree structure in Latvian higher education

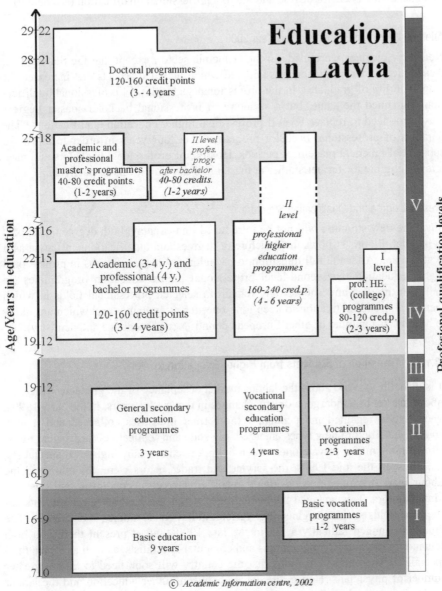

© *Academic Information centre, 2002*

Relatively short professional programmes provided professional training to holders of an academic bachelor degree and led to a professional qualification (see below).

After the Law's Amendments of the Year 2000

Not many changes were made in the academic sector, except that the Standard for Academic Higher Education was adopted which included aspects that increased the employability of graduates. In the professional sector, level I professional qualifications remained the same, but a structure of professional bachelor–master degrees was introduced to replace level II professional higher education qualifications.[1] The duration of professional bachelor programmes is four years in order to allow for substantial practical placement periods. Holders of professional bachelors and masters are eligible for further studies at master and doctoral levels respectively.

Present Degree and Qualification Structure

Since the new structure will not be introduced immediately, both degree types exist in parallel. Figure 1 shows the structure of degrees and qualifications in Latvia as it is at present. After the full transition to bachelor and master degrees in professional higher education the second-level professional higher education programmes (in italics in the diagram) should only remain in selected professional fields in which there is a strong motivation to keep long one-tier programmes and which are likely to be kept in a number of other European countries (e.g. medicine and dentistry).

13.1.4   Transition of Students from Higher Education to Work

It is difficult to write about the labour market acceptance of the graduates since the labour market has undergone drastic changes in the last ten years. In the early 1990s, when Latvia regained independence, the former industries collapsed and it took several years before new types emerged; big state and 'collective' farms were transformed into smaller private ones which did not need so many high-level specialists, etc. Thus, in the mid-1990s, the service and trade sectors were blooming and the labour market mainly needed highly qualified lawyers, economists and business administrators. This changed the mentality of young people and fewer students applied for fields such as engineering, agricultural, medical studies and sciences. The situation changed radically again in the late 1990s and at present there is a high demand for engineers, programmers and computer specialists, as well as agricultural specialists. There are indications that the country will soon need to train a greater number of physicians. Hence, the debate between higher education and the labour market was strongly influenced by the trends of each particular period.

---

1   Medicine, dentistry and pharmacy remained long one-tier programmes.

Attempts to improve the labour market relevance of graduates are being made through the introduction of professional higher education standards, and evaluation of programmes against the standards of the professions. The professional standards are developed by labour market representatives (usually in co-operation with educators).

As regards 'professional accreditation' and *effectus civilis*, professional bodies issue professional certificates in medicine, veterinary medicine, pharmacy, architecture, engineering and other regulated professions where the higher education credentials (like in pre-2004 EU member states and many other countries) are usually a prerequisite but additional. Specialist training is needed before one is issued a professional certificate for independent practice. The unemployment rate of academics or people having higher education in general is smallest amongst those who have several levels of education.

13.1.5 Governance and Steering of Higher Education

The state steering of higher education is basically through the allocation of the (insufficient) state budget. Attempts are made to allocate more funding (i.e. to create more state-financed study places) in the priority areas. Steering by the political parties *per se* is not possible: it can only be done through government or parliament. Private sector organisations, employers, trade unions, etc., influence steering by their representation in the Higher Education Council.

13.2   Accreditation and Approval Schemes in Latvia

The accreditation scheme in Latvia scheme involves *both* programme and institutional accreditation. Accreditation is a prerequisite to award state-recognised degrees or diplomas. Although there are certain differences between institutional and programme accreditation, it seemed easier to describe the two together, since the ownership, stakeholders, procedures and institutions involved are basically the same. The difference begins with decision-making: according to the Accreditation regulations,[2] the decision concerning the accreditation of programmes is taken by the Accreditation Commission, whilst that concerning institutional accreditation is taken by the Higher Education Council.

The licensing scheme will be described separately. It should only be noted here that the licensing of higher education institutions and programmes was introduced in the early 1990s together with legal provisions allowing for the creation of private higher

---

2   *Regulations for accreditation of higher education institutions.* Cabinet regulation No 442 adopted October 16, 2001.

education institutions and programmes and was initially only applied to the private sector. In short, a *licence* is the legal permission to start admitting students.[3] When a new institution is being established, it must obtain a licence as an institution and for each programme to be able to open. Opening a new programme in an existing institution also requires a licence. Thus, the Latvian licence means 'right to legally exist', whereas accreditation means the recognition of degrees or qualifications within the national system.

13.2.1 Accreditation of Higher Education Programmes and Institutions

Types of Institutions, Degrees and Programmes Covered by the Accreditation

The accreditation scheme in Latvia is designed for the whole higher education system. Institutionally it means that it applies to all universities and all other higher education institutions, including the relatively new type of institutions called *koledžas* (colleges), which are only entitled to deliver short, 'first-level higher professional education programmes'.

All disciplines or subjects are covered by a single accreditation framework and similar procedures. Of course, the selection of experts, as well as the criteria used depend on the subject or discipline to be assessed. It should also be noted that the composition of the Accreditation Commission can be adapted to the profile of the programme: while most of the Accreditation Commission members are permanent, specialists of the particular field are invited to participate in decisions on accrediting the appropriate programmes.

Higher Education Functions Accredited

The official documents do not specify a teaching or research orientation for the accreditation system. However, when establishing the system, the main aim was to ensure the quality of the credentials awarded. Thus, the main emphasis is on teaching.

At the same time, there are three aspects that engage evaluators in the assessment of research. First, criteria include an assessment of the relevance of research carried out by staff and students for the programme in question. Second, the qualification of academic staff is an important element in accrediting programmes and institutions. It should also be noted in this regard that no staff positions (including full professors) are 'lifetime positions'. Thus, every six years, staff members go through an open contest to be (re-)elected. The staff research activities are assessed individually

---

3   But this is not a guarantee that the degrees conferred will be state-recognised. They are only recognised following *accreditation*.

through the staff selection process. Third, the accreditation scheme also includes doctoral programmes where the procedures inevitably include an evaluation of research.

Actors and Institutions Involved in the Creation of the Accreditation Scheme

The accreditation scheme in Latvia was created jointly by the state and by higher education institutions. The need to establish an accreditation scheme for higher education institutions and programmes arose in the mid-1990s for three main reasons. Firstly, the major restructuring of programmes that began in 1991 and led to the replacement of the former unitary one-tier higher education system with mainly five-year programmes by a binary system with academic and professional programmes and a two-tier degree structure in the academic sector. This major change raised a question: are all the new programmes of sufficient quality? While the higher education institutions themselves were generally convinced that what they had done in terms of reforms led to good quality, government and society were ready to check the quality.

Secondly, the Education Law of 1991 allowed for the creation of private higher education institutions and they started to mushroom. While this was generally considered as a progressive move, many stakeholders (state, society and also the state higher education institutions) were sceptical about the new, usually small, business-oriented private higher education institutions. When allowing the establishment of private higher education institutions, it was already stipulated in the law that no institution or programme could be opened without a licence and that the degrees or diplomas awarded could not be state-recognised before accreditation.

Stakeholders and Types of Institutions Involved in the Accreditation Scheme

The main stakeholders of the accreditation scheme are the state (Ministry of Education and Science) and higher education institutions themselves (through their participation in the Higher Education Quality Evaluation Centre, HEQEC, and ownership and representation in the HEQEC board, the Higher Education Council and the Accreditation Commission). Employers and trade unions are involved because of their representation in the Higher Education Council and the Tripartite Co-operation Council of Professional Education and Employment and their involvement in the elaboration of professional standards. Students find their place in the scheme through their representation in the Higher Education Council and the Accreditation Commission.

Ministry of Education and Science. Since accreditation leads to state recognition of the degrees or qualifications conferred (and is necessary to use the state coat of arms on documents) and since it is the Minister of Education and Science who signs the accreditation papers for programmes and institutions, the Ministry of Education and Science is the main actor in the administration of the accreditation scheme.

The *Higher Education Quality Evaluation Centre (HEQEC)* organises the entire process. It:

- receives the applications for accreditation of programmes and institutions and checks if the information provided is sufficient,
- consults the higher education institutions or programmes when compiling the self-assessment reports,
- seeks suitable candidates to act as experts in the assessment of each institution or programme and later co-ordinates the work of experts,
- organises expert evaluation and receives expert evaluation reports;
- prepares the document package for the Accreditation Commission (for programmes) and Higher Education Council (for institutions),
- organises the publication of the accreditation outcomes (decisions, self-assessment and expert reports).

HEQEC is partly owned by the Ministry of Education and Science and partly by the higher education institutions. According to a decision of the Rectors' Council, the higher education institutions are represented in HEQEC ownership by five members: four state universities (University of Latvia, Riga Technical University, Latvian Academy of Medicine, Daugavpils Pedagogical University) and one private institution (Turība Business School). According to the statutes, the HEQEC board consists of five members. One is appointed by the Ministry, one by the University of Latvia and one by Riga Technical University, whilst the other two are elected by the meeting of the shareholders.

The *Accreditation Commission* takes decision concerning the accreditation of programmes. It is approved by the Minister of Education and Science. It comprises three members from the Ministry of Education and Science; one member from each Higher Education Council (Latvian Rectors' Council, Latvian Science Council, and Latvian Student Union); one representative of the Professional Education Co-operation Council and two representatives of the Tripartite Sub-Council on Professional Education and Employment. In addition, for the accreditation of a particular programme, one representative of the ministry supervises the particular professional field and, if necessary, experts from the professional field in question are added to the Accreditation Commission.

According to the Accreditation Regulations, the Accreditation Commission:

- considers the application for the accreditation of a programme,
- approves the experts who will be included in the evaluation commission of a particular programme and appoints the chairman of the expert team,

- having considered the expert evaluation of the programme and analysed the information submitted in the application for accreditation, it decides on programme accreditation.

The *Higher Education Council* has the mandate to decide on institutional accreditation. Its members include one representative of each of the following: the Latvian Academy of Sciences, the Latvian Rectors' Council, the Association of Art Higher Education Institutions, the Council of College Directors, the Latvian Student Association, the Latvian Association of Education Managers, the Chamber of Trade and Industry, the Latvian Employers' Confederation, the Trade Union of Education and Science Employees, and a representative of higher education institutions established by local governments and other legal entities. The Minister of Education is an *ex officio* member of the Higher Education Council. The head of the Ministry of Education and Science's Higher Education and Research Department participates in all Higher Education Council meetings but does not have a voting right.

The Higher Education Council has the following functions in the accreditation scheme:

- it may recommend experts for the evaluation team of a particular higher education institution,
- having considered the expert evaluation of a higher education institution and analysed the information submitted in the application for accreditation, the Higher Education Council decides whether to accredit the institution.

The *Evaluation commission* is an ad-hoc expert team appointed for the assessment of a higher education institution or programme. Each evaluation team should consist of at least three experts. Only one can be from Latvia. Foreign experts are sought upon recommendation by the body responsible for higher education quality assurance in the respective foreign country. In practice, most evaluation teams comprise one expert from Latvia, one from Estonia or Lithuania and one from Western Europe or North America. This enables the expert team to pursue the following goals:

- evaluation of Latvian programmes and institutions in a broader European context (particularly the 'Western' expert),
- looking at Latvian programmes or institutions from outside but with a good knowledge of the Latvian system and having similar developments and problems at home (in particular the Baltic expert),
- ensuring assessment against Latvian standards and regulations (the Latvian expert).

The functions of the Evaluation Commission in the accreditation scheme are the following. It:

- considers the self-assessment report and other information submitted by the higher education institution or programme,
- visits the higher education institution or programme and analyses their functioning *in situ,*
- prepares individual expert evaluation reports,
- formulates an overall opinion in the name of the expert team,
- submits the opinion and the individual expert reports that are forwarded to the Accreditation Commission (programme accreditation) or Higher Education Council (institutional accreditation).

Ownership, Initiative, Control and Review of the Accreditation Scheme

The introduction of the accreditation scheme in 1996 was initiated by the Law on Higher Education Establishments adopted at the end of 1995. This law was the result of long discussions and consultations between the state and the higher education institutions. The accreditation scheme is owned jointly by the state and the higher education institution. While greater decision-making power is still on the state side, the ownership by higher education institutions is embodied in both shares in the capital and participation in the board of the Higher Education Quality Evaluation Centre and in all decision-making bodies (especially the Accreditation Commission and the Higher Education Council).

Accreditation is embedded in the legislation as a recurring process. After the first accreditation round, completed in 2002, each programme and institution must be accredited anew every six years. Initiation of accreditation is only possible if it is felt that a programme or an institution does not perform according to standards and expectations. In these cases, according to the Accreditation Regulations, the Higher Education Council has the right to propose an extraordinary accreditation and the Minister of Education and Science then decides whether to initiate it.

While the laws and regulations do not provide details on how the accreditation scheme should be controlled, the practice is the following. First of all, the Director of HEQEC regularly reports to the Higher Education Quality Evaluation Centre board (consisting of representatives of many stakeholders, see above). The Higher Education Council and the Rectors' Council also periodically invite the HEQEC leadership to discuss the results and possible constraints of the accreditation process.

The scheme was intensively discussed between the end of 2002 and early 2003. The first accreditation round had been completed. The experience gained helped to indicate which aspects of the regulations needed amendments. It was also felt that the first accreditation round had helped higher education institutions to understand how they could better manage their own quality and this led to the establishment of simplified procedures for the repeated accreditation. Finally, in preparation for the Berlin ministerial conference, Latvian higher education wanted to establish its achievements in quality assurance and how to move forward. These discussions led to the preparation of new Accreditation Regulations and new practical guidelines and recommendations for the experts which were approved in early 2003.

Customers and Stakeholders

In addition to academia, the accreditation scheme also affects several other groups of stakeholders.

Students and (indirectly) *parents.* As the accreditation results are directly related to the state-recognition status of the degrees or qualifications conferred, they also have several other effects. For male students, the obligatory military service can be postponed while studying in accredited programmes (and they can be fully exempted of military service if awarded a recognised master's degree).

Students are only entitled to receive state loans, i.e. the 'study loan' to cover tuition fees (if charged) and the 'student loan' aimed at social needs, when a programme or institution is accredited. The same goes for state scholarships (there are very few).

Where employment requirements include a higher education degree or diploma, it should be from an accredited institution or programme. In practice, employers increasingly demand state-recognised degrees and diplomas even in non-regulated professions and in the private economy.

Employers and trade unions. The introduction of the accreditation scheme has clarified the issue of 'who is who' in higher education for the employers and trade unions, thus allowing to distinguish between trustworthy education providers and others. It has also given new tasks and responsibilities to both groups with regard to the elaboration of professional standards which are used to draft educational standards for professional curricula.

Rules and Regulations

According to the Law on Higher Education Establishments (article 9), state-recognised degrees or diplomas can be awarded after accreditation of both the higher education institution and the programme concerned. At the and of each academic year, a list of the higher education institutions that are entitled to issue state-recognised credentials (indicating all the accredited programmes in each of these institutions) is published in the official government newspaper *Latvijas Vestnesis*. If accreditation of a higher education institution or programme is annulled, the information must be published in both the government newspaper and in the educational newspaper *Izglitiba un Kultura*.

The main document regulating the accreditation scheme of programmes and institutions is the *Regulation for accreditation of higher education institutions* (Cabinet regulation No 442 adopted October 16, 2001), as explained above. The Accreditation Regulations are accompanied by two other documents approved at lower level, the *Guidelines for the accreditation of higher education institutions and programmes* and the *Questionnaire for the evaluation experts*.

The standards for higher education programmes are laid down in two other Cabinet regulations, the *Standard for academic higher education*[4] and the *Standard for professional higher education*.[5]

Financing

According to sections 52 to 56 of the Accreditation Regulations, the financing of the accreditation scheme is as follows. Expenses for the assessment of higher education institutions and programmes are covered by the higher education institutions themselves. State higher education institutions cover these expenses from the overall funds they receive from the state (no funds are earmarked for accreditation costs, though), while private higher education institutions cover accreditation costs with their income from tuition fees.

The method for calculation of costs of services comprising the accreditation package are approved by the Minister of Education and Science. Basically, the accreditation costs include costs of expert evaluation, maintenance costs of the HEQEC, as well as the costs for the publication of accreditation results. The breakdown of costs for each particular accreditation case is based on this method, and it is co-ordinated with the higher education institution or college concerned. The costs should be paid by the higher education institution before the evaluation commission starts its work.

Stages of the Procedure and their Duration

Accreditation procedures of both institutional and programme accreditation include the following formal stages:[6]

---

4   Regulations on state standard of academic higher education, Cabinet Regulation No 2, adopted January 3, 2002.

5   Regulations on state standard of second-level professional higher education, Cabinet Regulation No 481, adopted November 20, 2001.

6   A higher education institution can apply for institutional accreditation when at least 50 % of its programmes have been accredited.

- Preparation of application for accreditation. Timing of this phase depends solely on the higher education institution (usually this takes three to six months).
- Within 30 days after receipt of an application, HEQEC checks whether the information complies with the requirements. Should some of the information listed in Accreditation Regulations be missing, HEQEC asks the institution to supply this information. The higher education institution should supply it within one week. Checking whether the information regarding the higher education institution and programme complies with the data available at the State Enterprises Register and other state institutions takes no more than two weeks. Checking the application for accreditation and whether all the necessary information is provided, takes no more than 30 days and it is done in parallel.
- An expert team ('evaluation commission') is formed. It studies the self-evaluation report and other information submitted.
- A two-day expert visit is organised to the higher education institution or programme. Experts submit their individual assessments and compile an overall assessment report in the name of the Evaluation Commission.
- The assessment report is discussed at an open conference.
- After the conference, the expert team finalises the evaluation report and submits it to the Accreditation Commission or to the Higher Education Council, as appropriate.
- Within six months after receipt of the application, the Higher Education Council or the Accreditation Commission decides about accreditation[7] and submits its decision to the Ministry of Education and Science. In exceptional cases, the Minister of Education and Science may issue a motivated ordinance to prolong the particular accreditation case, but not longer than for another six months.
- The Minister of Education and Science issues an accreditation paper.

After the first accreditation round was completed, it was decided that the recurrent accreditation could be simplified, provided there were no substantial changes[8] in the programme and that a self-assessment report had been submitted each year. The simplified procedure includes an analysis of the self-assessment reports and site visit by one expert, after which the Accreditation Commission decides.

The actual time frames for the procedures do not differ much from the official timeframe, with one exception, namely the professional programmes, because of a lack of professional standards. Since 2000, the Latvian legislation requires that professional higher education programmes must comply with the professional standards to be accredited. The professional standards must be elaborated by the labour market

---

7   In principle, the HEC or the Accreditation Commission can visit the higher education institution to clarify additional issues *in situ*.

8   'Substantial changes' are flexible enough to allow for further development of the programme.

side (in co-operation with educationalists). The problem is that the labour market is slow in developing these standards. As a result, if a higher education institution wants to present a professional higher education programme for accreditation, but no professional standard has been approved, the higher education institutions them- selves have to take the initiative, organise working parties, and help to elaborate the professional standard. It is evident that this is an additional burden for higher educa- tion institutions and that it causes delays in accreditation.

Rules for Objection

There are no rules concerning objection to the procedures. In practice, this means that, since all the bodies involved in the accreditation scheme are subordinated to the Minister of Education and Science in one way or another, an appeal can be submit- ted to the Minister. In practice, it will be the legal department of the Ministry of Education and Science that will have to verify whether the procedures have been carried out according to the legal regulations. In case of further dissatisfaction with the results, the higher education institution can apply to court.

In practice, all procedural problems are usually solved without formal applications to the minister. Issues are settled in discussions between the programme or institu- tion concerned, HEQEC (which is the body that should help higher education insti- tutions to settle organisational problems of accreditation), and sometimes representa- tives of the Ministry of Education and Science or the Higher Education Council.

Links Between Accreditation and Approval Schemes

The main formal link is between accreditation and recognition of the degrees or qualifications awarded. In order to be entitled to award state-recognised degrees or qualifications, both the programme and the higher education institution must be accredited.

There are no formal links between the accreditation status of a programme in a state- sector higher education institution and the state funding allocated to that programme. In practice, however, there could be consequences.

Effects of International Experts

Assessment that includes international experts has benefits and drawbacks. The benefits are obvious, and they are the reason why Latvia decided to pay the addi- tional costs and overcome difficulties to get an 'outside view' on the international credibility of Latvian accreditation; 'European dimension', strong arguments in national debates with employers, parents, other stakeholders and society at large; finally, reducing 'small country effects' where the higher education system is closely interrelated (an issue here is finding a competent yet independent expert for each field).

There are, however, some possible drawbacks. Although in most cases the experience has been positive, it could be interesting for other countries that are thinking of introducing evaluation by foreign experts to analyse Latvia's experience:

- *High costs.* Even if enthusiastic foreign colleagues are ready to work as experts for fees they consider symbolic, travel and subsistence costs plus expert fees are a heavy burden for the higher education institutions (state as well as private).
- *Language.* Because foreign experts are called upon, all the main documents submitted with the application for accreditation must also be translated into English, adding workload and costs to the institution. The need to speak in a foreign language during the assessment visit and at the conference following it is an additional problem, since not all staff members speak good English, even if they are fluent in another foreign language. The use of a foreign language when being assessed increases the probability of misunderstandings.
- *Knowledge of the Latvian system.* Each country has its own balance among educational, employment and administrative systems, where the labour market and education system have (more or less) adapted to each other. It is not easy for a foreigner to immediately grasp the features of a different education system; hence misunderstandings happen every now and then. Yet, there are many positive experiences when experts have been invited repeatedly.
- *Measuring against national standards and legal regulations.* This issue is partly related to the previous one. It is essential that the expert team has a good knowledge of the requirements of Latvian legislation and educational standards, something that is again not easy to attain. In practice, it sometimes means that the Latvian expert on the team has to verify compliance with Latvian standards and regulations alone. Unfortunately, this can also lead to diverging views inside the expert team or, in extreme cases, to disagreements between the expert evaluation report and the decision taken by the Accreditation Commission or Higher Education Council.
- The last point is very subjective but interesting. In some individual cases the *judgements of foreign experts can be over-forgiving or over-demanding*. The former has been observed more frequently and can be summarised as: 'the programme (or institution) is on the right way, let's accredit it', ignoring that it does not yet comply with the requirements and standards. In these cases, the final decision made by Accreditation Commission has sometimes been the opposite of the team's opinion.

Dissemination of Outcomes

Information dissemination takes place in the following ways:

1. Compulsory actions foreseen in legislation:

- Annual publication of lists of accredited programmes before the beginning of admission to higher education institutions in the official government newspaper *Latvijas Vestnesis* and in the educational newspaper *Izglitiba un kultura.*
- If the accreditation of a programme or institution is refused, publication in the official government newspaper within two weeks.

2. Additional information dissemination:

- Publication of both the programme and institutional evaluation reports and decisions by Accreditation Commission and Higher Education Council in the educational newspaper,
- Publication and regular updating of all the above information on the Higher Education Quality Evaluation Centre homepage (www.aiknc.lv).

13.2.2   Licensing of Higher Education Programmes

In the Latvian higher education system licensing of a programme means granting a right to start student admission with no guarantee that the qualification awarded at the end will be state-recognised.

Range, Actors, Stakeholders, and Ownership

A licence is required to start a new programme in the entire higher education system, regardless of the discipline, the type of institution or its ownership (state or private). Equally, licensing covers programmes countrywide. Basically, licensing is oriented to teaching and resources for it. However, checking the qualification of academic staff includes analysing their research biographies. Licensing was introduced and owned by the state. The stakeholders of the licensing scheme are the Ministry of Education and Science and higher education institutions themselves (by delegating representatives to the licensing commission).

The scheme was initiated in the Education Law of 1991 simultaneously with the permission to establish private higher education institutions. Society felt a need for an initial check to know whether new programmes established by the mushrooming private institutions were relevant. In the Law on Higher Education Establishments of 1995, the licensing procedure was extended to newly established programmes in state institutions to prevent duplication and to ensure better use of state funding. Compared with accreditation, the difference is that licensing is required to demonstrate that the higher education institution or programme is capable of reaching the achievements or indicators that become mandatory for accreditation. To ensure that the state and higher education institutions share control over the scheme, the Licensing Commission is composed of two members from the Ministry of Education and Science and one each from the Higher Education Council, the Rectors' Conference and the association of private higher education institutions.

Rules and Regulations

The main document that regulates licensing is the *Regulations for licensing programmes delivered by higher education institutions* (Cabinet regulation No 3, adopted January 3, 2002).

The licensing procedure includes the following stages:

- Preparation of the application for accreditation. Timing of this phase depends solely on the higher education institution itself.
- Within 30 days after receipt of an application, the Ministry of Education and Science checks whether the information complies with the requirements. Should some of the information listed in Accreditation Regulations be missing, the Ministry of Education and Science asks for this information to be supplied within one week.
- The decision should be taken by the Licensing Commission within 30 days after receipt of an application with all the necessary documents. The LC can refuse a licence, if:
  - documents submitted do not comply with requirements of legal acts and regulations,
  - staff qualification requirements are not met,
  - technical and informative support is not sufficient,
  - the content and delivery mechanisms of the programme are not sufficiently elaborated.
- The Ministry of Education and Science issues a licence to the programme.

The actual time frames for the procedures do not differ much from the official time frame. At the same time, the same problem of developing professional standards for licensing professional programmes exists as for accreditation (see above).

Formal Rules for Objection Regarding the Licensing Procedure. There are no formal rules concerning objections, but an appeal can be submitted to the Minister and an answer should be received within two weeks. In case of further dissatisfaction with the results, the higher education institution can apply to court.

Formal Rules for Information Dissemination Regarding the Outcomes. There are no formal regulations regarding the publishing of results. In practice, a list of licensed programmes is published in the educational newspaper before the admissions period to higher education institutions begins, and it is also available on the webpage of the Higher Education Quality Evaluation Centre.

Formal Links between Licensing and Other Higher Education Policies. Once they have obtained a licence, higher education institutions are allowed to start student admission. It was difficult to quantitatively prove that criteria were being met when the potential to fulfil requirements rather than their actual fulfilling was under review. This often leads to difficult discussions with licence seekers. At the same time, students, parents and society at large made it clear that programmes that did not lead to decent qualifications should not be allowed.

Actual Information Dissemination of Outcomes

Information dissemination takes place as follows.

*   Annual publication of lists of licensed programmes before the beginning of admission to higher education institutions in the educational newspaper *Izglitiba un kultura.*
*   Publication and regular updating of this information on the Higher Education Quality Evaluation Centre's homepage.

13.3   Driving Forces for Accreditation and Licensing

International and national credibility of the qualifications should come first, followed by customer protection and a guarantee that the credentials are of quality, introducing continuous improvements in higher education, with a view to labour market relevance, but also competition for students.

International credibility of awards is probably the most important point that helped to reach a consensus between higher education institutions, the state and other stakeholders on the introduction of quality assurance in Latvia. After opening up to European and wider co-operation in the early 1990s, the change to a bachelor–master system and the curricular reform following the 1991 Education Law, all Latvian stakeholders were in favour of measures that would support the international credibility of the Latvian credentials that were not well-known abroad, first of all in Europe. International credibility was the main reason why the higher education institutions, which initially considered external quality assurance schemes an infringement on their autonomy, agreed to the establishment of an accreditation scheme which involved foreign experts. In this sense, the introduction of the scheme has been successful. Now that all the state-recognised programmes have been assessed by international teams, Latvia can discuss the mutual recognition of accreditation results in the European forum (i.e. ENQA).

Credibility in the eyes of potential students and their parents and customer protection are equally important. Since between 1991 and 1995, the creation of private higher education institutions was allowed and the entire higher education system had undergone a curricular reform with the change to the bachelor–master structure that replaced traditional long one-tier programmes, the need was felt to 1) check whether the newly-established private institutions offered higher education of sufficient quality and 2) make an inventory of the whole system.

In this respect, the introduction of the two-stage licensing or accreditation scheme has been a success. Licensing allows for the filtering of cases when the institution that is willing to open a programme is, in fact, not capable of bringing it up to the standards and requirements within the period before accreditation.

Accounting to society. Assessment by international peers followed by accreditation is, on the one hand, the way the state can monitor the use of the funds it allocates to the state institutions, and the way students (or their parents) who pay tuition fees[9] can monitor how the money they pay for their studies is used.

Labour market relevance of qualifications. It is self-evident that assessment of professional higher education programmes against professional higher education standards and the professional standards of the profession in question ensures the labour-market relevance of the programmes. At the same time, the presence of employers' representatives in the Accreditation Commission, Higher Education Council and the bodies that control the quality assurance system ensures a feedback from the labour market to the higher education institution.

Involvement of labour market representatives in standard-setting. For accreditation, higher education programmes, and especially those targeted at a particular profession, are evaluated against professional standards which should be elaborated by the employers and professionals of the profession and approved by the Cabinet. Even if in practice the labour market side is slow in developing professional standards and therefore the higher education institutions that wish to accredit their programmes have to take the initiative themselves, the above legal requirement stimulates co-operation between labour market and higher education and in the end leads to better labour-market acceptance of graduates.

13.3.1   Relationships between Accreditation Schemes and Evaluation Schemes

At present, there are no specific evaluation schemes in Latvia. However, as the higher education institutions stated in their answers to the EUA questionnaire for the Trends III report, in the course of the first accreditation round they were ready to carry out a permanent internal evaluation and improvement.

---

9   Tuition fees are also paid by some of the students at state institutions. In addition to the study places which are financed by the state (and for which there is a competition to be admitted), state institutions may admit more qualified candidates who pay tuition fees.

It is not likely that Latvia will give up accreditation in a foreseeable future, but possibilities for using it as an external approval of the internal quality assurance procedures is foreseen in the new accreditation regulations of 2002.

13.3.2   Relationship between Accreditation and Licensing

A licence is a 'green light' for student admission to a programme. It is needed to prove that the higher education institution is capable of bringing the programme up to accreditation standards within two years. Thus, it is a prerequisite for accreditation.

13.3.3   Consequences of the Creation of the Accreditation Scheme for the Higher Education Institutions, Departments and Scholars

As regards new or private programmes, accreditation is a guarantee for the staff that the programme has been approved and has fully gained 'the right to exist'.

For all staff it means more work. Compared to the situation before the accreditation scheme was introduced, it led to much greater staff involvement in quality monitoring, a feeling of responsibility and ownership regarding programme as a whole (compared to own field only), deeper insight into overall curriculum development, a comparative approach (with similar programmes in the EU countries), and a better understanding of the higher education-labour market links and labour market requirements. According to the answers of the Latvian higher education institutions to the Trends III questionnaire, the introduction of accreditation has consolidated an internal quality culture and continuous improvements. Since professional programmes are assessed against profession standards (developed by or in co-operation with the labour market), it provides arguments for the never ending and often bitter debate with the employers regarding the labour market relevance of graduates. Existence of the professional standards are of great importance here, since the professional standard is a document where the employers have formulated their requirements. Assessment procedures prior to accreditation have stimulated the debate about priority of learning outcomes over the input characteristics of programmes.

13.3.4   Consequences of the Creation of the Accreditation Scheme for Students

Students and (indirectly) *parents.* First of all, for students accreditation is the guarantee of a programme's quality. The involvement of employers in accreditation is also reassuring with regard to future employment perspectives. As the accreditation results are directly related to the state-recognition status of the degrees or qualifications conferred, they also have several other effects.

Students will be better served. The accreditation scheme enables a reorientation from the educator-driven development of programmes towards the development of the programmes orientated towards the professional field, comparability to similar programmes in other European countries and meeting standards set for academic and professional higher education programmes. This also means a switch to output-oriented curriculum development.

Finally, the self-assessment phase of the accreditation scheme inevitably leads to continuous improvement in the higher education institutions.

13.4   Relation to the Bologna Process and Previous European Experiences

The quality assurance system in Latvia was *not* created by or because of the Bologna process. In 1999, when the Bologna Declaration was signed, it already functioned and had gained momentum in Latvia. The first round of accreditation was completed at the end of 2001.

Asked how they see the further co-operation in quality assurance in Europe for the *Trends III* report, Latvian key players in higher education showed a unanimous view: European co-operation in quality assurance should take place as co-operation of national higher education quality agencies through ENQA; not through establishing a European accreditation body.

There is also a clear view among Latvian stakeholders that using ENQA as a platform for exchange of information and experiences will help establish mutual trust among the higher education quality assurance systems of different countries and will thus promote mutual recognition of qualifications.

The starting point in establishing a quality assurance system higher education in Latvia was the international seminar on this topic, organised by the Council of Europe in Riga October 24–25, 1994. Well-known European quality assurance experts spoke at this seminar and participants were selected from the leadership of higher education institutions and high-ranking ministry officials from Estonia, Latvia and Lithuania. The need to establish quality assurance schemes was widely discussed and it was agreed that the Baltic states should co-operate in this, with a view to establish comparable criteria and procedures in all three countries and to further use each others' experts in evaluation teams.

At the end of the seminar, Ministers of all the three states signed a protocol on Baltic co-operation in higher education quality assurance. For further co-ordination in quality assurance systems and – making from the start a link long missing in other European developments – recognition of foreign qualifications, the ministers also decided to establish Baltic Higher Education Co-ordination Committee (BHECC). The BHECC included representatives from the Rectors' conferences, ministry representatives, and heads of the recognition centres (ENIC or NARIC). Co-operation in the BHECC helped establish comparable quality assurance systems in the Baltic states. Moreover, the BHECC drafted a Baltic recognition agreement to complement the Lisbon Convention. To speed up implementation, it was first signed in 1999 as a protocol between the heads of the recognition centres, but in 2000, the Heads of States signed it as a formal agreement between states.

Looking at European models, initially three European quality assurance systems were widely studied: the British, Dutch and Danish systems. With the assistance of the British Council (1994–1996), several Latvian key players had possibilities to visit the British Higher Education Quality Council (HEQC) and Funding Councils, and at a later stage a project was carried out where British representatives provided training to the Latvian future exerts for evaluation of study programmes and institutions. A TEMPUS CME project was carried out (1995–1996) in which representatives of the Latvian Ministry, the Rectors' Council and the newly appointed management of the Higher Education Quality Evaluation Centre studied the Dutch quality assurance system, and Dutch experts gave several seminars to a wider group of Latvian higher education leadership, government representatives and invited delegations from Estonia and Lithuania. Another TEMPUS CME in 1996–1997 was used to train HEQEC staff and higher education leadership in drawing up self-evaluation reports.

The PHARE Multi-Country Project (1997–1998) in higher education, which covered eleven Central and Eastern European countries, in a way came late for Latvia. The accreditation scheme was already up and running and the basic principles were already clear. Still, of course, it was useful as it helped training a wider group of stakeholders and the quality assurance manual produced in the project could serve as a good reference.

Was the Latvian scheme derived from European models? In fact, in the mid-1990s, when Western European experts advised to introduce accreditation in Central and Eastern European countries, most Western European countries themselves used schemes other than accreditation. So the answer is *yes and no*:

- Yes, the ideas brought by Western European experts were appreciated and used,
- Yes, the sequence self-assessment – peer assessment – decision – publication was adopted,
- No, there was no exact model copied from a Western European country and directly applied in Latvia.

13.5   Other Quality Assurance Activities

13.5.1   Internal Approval of Programmes and Courses Inside Higher Education Institutions

A number of institutions, especially the bigger and multi-faculty ones, have internal mechanisms of approval of programmes and individual courses (mainly for new ones). The practical realisation of these mechanisms differs from institution to institution. An example could be that to start a programme the department has to draw up a detailed description similar to self-assessment reports used at accreditation and to present it to the university senate, which decides on approving the programme. At an even smaller scale, each new subject course has to be submitted for approval at institutional (or faculty) level.

13.5.2   Staff Performance Assessment at Election or Re-election

In Latvia, staff positions are not lifetime appointments. Each staff member is subject to (re-)election every six years. At that point, the previous teaching and research activities are assessed, using as indicators:

- types and intensity of teaching activities,
- participation or leadership in research projects,
- number and level of scientific and other publications,
- international activities such as guest lecturing,
- participation in international research or higher education development projects,
- participation in curriculum development,
- writing textbooks and developing teaching aids,
- organisational activities at institutional, state and international level etc.

14 Multipurpose Accreditation in Lithuania: Facilitating Quality Improvement, and Heading towards a Binary System of Higher Education

BIRUTĖ VICTORIA MOCKIENĖ

14.1 The Higher Education System

Since 1999/2000, the higher education system in Lithuania has been diversified. In September 2002, it consisted of 43 institutions which were of two types: 19 university-type (academies, colleges, seminaries, and universities) and 24 non-university-type called *colleges* (*kolegijos*).

Higher education institutions may be state owned or private (not belonging to the state). Currently, there are four private university-type and nine private colleges.

During the years of Independent Lithuania, student enrolment fluctuated. There were more than 63,000 students in 13 institutions in 1990/91. The numbers dropped in 1995/96: the student body then consisted of 54,000 persons. As from 1996, an incremental growth was observed (Education and Culture, 2001). In 2001, overall enrolment reached 115,000 students. 105,000 students (except doctoral) were enrolled in university-type institutions. In addition, 10,000 were enrolled in colleges.

Statistical data show that in the last five years the overall admission to universities and post-secondary education institutions (*aukštesnioji mokykla*) grew. In 1996, over 20,000 students were admitted to university-type institutions, and over 11,000 to Post-secondary Education Institutions. In 2000, universities admitted more than 34,000 students; however, admission to Post-secondary Education Institutions dropped to 10,000 (Lietuvos švietimas, 2000). This change is explained by the restructuring of the higher education system, when a number of Post-secondary Education Institutions became colleges. Therefore, we may conclude that the number of student admissions grew significantly.

Furthermore, the enrolment in undergraduate programmes grew substantially from 14,800 in 1996 to 22,700 in 2000. This growth is explained by two factors: the additional student admission in colleges (3,400) and growing access to education because of new entrants who pay tuition fees. Since in 2000 there were less than 37,000 secondary schools graduates, almost all of them could be admitted to either a higher education institution or to a Post-secondary Education Institution.

299

S. Schwarz and D.F. Westerheijden (eds.),
Accreditation and Evaluation in the European Higher Education Area, 299–322.
© 2004 *Kluwer Academic Publishers. Printed in the Netherlands.*

By allowing commercial studies (i.e. with full costs covered by the student), Lithuanian authorities improved access to higher education. Moreover, in the summer of 2002 the *Seimas* (Parliament) approved two amendments to the Law of Higher Education that introduced a symbolic obligatory tuition fee, 500 Litas (approximately € 120) for newly admitted students. In 2000, universities admitted 13,179 students to undergraduate places financed by the state, and 9,517 to places with tuition costs to be borne by students. At the same time, more than 30 % of graduate students paid for their studies (Lietuvos Švietimas, 2000, p. 59). In the future, the Government plans the admission of almost 43,000 new higher education students supported fully or partially by the state; 25,600 undergraduates, 9,355 graduates, and 683 postgraduates at universities, and 6,325 at colleges. The remaining students will be admitted to programmes that require students to cover costs of tuition and fees (Decision of the Government, 2002). The additional revenues should help universities to improve the quality of studies by providing more funds for human resources and by renovating material resources.

Lithuanian higher education institutions provide the following types of programmes: consecutive and non-consecutive university programmes, and consecutive non-university programmes. Universities organise sequential studies in three stages: undergraduate, graduate and post-graduate (doctoral).

A university-level undergraduate study programme in Lithuania comprises 140–180 credit points (one credit corresponds to 40 hours of student work – in classes, independently, etc. – or 1.5 ECTS credits) and lasts between three and five years. Two-thirds of the subjects must be studied at the same higher education institution. There are three blocks of subjects: comprehensive humanitarian and social studies (at least 30 % of all credits); fundamentals of the branch of studies (at least 30 % of all credits); and specialised subjects (at least 30 % of all credits). Graduates at this level are awarded a *bakalauras* (Bachelor's degree) or *profesinė kvalifikacija* (diploma of vocational qualification and certificate of graduation from a higher education institution). At the non-university level study programmes consist of at least 120 to 160 credits and last for at least three to four years. A professional qualification and diploma of higher education are obtained after successful completion.

Graduates with undergraduate degrees may apply for *Magistrantūra* (Master's) or *Specialiosios profesinės* (Specialised professional) studies. Those who are admitted to the second stage programme may pursue specialised vocational studies (lasting for one to two years and comprising 40 to 80 credit points) or studies leading to a Master's degree (lasting for 1.5 to 2 years and comprising 60–80 credit points). Master's graduates have to defend a thesis or a diploma project. Upon obtaining this degree, the recipient can start doctoral studies or practical activity. After completing a professional, specialised professional programme, students obtain a professional (e.g. teacher, engineer, economist, etc.) qualification.

Another type of programme, integrated studies, may be offered by Lithuanian university-type institutions. Their duration is at most six study years (240 credits) and no less than 4.5 to 5 study years (200 credits). Studies of the first four years (160 credits) are attributed to the first stage of undergraduate studies, and studies of the remaining one to two years (40–80 credits) are attributed to the second stage of sequential studies. After successful completion of these studies the professional qualification or Master's degree is awarded. In addition, vocational post-graduate study programmes of one to two years duration may be organised. These programmes are very popular and are becoming even more so in the field of engineering.

After completing graduate studies, students may apply for the third stage or postgraduate studies leading to the *Daktaras* (Doctor) research degree or the *Rezidentūra* (Residency, a specific form of training for medical doctors) or the *Meno Aspirantūra* (the highest training level of artists' or postgraduate art studies). These doctoral-level studies last for at least three years for those with Master's degree and up to four years for those who have completed either specialised professional or integrated (continuous) university level studies. The doctoral courses comprise up to five subjects and final examinations, each subject comprising at least 45 hours. Upon completion of the courses, a doctoral thesis must be prepared and defended publicly to qualify the candidate for the doctorate. Doctoral studies may be jointly organised by higher education and research institutions. *Meno aspirantūra* studies are designed for the preparation of lectures in the field of arts and for specialisation of artists or defence and preparation of an art project. After the successful completion of studies, students obtain the qualification of *Meno Licenciatas* (licentiate in arts).

The number of graduates from higher education institution grew steadily in the last decade. There were 9,472 graduates from university-type institutions in 1990. Following growth in 1995 (12,366 graduates), there was a slight drop in 1996 (12,280) and in 1997 (11,690). Since then, the number of university graduates increased again: 13,142 in 1998, and 14,889 in 1999 (Švietimas ir kultūra, 2001).

The market absorbs almost all graduates. Unemployment rates among higher education graduates are relatively low. Highly educated persons are obtaining employment in a variety of services, commerce and industries. In recent years, an oversupply of medical doctors forced medical schools to reduce admission. Moreover, higher education institutions produced more engineers than the market could absorb.

One of the priorities of the Government policy is to steer the system of higher education towards a balanced supply of highly qualified graduates for the labour market. These priorities are embedded in legal documents. For example, according to Article 4 of the Regulations on Programmes of Consecutive Studies (October 26, 2000 – emphasis added):

A higher education institution organising or striving to organise a study programme has to ensure the content and structure, teachers' qualification, material facilities and methodical framework necessary for studies regulated by these Regulations, and other conditions for the acquisition of higher education and professional qualification in conformity with the demand of the *labour market*.

The Lithuanian Ministry of Education and Science regularly conducts research on the market for higher education graduates. Results of this research help the Ministry to define priorities. The market demand for specialists with higher education degrees became one of the most important indicators in reshaping the structure of higher education programmes.

Public higher education institutions are established by Parliament (*Seimas*); private higher education institutions are licensed by the government. Parliament approves budget allocations for the higher education system every year. In recent years, the higher education community experienced a significant shift from self-regulation towards central control by the government. The Ministry of Education and Science, and more specifically its Department for Science and Higher Education, is in charge of the policy implementation in the fields of higher education and research. The government, which in 2002 was formed from a coalition of left-wing parties, prepared a proposal for funding higher education. The Science Council of the Republic of Lithuania launches discussions and prepares recommendations to the Parliament and the government on all major issues in higher education and research. Most important amongst the other interest groups that influence strategic policy and lobbying in higher education are the following: the Lithuanian Universities Rectors' Conference, The Directors' Conference of Lithuanian Colleges, The Conference of the Chairmen of the Senates (Councils) of Institutions of Higher Education and Science of Lithuania and the State Research Institute Director's Conference.

The Lithuanian Universities Rectors' Conference is a public organisation, which plays a role in analysing draft decrees prepared by the Department of Science and Higher Education. It also makes recommendations concerning the registration of new higher education institutions that provide Master's and Doctoral study programmes. It prepares various scientific and study projects and programmes and co-operates with its international counterparts.

The Directors' Conference of Lithuanian Colleges is a public organisation which brings together all the directors of Lithuanian colleges. The main objectives include the development of higher non-university education, sharing best practices within the non-university sector, representation of Lithuanian colleges nationally and internationally, co-ordination of efforts for quality assurance in the colleges, integration of Lithuanian colleges into the common European Higher Education Area and the promotion of a European dimension in higher education.

The Conference of the Chairmen of the Senates (Councils) of Institutions of Higher Education and Science of Lithuania is an independent public organisation formed by a majority of the chairmen of the Senates (Councils) of institutions of higher education and science of Lithuania.

The State Research Institute Director's Conference determines the development of fundamental and applied science, evaluates scientific programmes and helps scientists to develop international relations. The Conference is a scientific expert on new technology and projects. (Links to above mentioned associations available on http://www.mokslas.lt.)

The Lithuanian Students' Association plays a significant role in higher education reform. Students discuss not only national quality assurance policies, but also invite international colleagues to discuss developments in the field. In 2000, the forum of the European students associations (ESIB) was held in Vilnius; it focused on quality of higher education.

14.2   Accreditation Schemes

14.2.1   Accreditation

Two types of accreditation should be established in Lithuanian higher education: accreditation of programmes and accreditation of institutions. But only accreditation of study programmes is institutionalised. The Centre for Quality Assessment in Higher Education (see also section 14.2.5) is currently deliberating plans on accreditation of universities and colleges. Institutional accreditation will be a part of quality improvement and monitoring system in education, which in the future will embrace all levels of education.

The accreditation scheme, as depicted in Figure 1, includes processes organised by the Centre and the Ministry. The Centre prepares a project of external evaluation, conducts the evaluation, ensures that peers prepare reports on the quality of programmes, and, finally, submits the report together with recommendations to the Experts' Council. The Experts' Council examines the final reports and presents recommendations on accreditation to the Ministry of Science and Education. Based on these recommendations, the minister issues a decree on the following types of accreditation of evaluated study programmes:

- Full accreditation: valid until next exhaustive external evaluation;
- Provisional accreditation: Valid for no longer than two years;
- Limited accreditation: Valid for no longer than three years;
- Non-accreditation: Programme is terminated.

Figure 1. Accreditation scheme

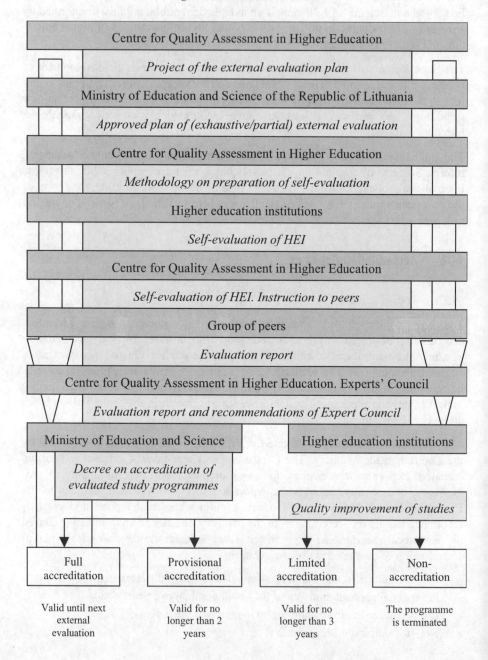

A regular programme evaluation for the purposes of accreditation was initiated by the Centre in 1999. The first recommendation on accreditation was issued by the Experts' Council on February 14, 2000; it included programmes in construction engineering. Formal accreditation of programmes emerged in spring 2002 when the first Ministerial order was issued on the accreditation of 220 university-type programmes and two programmes of Alytus College (Dėl aukštojo mokslo studijų programų akreditavimo, April 30, 2002). The accreditation of those programmes is valid for approximately seven to eight years, if other legal acts do not decide otherwise. 45 study programmes were accredited provisionally (for a period of two years) and four obtained limited accreditation. Admission of students to the latter programmes is forbidden. If on re-evaluation (in 2003) experts find that the quality of the programmes has improved, student admission will be allowed. If not, these programmes will be terminated.

The Law on Higher Education of the Republic of Lithuania does not prescribe procedures of accreditation or evaluation. The evaluation procedures are prescribed in the *Rules of assessment for institutions of research and higher education* which were approved by the Minister of Education and Science on 29 December 2000. The Ministerial decree of March 18, 2002 on decisions regarding evaluated programmes provided the legal grounds for accreditation.

14.2.2   Approval

Two processes of approval were established: for programmes and for institutions. The difference between evaluation for approval and evaluation of existing programmes lies in the focus of the evaluation. In the case of approval, experts look at the input and environmental indicators. They seek evidence of whether the initiators of a new programme or institution are capable of organising higher education studies. Moreover, the experts want to see proof of market demand for a specific programme or institution. Finally, they draw attention to the competitive environment; a new initiative may duplicate already existing programmes and fail to create added value.

New programme approval by the Centre leads to formal recognition of the programme by the Ministry of Education and Science. The Ministry includes positively evaluated programmes in the Register of the Study and Training Programmes, which is maintained as a database that is accessible to the general public, potential students and other stakeholders (Studijų ir mokymo programų registravimo tvarka, 1999). In fall 2002 the register maintained data on 970 university-type programmes and 200 non-university-type programmes; 412 are undergraduate, 421 graduate, and 126 specialised professional (Studijų ir mokymo programų suvestinė, 2002).

Figure 2. Approval of state higher education institution

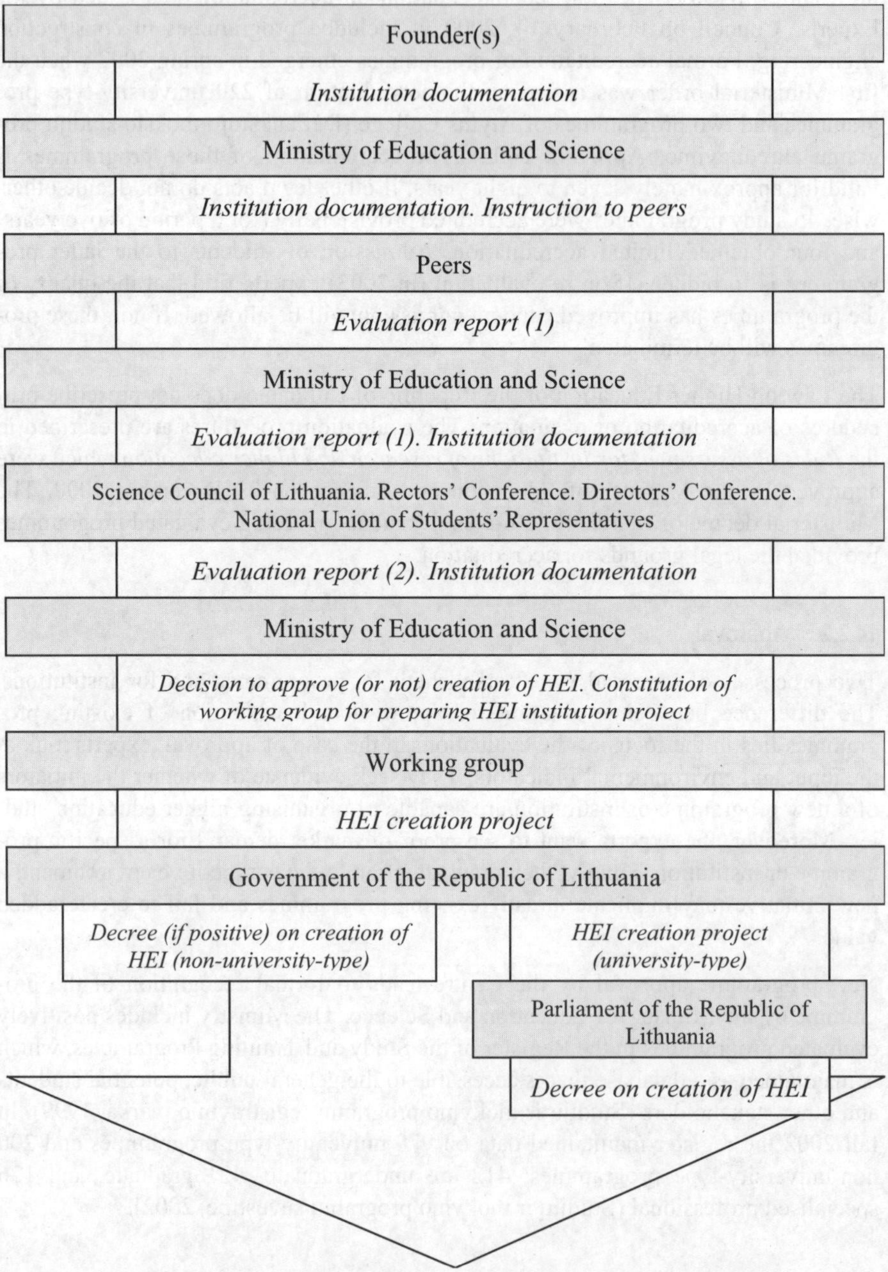

Founder(s)

Institution documentation

Ministry of Education and Science

Institution documentation. Instruction to peers

Peers

Evaluation report (1)

Ministry of Education and Science

Evaluation report (1). Institution documentation

Science Council of Lithuania. Rectors' Conference. Directors' Conference. National Union of Students' Representatives

Evaluation report (2). Institution documentation

Ministry of Education and Science

Decision to approve (or not) creation of HEI. Constitution of working group for preparing HEI institution project

Working group

HEI creation project

Government of the Republic of Lithuania

Decree (if positive) on creation of HEI (non-university-type) / *HEI creation project (university-type)*

Parliament of the Republic of Lithuania

Decree on creation of HEI

Figure 3. Approval of private higher education institution

Founder(s)
Institution documentation
Center for Quality Assessment in Higher Education
Institution documentation. Instruction to peers
Peers
Evaluation report (1)
Center for Quality Assessment in Higher Education
Evaluation report (1). Institution documentation
Founder(s)
Evaluation report (1). Institution documentation
Ministry of Education and Science
Institution documentation. Evaluation report (if positive)
Science Council of Lithuania. Rectors' Conference. Directors' Conference. National Union of Students' Representatives
Evaluation report (2)
Ministry of Education and Science
Decree (if positive) on creation of HEI (project). Evaluation reports (1 and 2)
Government of the Republic of Lithuania
Decree on creation of HEI. Licence

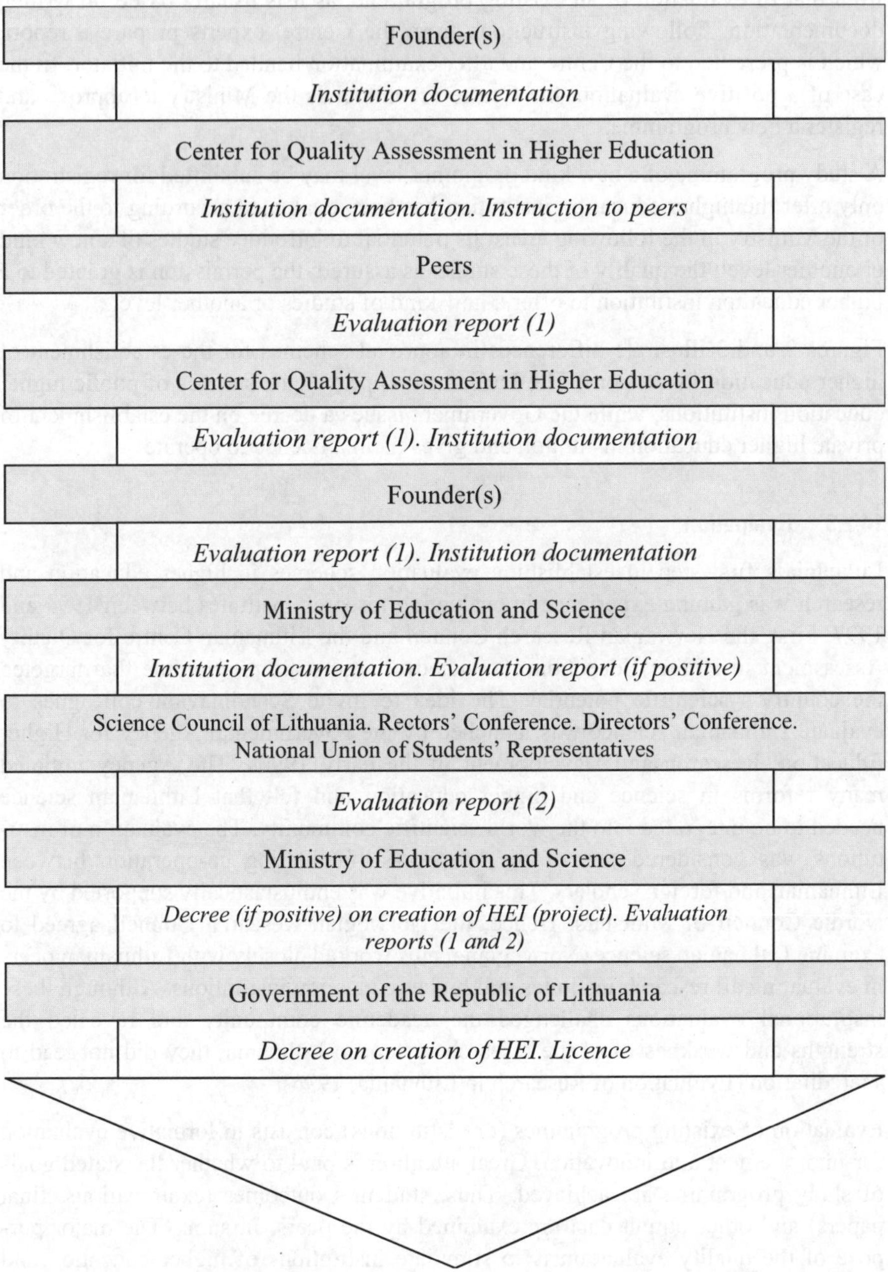

Approval of a new programme is less complex than evaluation, and the result differs from that of evaluation of an existing programme, as it is usually based on written documentation. Following instructions from the Centre, experts prepare a report, which is presented to the Centre and after examination handed to the initiator. In the case of a positive evaluation, the Centre recommends the Ministry to approve and register a new programme.

A study programme of a new kind or another level may be submitted for registration only after the higher education institution has been evaluated according to the order of the Ministry in the following areas: its potential to introduce studies of a new kind or another level; the quality of these studies is assured; the permission is granted to a higher education institution to offer a new kind of studies or another level.

Figures 2 and 3 illustrate differences in approval schemes for the establishment of higher education institutions. The Parliament approves the statutes of public higher education institutions, while the Government issues a decree on the establishment of private higher education institution and gives them a licence to operate.

14.2.3   Evaluation

Lithuania's first step in establishing evaluation schemes in higher education and research was gaining experience in evaluating research institutes between 1994 and 1997. First, the Norwegian Research Council and the Lithuanian Centre for Quality Assessment in Higher Education conducted a large-scale programme that targeted the country's scientific potential. The idea to invite Scandinavian colleagues to evaluate Lithuanian science was launched by the governmental Agency for Higher Education, Research and Development in the early 1990s. The Agency initiated many reforms in science and higher education and felt that Lithuanian science needed to be integrated into the world scientific community. The evaluation of institutions was considered one of the 'windows' facilitating co-operation between Lithuanian and foreign scholars. This initiative was enthusiastically supported by the Nordic Council of Ministers. Hence, the Norwegian Research Council agreed to examine Lithuanian science. Norwegian teams worked closely with Lithuanian peers in evaluating all research institutes and higher education institutions. Although these institutional evaluations challenged the academic community and revealed the strengths and weaknesses of the research system in Lithuania, they did not lead to accreditation (Evaluation of Research in Lithuania, 1996).

Evaluation of existing programmes (or institutions) consists in formative evaluation for improvement and innovation. Great attention is paid to whether the stated goals of study programme are achieved. Thus, student's outcomes (examinations, final papers) and other output data are examined by the peers. In sum: 'The major purpose of the quality evaluation is to stimulate institutions of higher education and research, their subdivisions and all the scientists too seek clear perception of the need of Lithuania, the mission, objectives and tasks of the institution, to help institution reveal its weaknesses and strengths, and to facilitate its effectiveness' (Rules, Article 3).

Article 44 of the Law on Higher Education, on registration and evaluation of study programmes, states that the Ministry may take into account results of evaluated programmes for funding decisions (Law on Higher Education, 2000). The funding decision is defined by the contract between the higher education institution and the Ministry.

The evaluation scheme, which was used from 1996 through 2002, involved similar processes to the current accreditation scheme. Previously, all formally recognised higher education institutions were part of the quality evaluation scheme, i.e. the element of accreditation at the end of the scheme was not included. A higher education institution had to participate in the evaluation process by presenting self-evaluation reports on the programmes included in the list belonging to a particular field of study or subject.

14.2.4   The Range of Application of the Schemes

Lithuania is a small country and administratively higher education institutions are not divided into regions. However, for the sake of efficiency, and in order to save time and resources, the Centre can split the team of experts into two or three groups. For example, when law programmes were evaluated in Vilnius, Kaunas and Utena, two groups of experts (including international peers) divided their tasks. All groups focused on programmes at university-type institutions. For the site visits to non-university-type institutions the group was split into two smaller groups. But the final report is always prepared and signed by all group members, even if they did not visit the institution.

Integration of research and teaching is a keystone of Lithuanian higher education. Therefore, institutions have to address this issue in their self-evaluation reports. For example, they must specify how research results of the academic staff are integrated into the study process and indicate whether students' research projects are related to the research areas of the department.

As mentioned in section 1, research institutes are involved in post-graduate studies, but their main mission is research and development. A separate methodology is applied for assessing these institutes. Starting in 1994, research capacity was evaluated in all 29 state research institutes. Moreover, from 1995 through 1997 experts of the Centre analysed the productivity of the research institutes. One of the aims of these evaluations was to identify the most advanced areas of science in Lithuania and to provide suggestions as to how to integrate scientific achievement into Lithuania's market and industries. Another aspect of evaluation was the identification of achievements in the field of co-operation between research institutes and universities, both in research and study areas. Although in some areas, such as physics, chemistry, philosophy, cultural studies, linguistics and Lithuanian literature, co-operation was very fruitful, in other areas there was no integration. The tension between research institutes and universities has its roots in the former Soviet system that split research and studies. Despite many attempts, interaction between the two sectors remains insufficient. In recent years, following the recommendations of quality evaluation teams and suggestions by the governmental officials, a new strategy to attain integration has been adopted, viz. a model of research institutes within universities has been proposed. This has already led to several research institutions integrating their activities into universities.

Higher education institutions are responsible for the evaluation of individual subjects or disciplines. They establish procedures for the development and approval of curricula that include evaluation of the syllabi of individual courses. Many universities and colleges encourage the introduction of interdisciplinary courses. Furthermore, all institutions develop internal student evaluations of instructors. Department heads and deans discuss regularly the results of those evaluations, which may have an impact on employment relationships.

Thus, none of the buffer organisations which evaluate the quality of programmes and institutions are involved in the evaluation of individual subjects and disciplines. However, while evaluating programmes, the Centre's peers study documentary evidence of existing internal institutional quality mechanisms that should include the evaluation of syllabi and the improvement of instructional processes. For example, the Vytautas Magnus University regulations of studies state the following: 'Studies in each subject should be evaluated at the end. A questionnaire, which is approved by Rector's office, is used. Departments and deans conduct the analysis. Councils of faculties and rector's office staff analyse the results.' (Vytautas Magnus University, 2002.)

14.2.5   Organisations

Two buffer organisations, the Centre for Quality Evaluation in Higher Education (the Centre) and the Quality Evaluation Unit of the Methodological Centre for Vocational Education and Training (the Unit), are engaged in implementing schemes of accreditation, evaluation and approval of new programmes and institutions. There is a division of functions between the Centre and the Unit.

The Centre:

- Evaluates new programmes of university-type institutions; this evaluation leads to registration.

- Organises exhaustive evaluation of university-type and college-type programmes; this evaluation leads to accreditation. Alternatively, evaluation can be carried out to assess the situation or to address specific issues.
- Evaluates applications for the creation of higher education institutions.
- Evaluates research institutions.

The Unit:

- Evaluates new programmes of colleges; this evaluation leads to registration (in the near future this function will be transferred to the Centre).
- Carries out institutional evaluation of colleges for institutional accreditation purposes (anticipated to start in 2004).

The Centre was established in 1995 to maintain a high level of higher education in Lithuania. In September 2002, it assumed a new function: According to Article 8 of the Governmental Decision it started to evaluate applications of new private and (probably) state higher education institutions. (Aukštųjų mokyklų steigimo tvarka, 2002.09.13). The basic goals of the Centre are as follows:

- To co-ordinate and methodically guide the regular self-analysis process of scientific and pedagogical activity of the state and non-state institutions of research and higher education,
- to organise expert evaluation of that activity,
- to gather and publish information about the quality of that activity,
- to offer suggestions about the improvement of that activity.

The Centre is also involved in the evaluation of research and higher education institutions, as mentioned above. It acts as the secretariat of the Expert Council of the Quality Assessment of Research and Higher Education Institutions (Expert Council), which started its activities in 2000. The Centre co-ordinates its programme of evaluation with the Department of Science and Higher Education of the Ministry of Education and Science. In fulfilling its tasks, the Centre co-operates with the Science Council of Lithuania, the Lithuanian Academy of Science, the Conferences of heads of research and higher education institutions, vocational and employment associations and other public institutions. Some of these non-profit institutions or interest groups help to monitor quality in higher education and research. For example, the Lithuanian Universities Rectors' Conference makes recommendations concerning the registration of new higher education institutions that offer Master's and Doctoral study programmes, while the Directors' Conference of Lithuanian Colleges co-ordinates quality assurance in the colleges. The State Research Institute Director's Conference evaluates scientific programmes and helps scientists to develop international relations.

The Unit of Study and Teaching Quality Evaluation was established in 1999 in the framework of the EU technical and financial support programme 'Institutional Building in Education Reform'. Since 2000, the Unit has been continuing its activity in the creation of a Methodological Centre for vocational education and training. The aim of the unit is to evaluate the quality of study/training programmes and to audit schools' activity, and to inform society about the results of evaluation. The Unit's functions are as follows:

- Act as Secretariat for the Council and the Commission. The Council of vocational education and training quality evaluation is an expert institution. Its members are appointed lecturers/teachers of higher schools, social partners and representatives of other institutions. The Commission is the central vocational education and training expert. It acts under the rule of the Methodological Centre for Vocational Education and Training.
- Create a database on review experts and organise experts' training.
- Organise the external evaluation expert groups.
- Consult Schools on issues of evaluation and assist them in teaching personnel to effectively evaluate quality internally.
- Implement initial evaluation of vocational training programmes' in accordance with the governmental and ministerial regulations concerning vocational education and training.
- Co-ordinate the preparation of vocational schools' external evaluation reports and organise their publication.

The Ministry of Education and Science approves the regulations of the Centre and the Unit, and provides basic funding for their operations. Their leadership is financially accountable to the ministry.

The Centre contracts local experts and foreign experts. The policy of the Centre in forming groups is flexible: foreign experts can work together with the Lithuanian experts or form separate groups. In 2001, the first international peer team (including one local expert) assessed law programmes. The involvement of international peers largely depends on the availability of financial resources. Experts are proposed to the Centre by:

- the institutions of research and higher education, the Science Council of Lithuania, the Lithuanian Academy of Sciences;
- boards or councils of professional societies (e.g. doctors' unions, engineers' unions, scientists' unions, students' unions of research and higher education institutions), creative organisations;
- ministries or other state institutions concerned with higher education or research;
- scientists and other experts with experience of evaluation;

- foreign quality assurance agencies.

The experts proposed to the Centre should have been active in research and pedagogy for the last five years, i.e. they have to have published a sufficient number of articles in research publications that are on the list of the Institute of Scientific Information and on a list approved by the Department. Other proposed experts must be familiar with higher education and research in Lithuania and with foreign experience in respective subject areas. The recommendation of experts is based not only on their professional competence, but also on such personal qualities as adherence to principle, goodwill, fairness and ability to make impartial evaluations, readiness to implement progressive ideas. Scientists from other subject areas than the evaluated subject area (field) can be involved in expert groups. Elimination or reduction of potential conflict of interest of the experts through relations with the evaluated units is sought. The leader of the expert group must be impartial. Research and higher education institutions to be assessed can propose candidates to an expert Group to the Centre beforehand, defending their suitability. The Centre informs all the institutions to be evaluated about the planned composition of an expert group. Institutions have the right to contest refusal of proposed experts.

The Centre organises workshops during which the experts and the officials of the institutions concerned with the internal evaluation get acquainted with the aims, tasks and procedures of the evaluation, as well as with the practice of other countries. (These guidelines are available on: www.skvc.lt).

Both the Centre's and the Unit's formal rules in quality evaluation are legal documents, approved by the Ministry.

Funding. The budget allocations for the Centre's operations and evaluation projects come from the government's 'appropriations for the general needs of higher education', which also support international co-operation programmes (such as Socrates, bilateral agreements of academic mobility, EUREKA) and the Lithuanian Fund of Science and Studies. The Department of Science and Higher Education, after discussions with the Lithuanian Science Council and the Lithuanian Rector's Conference, drafts a proposal to the government. Thus, the academic community reaches a consensus in the allocation of general funds for improvements of the higher education system.

In addition, The Centre receives funds from the British Council and the Open Society Fund (Soros Foundation). They are used for partial coverage of costs of peers during their stay in Lithuania and to organise conferences. Finally, in a number of European Commission's projects on quality assurance and higher education reform, the Centre received support from the PHARE grants.

14.2.6   Implementation of Rules

The process of implementation of accreditation schemes is robust. All procedures foreseen in the rules are followed. Some flexibility is allowed in determining schedules and time frames of evaluation. However, there are no specific rules for self-study of higher education institution in terms of the duration of preparation. Since the idea of quality improvement is embedded in schemes, institutions are expected to produce information for their self-study on a regular basis while implementing their internal quality assurance procedures.

The duration of the actual evaluation of a programme depends on the number of programmes included in the project and the specificity of the project (national, international). Higher education institutions are given three months to prepare a self-study report. Experts have at least two months to familiarise themselves with the self-evaluation reports. Then the expert group conducts a site visit to the higher education institution (an institution is usually visited in one day). After the site visits the experts draft a report and send it to the higher education institution. Within ten days the higher education institution corrects factual errors and may argue for changes in certain conclusions and recommendations of the assessment. On receiving these remarks the experts prepare the final external assessment report and submit it to the Centre. A summary of the final conclusion of the evaluation is published by the Centre. If the heads of the institution have special comments about the summary, those comments are published as well.

Seven days are given for institutions to respond to the Minister's draft decision regarding accreditation. These comments are expected when the decision is provisional or limited accreditation of programme.

Approval of new study programmes is organised in cycles defined by the plan issued by the Ministry. The Centre has to conduct evaluation of new programmes in 2.5 months. However, it often takes longer for the institution to meet all the requirements of the Centre. New programme documentation often needs improvement. Hence, the evaluation might take 3.5 months. When all the programmes listed in the plan are evaluated, the Centre receives the conclusions of the Expert Council and sends final recommendations (i.e. the summary issued by the Council) to the Ministry.

14.3   Analysis of Accreditation and Evaluation Schemes

Seeking to respond to the many voices that supported non-intrusive quality control, Lithuania developed an original model of quality assurance in higher education. These voices represented state higher education institutions that wanted to implement dominant ideas of university autonomy and academic freedom. Private higher education establishments only emerged at the end of the 20th century. While neighbours in Latvia and Estonia, forced by a mushrooming private sector, established accreditation schemes, Lithuania's policy had elements of caution and resistance to speeding-up the development of private higher education. In the case of the established public sector, accreditation schemes did not seem appropriate. Institutions received a legitimate right to operate and they promised to implement quality assurance mechanisms. A collegial external evaluation process, involving activities of a buffer organisation, the Lithuanian Centre for Quality Assurance in Higher Education, was acceptable for all public institutions.

Two alternatives, quality assurance for improvement purposes versus accreditation for accountability purposes, have been on the table since debates on higher education quality began. In 1995, teams of higher education experts proposed to implement the first approach. Four teams involving experts from universities created rules for quality evaluation.

In addition, a strong sense of securing quality, and a firm notion of maintaining some sort of control in higher education are embedded in the culture of Lithuanian society. The legacy of a high prestige of educated people is linked to rigid requirements of higher education. Moreover, the legacy of Soviet control mechanisms often plays a positive role in a continuous accountability process; it features bureaucratic routines with which many in academe are familiar. However, borrowing models from abroad was unacceptable. The academic community looked for schemes that best fitted its identity and the needs for reform in higher education.

Two tensions may be distinguished that are related to evaluation that is not based on accreditation. First, there is tension about the standardisation of programmes. The Constitution of the Republic of Lithuania and the Law on Science and Higher Education (1991) provided legal foundation of autonomy and academic freedom for universities. This legal foundation was recently challenged by the standardisation of study trends. The minister approves the regulations. Universities, while designing their curricula, have to comply with structural norms and requirements prescribed for programmes. These regulations will be used in approval quality evaluation and accreditation schemes. Although standardisation is aimed at more clarity and transparency of the programmes, it will force universities to apply more bureaucratic procedures in curricular design. Moreover, standardisation may invoke passive compliance among academics and result in less creativity in the study process. Working groups that are currently involved in this process should secure values of academic freedom and provide sufficient room for innovation in programme design.

Second, there are tensions caused by the dissatisfaction that traditional forms of academic authority failed. External quality evaluation of institutions and programmes was suggested by academics themselves. In the transitional post-Soviet period innovators understood that traditional forms of academic authority had failed. Universities suffered from slow reforms and from corruption. Innovative new leaders proclaimed openness and transparency of policies by introducing evaluation of institutions and programmes. External evaluations helped institutions to look at themselves in the mirror, to understand their weaknesses and to get rid of old traditions that hampered change.

Both accreditation and evaluation schemes use similar conceptual frameworks, which are improvement-oriented. Moreover, the sequence of evaluation procedures is similar. All schemes that are applied for university-type higher education institution are implemented by the same buffer organisation.

Although there is no direct legal link between accreditation schemes and approval schemes, both processes include elements of control, recognition and accountability. Basically, the Ministry has the authority to approve or terminate the programme, based on the evaluation. Therefore, centralised decision-making makes accreditation schemes and programme approval schemes similar.

Universities experienced several positive consequences of the accreditation schemes. First of all, self-analysis helped to establish procedures for regular collection of information about an institution's inputs and outputs of research and education. Furthermore, external evaluation proved successful because it facilitated the reshaping of old courses. In many cases, internal critique did not have as much impact as the external view. Academics, seeking to be innovative, in most cases agreed with the recommendations of the reviewers. This process of positive change enabled universities to co-operate with foreign partners. Some of the partner institutions in Europe saw an accreditation label as a sign of good quality.

Lithuanian policy emphasises widening access to students and preparing them for jobs on the market. The non-university sector widened access of secondary school graduates to tertiary education. A formal decision on accreditation indirectly linked recognition of education by the market and by other educational institutions (both in the country and abroad). The rights of students for recognition are secured if they graduate from officially recognised programmes (or institutions).

Another important consequence is the system of student loans. Only students enrolled in recognised, registered programmes, are entitled to apply for a loan from the State Fund for Studies and Research. While public funds for loans are limited it is likely that in the future the State Fund will support students who are enrolled in accredited programmes.

The policy debate around accreditation catches the attention of the general public. Citizens are concerned about the value of higher education credentials. When accreditation of a popular Law programme at Vilnius University was questioned, the general public and the media reacted strongly. However, since accreditation was established only for a couple of years, there was no tension between established schemes and society. In fact, society needs more information about the benefits of evaluation and the value of accreditation.

Changes in the scheme concerning costs and benefits of accreditation can be anticipated. First of all, the vocational sector will establish an accreditation scheme for colleges by 2004. Second, similar developments, involving evaluation and audit of institutions, are legitimised in secondary education sector. Costs of accreditation will grow because all sectors of education will be included in the process. The Government is interested in cost-saving innovations. Private institutions are concerned about their spending for formal approval and accreditation. Investments in the system of quality monitoring can be costly; therefore, the effect of those schemes should be visible and the benefits should outweigh the costs. Hence, a cost-benefit analysis is needed to provide some feedback. Research is needed on benefits of accreditation. Focus groups and survey techniques could be used to identify key issues of accreditation in higher education.

14.4 External Influences

The Bologna process did not play a significant role in the establishment of accreditation schemes in the country. The process of setting up schemes of quality evaluation in higher education took place in Lithuania almost five years ago. By the time the Bologna meeting was held, Lithuanian higher education institutions had established their procedures of evaluation. Rather to the contrary, the developments in Eastern European countries, especially in the Baltic States, in the field of quality assurance were exemplary and influenced innovations in the region.

Politically, the Bologna process meant a step forward in bringing Western Europe and Eastern Europe to a closer dialogue on higher education. Some aspects in favour of the Bologna process can be mentioned. First, when the ministers of education from 29 countries were invited to sign the Bologna declaration in June 1999, they were exposed to the importance of internationalisation in the field of higher education. Internationalisation included the following areas: academic mobility, recognition of qualifications, introduction of the Diploma Supplement, and quality assurance. Having signed the Declaration, ministers committed themselves to support developments in these areas in their respective countries. Second, representatives of Eastern European countries gained more visibility vis-à-vis Western European partners. This was useful for further developments of the enlargement of the European Union.

Although the Bologna process did not directly impact on evaluation developments in Lithuania, the Declaration facilitated diversification of the higher education system. Non-university institutions of higher education were legitimised; the system of higher education thus became binary. Furthermore, different interests groups came to a compromise in allowing short higher education programmes, of at least three years, which were registered as non-university-type higher education programmes. Consequently, students have a wider choice of options for their studies. However, articulation between the non-university sector and the university sector needs to be achieved. For students seeking admission from one sector to the other, there may still be barriers of transferability of studies and recognition of credentials.

Lithuania joined the World Trade Organization (WTO) in 2001 and signed the General Agreement on Trade and Services (GATS). The country committed itself to free service provisions in all sectors of trade. Higher education, as one of those sectors, is included in Chapter 5C of GATS. No restrictions have been established in market access and in national treatment provisions (Articles 1, 2, and 3). However, Lithuania did not make specific commitments regarding provision of services of physical persons (Article 4). This implies that national authorities have the right to restrict market access to persons and to impose national regulations on the services of physical persons. What does that mean for the higher education system? Although the country allows the establishing of foreign or trans-national higher education institutions and does not discriminate against these institutions, it has the right to exclude from GATS all persons that work without a formal contract. By signing GATS and opening the higher education market to foreign providers, Lithuania entered a phase of globalisation. Although the consequences of this competitive process on higher education will be seen in the future, quality standards will be an issue. We might anticipate that the nation's higher education institutions will have to improve quality in order to compete successfully for students. Otherwise, a stream of students may drift to colleges and universities established by foreign providers.

Another possible development as a consequence of globalisation may occur in the accreditation field. If transnational bodies for accreditation will be established, alternative policies might have to be debated in the field of quality evaluation. Will accreditation be national or transnational? So far, international teams have started evaluating law, medicine, and education programmes. This shows that Lithuanian quality assurance schemes already include some globalisation aspect.

Many ideas and concepts of quality assurance and accreditation have been taken from Western models. The applicability of those models has been widely discussed in Lithuania. At least four external influences can be distinguished in the development of quality assurance and accreditation schemes:

- Integration into supra-national governmental organisations, such as UNESCO, Council of Europe, European Commission, and OECD;
- Growing international academic mobility and, as a consequence, the need for comparison of degrees and qualification in higher education:

- Participation in networks of quality assurance agencies, such as the International Network of Quality Assurance Agencies in Higher Education (INQAAHE);
- Co-operation with international specialised organisations of higher education, such as the association of engineering schools.

We wish to make some observations on the first point. First, in the early 1990s, UNESCO-CEPES (the Centre for Higher Education, Bucharest) organised a series of events and published papers on quality assurance in higher education. Experts from the United States and Western Europe shared their ideas with representatives from Central/Eastern Europe on the strengths and weaknesses of the accreditation model. Professor Algirdas Cizas, who later became the first director of the Centre for Quality Evaluation in Higher Education, was an active participant, and he published a number of articles about idiosyncrasies of quality assurance in a small country like Lithuania (see list of publications at www.skvc.lt)

In the mid-1990s, the Council of Europe launched a programme to support innovations in higher education in the new member-states. Quality assurance became one of the central themes of the Legislative Reform Programme. The Council of Europe tried to provide expert advice based on the needs of individual countries and the problems emerging in a specific region, e.g. three Baltic countries. Therefore, series of workshops on the topic were organised in Riga, Tallinn, and Vilnius. This resulted in the creation of the Baltic Higher Education Co-ordination Committee (BHECC), which focuses on co-operation in quality assurance and recognition of credentials.

Together, UNESCO and the Council of Europe initiated the 1997 Lisbon Convention, which included provisions on quality assurance. Lithuania was amongst the first five countries that ratified this convention.

Two significant PHARE investments (a programme of the European Union for co-operation with Central and Eastern Europe) contributed to the development of quality assurance in Lithuania. First, one of the four components of the 'Multi-country programme in higher education' targeted quality assurance. Second, the national PHARE project 'Higher Education Reform' helped to restructure the higher education system and to establish evaluation schemes for non-university-type institutions. TEMPUS, a part of PHARE, helped universities to set up quality assurance mechanisms and to prepare some of the institutions for large-scale co-operation in SOCRATES exchanges. The PHARE programme also facilitated developments in quality evaluation in vocational, post-secondary sectors.

Several initiatives of OECD's IMHE (Institutional Management in Higher Education) programme involved Lithuanian experts from Vilnius University, Kaunas University of Technology and the Vilnius Gediminas Technical University. Events were held in Vilnius; and publications of the OECD/IMHE on quality assurance were important sources for institutional improvements.

Lithuanian experts joined the INQAAHE network in 1993, when the concept of evaluation was adopted by the Science Council. (Mockienė, 1993). Participation in the network opened ways of communication world-wide on issues of accreditation.

International associations of specialised higher education schools in engineering, arts, education, business and other fields helped to redesign curricula and reshape study processes in technical and engineering education. For example, in the early 1990s, Kaunas University of Technology launched an international evaluation of engineering programmes. This pioneering effort facilitated the reform of higher education in engineering towards a more holistic learning approach.

14.5   Other Evaluation Activities

In 2000, the government introduced audit requirements for all public institutions. The audit includes examination of institutional goals, efficient use of financial and human resources, as well as general effectiveness of the public organisation.

Moreover, institutions individually pursue strategic development policies that may include aspects of quality of teaching and research. For example, in the early 1990s, Kaunas University of Technology established *programme committees* in charge of curriculum redesign according to best practices in Europe and the world (Kaunas Technology University, no date). Vilnius University also created special leadership groups that devised internal policies of evaluation and improvement as a significant component of overall strategic management. For example, in 2002, Interfaculty (inter-school) committees of study programmes and the University's Academic Commission were responsible for quality assurance at this institution. These activities are related to growing participation in academic mobility within the SOCRATES programme. Any institution willing to participate in mutual academic mobility must comply with the requirements set by the EU programme. Consequently, participation in the SOCRATES exchanges can be used as a quality indicator of a programme.

Acknowledgements

This chapter would not have been completed without the assistance of Mr. Almantas Šerpatauskas, Programme Specialist of the Lithuanian Centre for Quality Evaluation in Higher Education, Mr. Darius Tamošiūnas, Acting Deputy Director of the same Centre, and Aušra Jančauskiene, Head of the Unit of Study and Teaching Quality Evaluation of the Methodological Centre for Vocational Education and Training. I am very grateful for their information, consultations, and numerous comments on the draft.

References

II etapo uždaviniai (2001). [Objectives of the second stage of the educational reform]. In Švietimo reformos rezultatai. Vilnius: Švietimo ir mokslo ministerija. P. 140-144.

Aukstųjų mokyklų steigimo tvarka (September 13, 2002). [Order of establishment of higher education institutions]. Patvirtinta Lietuvos Respublikos Vyriausybės 2000 m. Rugpjūčio 30 d. nutarimu Nr. 999; 2002 m. Rugsėjo 13 d. nutarimo Nr. 1441 redakcija. Vilnius.

Decision of the Government of the Republic of Lithuania No. 999. Concerning the Procedure of Establishment of Higher Education Institutions. August 3, 2000. Vilnius.

Dėl aukštojo mokslo studijų programų akreditavimo (Decree April 30, 2002). [Decree on accreditation of higher educaiton programmes]. Lietuvos Respublikos Švietimo ir Mokslo ministro 2002 m. balandžio 30 d. įsakymas. Nr. 785. Vilnius.

Dėl Švietimo ir mokslo ministro 2001 m. rugpjūčio 13 d. įsakymo Nr. 1194 'Dėl sprendimų dėl įvertintu aukštojo mokslo studijų programų priėmimo tvarkos patvirtinimo' dalinio pakeitimo. (March 18, 2002) [Decree on decisions regarding evaluated programmes]. Vilnius.

Evaluation of Research in Lithuania. (1996). Volume 1, 2. Oslo: The Research Council of Norway. Volume 1, 2.

Higher Education in Lithuania. (2000). Vilnius: Justitia.

Institucijos strateginis veiklos planas (2002). Mokslo ir studijų departamentas prie Švietimo ir mokslo ministerijos. Retrieved on October 30, 2002 from http://www.mokslas.lt

Jančauskiene, A. (2002-2003). Personal communication.

Kaunas Technology University. Programų komitetai. http://www.ktu.lt.

Law on Higher Education of the Republic of Lithuania. Official Gazette. No 27-715, 2000.

Leišytė, L. (2002). Higher Education Governance in Post-Soviet Lithuania. University of Oslo, Institute for Educational Research, Report No 8.

Lietuvos švietimas (2000). [Education in Lithuania]. Vilnius: Švietimo ir mokslo ministerija. P. 59-63.

Law on Science and Higher Education (1991).

Lukošiuniene, D. et al. (2002). Lietuvos aukštasis mokslas. [Lithuanian Higher Education]. Vilnius: Justitia. P. 55-62.

Mockienė, B., Frazer, M., Westerheijden, D. et al. (1998). A Comparative Review of Recent Legislation. In: Quality Assurance in Higher Education: A Legislative Review and Needs Analysis of Developments in Central and Eastern Europe. June 1998, European Training Foundation, PHARE. P. 9-22, 34-39, 48-59.

Mockienė, B. (1996). Baltijos aukštojo mokslo koordinaciniame komitete. [Baltic Higher Education Coordination Committee]. In: Mokslo Lietuva. [Scientific Lithuania], 1996 m. kovo 7 d. Nr. 5(120). P. 2 & 6.

Mockienė, B. (1993). Problems and Concepts of Evaluation of Higher Education and Research Institutions in Lithuania. In: QA, International Network for Quality Assurance Agencies in Higher Education. Issue No 5, October, 1993. P. 24-27.

Order of the Minister of Education and Science No. 1281 Concerning the Procedure of Evaluation of Readiness of Institutions to Implement Non-University Studies. October 18, 2000. (Amended by order No 1373, November 8, 2000.) Vilnius.

PHARE (2000). The European University: A Handbook on Institutional Approaches to Strategic Management, Quality Management, European Policy and Academic Recognition. June 2000. PHARE: European Training Foundation.

Regulations on the programmes of consecutive studies (2000): Order No 1326 of October 26, 2000. Minister of Education and Science of the Republic of Lithuania. Vilnius.

Regulations of the Centre for Quality Evaluation in Higher Education. http://www.skvc.lt.

Rules of quality evaluation for institutions of research and higher education. (June 28, 2001). Approved by order No 1055 of the Ministry of Education and Science of the Republic of Lithuania on June 28, 2001. http://www.skvc.lt.

Studijų ir mokymo programų registras (2002). [Register of programmes] Švietimo ir mokslo ministerija. Retrieved on November 18, 2002 from http://www.mokykla.smm.lt/statistika/SP_5-1.html.

Studijų ir mokymo programų suvestinė pagal mokymo sritis ir lygmenis. (2002). [The summary of the study and training programmes according to fields and levels]. Retrieved on November 18, 2002 from http://www.mokykla.smm.lt/statistika/SP_5-1.html.

Studijų ir mokymo programų registravimo tvarka [Order of the registration of programmes of studies and training]: Lietuvos Respublikos Švietimo ir Mokslo ministro isakymas (1999.12.10). Nr. 1233. Vilnius.

Studijų krypties reglamento sandara. (2001). [Structural composition of the regulations for the trend of studies]. Patvirtinta Švietimo ir Mokslo ministro 2001 m. balandžio 23 d. įsakymu Nr. 658. Vilnius.

Studijų programų išorinio vertinimo 2002 metais planas. (2002). [Plan of external evaluation of study programmes]. Retrieved on November 12, 2002 at http://www.skvc.lt.

Šerpatauskas, A. (2002/2003). Personal communication.

Švietimas ir kultura (2001). [Education and Culture]. Lietuvos statistikos metraštis. Retrieved on November 18, 2002 from http://www.smm.lt/statistika/s_stat12.htm.

Vytautas Magnus University (2002). Studijų kokybės vertinimas. [Evaluation of quality of studies. In:Regulations of studies]. In Studijų reguliaminas. http://www.vdu.lt.

The order of the Minister of Education and Science No. 2390: Regarding the changes in the procedure of the vocational training quality evaluation in vocational schools. January 18, 2001. Order No. 73. Vilnius.

15   The Netherlands: A Leader in Quality Assurance Follows the Accreditation Trend

MARGARITA JELIAZKOVA & DON F. WESTERHEIJDEN

15.1   The National System of Higher Education in the Netherlands

15.1.1   Place in the System of Education

The Dutch education system includes the following levels: primary education for children between the ages of four and twelve, secondary education as a continuation of primary education for pupils between twelve and (16 to) 18 years old, higher education for students aged eighteen and above, adult and vocational education and certified education (from 16 onwards). At the end of comprehensive primary education, pupils are assigned to general pre-vocational secondary education, senior secondary education or pre-university education. The general pre-vocational education (VMBO) lasts for four years and gives access to the senior vocational secondary education (MBO) and the apprenticeship system (LLW), which are both part of vocational and adult education. A third type of secondary education is the five-year senior general secondary education (HAVO), which can be directly accessed after primary education or after completing the VMBO. HAVO graduates can attend MBO or pre-university education (VWO). Pre-university education gives access to the university (WO), higher professional education (HBO) and to distance learning courses in higher education (Open University).

15.1.2   Size and Structure of Higher Education

The Dutch higher education system is a binary system and consists of 13 universities (including Wageningen Agricultural University, which is financed by the ministry of agriculture) and 56 institutions offering higher vocational education. The latter, the HBO-institutions, are somewhat comparable to the German *Fachhochschulen* or the British (former) polytechnics, although the official length of their study programmes is longer: four, instead of three years (full-time). Besides the 13 traditional public research universities, there is a limited number of small 'designated institutions': a university for business administration, four institutes for theological training and a humanistic university, as well as several international education institutes. The total number of these designated institutes is 61. They fall under the Higher Education and Research Act but do not receive government funding, and the students receive no

S. Schwarz and D.F. Westerheijden (eds.),
Accreditation and Evaluation in the European Higher Education Area, 323–345.
© 2004 *Kluwer Academic Publishers. Printed in the Netherlands.*

financial aid.[1] However, the degrees they issue are recognised. These institutions are often not included in the official statistics.

In addition to these two major sectors, higher education in the Netherlands is also provided through the Open University, located in Heerlen with a number of support centres around the country. The Open University offers a wide range of courses, leading to both formal university and higher vocational education degrees. (In statistics, it is often included in the public university sector.)

There are no other formal sectors of post-secondary education in the Netherlands. In addition, the 'designated' institutes and organisations offer a large number of recognised certificates, diplomas and degrees in various professional fields such as accountancy, business administration, etc. These are usually structured as 'external studies' in the sense of distance learning courses with limited face-to-face interaction.

15.1.3   Types of Degrees

The distinction between vocational education and university education still remains under the newly introduced bachelor-master system. For the universities, the bachelor-master structure is now becoming the norm. This means that the programmes are split in two parts:

- A bachelor's part consisting of 180 credits (in ECTS-equivalents);
- A master's part consisting of (as a rule) 60 credits.

For the higher vocational institutions, the existing first degree courses continue to be considered as a bachelor's course of 240 credits. The higher vocational institutions can also offer (professional) Master's courses. The courses offered at the moment will only be officially recognised if they obtain accreditation from the Netherlands Accreditation Organisation (NAO).

Access to master's programmes is based on the entrance requirements determined by the institutions. In general, students are admitted on the basis of their having completed a relevant bachelor's programme. The law specifies that every academic bachelor programme should give entrance to at least one academic master's programme. In those cases where the master's programme does not correspond to the bachelor's programme, admission may be selective. A master's degree will be required for entrance to doctoral programmes.

---

1   The new accreditation scheme will change this arrangement; any accredited programme, regardless of the institution's funding, will entitle students to receive financial aid.

15.1.4   Types of Programmes

Government-funded higher professional education courses cover the following seven areas: Education, Economics, Behaviour and Society, Language and Culture, Engineering and Technology, Agriculture and Natural Environment, and Health Care. Most HBO-institutions offer courses in several of these fields.

Of the 13 universities, nine carry out teaching and research in a broad range of disciplines spanning seven sectors: Economics, Health, Behaviour and Society, Law, Engineering and Technology, and Language and Culture. Three focus on engineering and technology. The Agricultural University in Wageningen provides courses in the field of agriculture and the natural environment.

In both higher education sectors, there are full-time and part-time courses. Dual courses combining learning and work were introduced on an experimental basis in 1998/99.

The total number of programme types listed in the Central Register of Higher Education Study Programmes (CROHO) is 117. Within these programmes, students are to some extent free to combine their own programmes. Equally, with the approval of the relevant examining board students may establish their own degree studies by selecting from different programmes.

15.1.5   Transition from Higher Education to Work

Close contacts between HBO institutions and the labour market are extremely important. They occur at both national and individual course level. Each year a national survey of HBO-graduates, known as the HBO-Monitor, is carried out on behalf of the HBO-Council.

Universities prepare students for research training and for occupations in which it is useful to have an academic background. Only a small proportion of graduates (around 10 %) are eventually employed in research. Like the HBO institutions, the universities monitor the position of their graduates on the labour market by means of an annual survey, which began in 1998.

15.1.6   Governance and Steering of Higher Education

The Dutch education system combines a unified education system, regulated by central laws, with decentralised administration and management of schools. Overall responsibility for the public-private education system lies with the State, represented by the Minister of Education, Culture and Science, and the legislative power of the Dutch Parliament.

The Ministry lays down the conditions, especially in primary and secondary education, relating to the types of schools that can exist, the length of courses, compulsory and optional school subjects, the minimum and maximum number of lessons to be given and their length, the norms for class division, the examination syllabus and national examinations, and standards of competence, salaries, status and teaching hours of teaching staff. The Ministry does not set up schools, but does determine the norms for their establishment. This applies to both public and private education.

The government establishes a framework within which HBO institutions have to operate, but it is the responsibility of the competent authority to expand on the Government framework concerning the teaching and examination regulations. In their education and examination regulations, HBO institutions are required to specify the teaching programme, the main subjects and the content and form of the different examinations.

The same legal framework applies for the universities. Their daily management is in the hands of the Executive board and the University Council. The Executive Board, which comprises three members, including the rector, is accountable to the Minister of Education, Culture and Science and to the University Council. The University Council comprises up to 30 representatives of the academic staff, students and the support and administrative staff.

The Information Management Group (IBG) is a semi-independent part of the Ministry of Education, Culture and Science that implements the Student Finance Act (WSF) and the study costs and allowance schemes. Its other duties include the collection of school and course fees, the provision of administrative support for examinations, the placement and registration of prospective students, the evaluation of diplomas and the implementation of benefit schemes for education personnel.

The Central Funding of Institutions Agency (CFI) is the executive agency responsible for funding the education system on the basis of legislation and regulations and in accordance with the established financial frameworks. Its duties also include providing information for policy-making and funding purposes. The CFI is responsible for the proper and efficient funding of institutions. Since 1 January 1996, when the CFI acquired agency status, it has formed an autonomous part of the Ministry of Education, Science and Culture.

There are several advisory and consultative bodies in the Netherlands that are entitled to make recommendations on educational policy. The Educational Council (*Onderwijsraad* , OR) is a permanent advisory board which was established in 1919. Its task is to ensure continuing equal financial treatment for public and private education, the coherence of educational policy and legislation and the freedom of education. The Royal Dutch Academy of Sciences (KNAW) and the Advisory Council on Science and Technology Policy (*Adviesraad voor wetenschaps- en Technologie-*

beleid, AWT) advise on science and science policy respectively. Advisory bodies that offer advice on other matters in addition to education are the Socio-economic-Council (SER) and the Advisory Council on Government Policy (*Wetenschappelijke Raad voor het Regeringsbeleid*, WRR).

With regard to higher education policy, the Minister also consults the Higher Education Consultative Committee, which includes the associations of HBO colleges, universities and teaching hospitals and the national teaching organisations. Consultation takes place within the Student Consultative Committee between the Minister and representatives of the national student organisation.

Negotiations with the trade unions on conditions of service and the staff's legal status take place at various levels within the education sector, but in the higher education sector, they are between the collective universities, respectively the collective HBO-institutions, and the relevant trade unions, since the higher education institutions have become (partially) autonomous in this respect too.

Higher Education and Research Act 1993

The Higher Education and Research Act (WHW) came into force on 1 August 1993. It regulates higher education (i.e. HBO-institutions, universities, the Open University and the 'designated institutions'), teaching hospitals and academic research. This Act replaced the University Act, the Higher Professional Education Act and numerous other regulations governing higher education and research (from over 2,000 to around 300 regulations).

The administrative relationship between the government and institutions of higher education and research, as defined in the Act, is based on the following principles:

- the government should only intervene to prevent undesirable developments when self-management by the institutions is likely to have unacceptable results;
- government intervention should primarily take the form of remedying imperfections in the system *ex post*;
- the instruments at the government's disposal should be characterised by a minimum of detailed regulation;
- the institutions must lay down norms to ensure legal certainty and proper administration.

The Act grants the institutions considerable freedom in matters of programmes. They are responsible in the first instance for maintaining quality, providing an adequate range of teaching and research programmes and ensuring access to education. Quality control is exercised by the institutions themselves, by external experts and, on behalf of the government, by the Inspectorate for Higher Education. In principle, the government assesses on an *ex post* basis only whether funds have been allocated efficiently and whether the intended results have been achieved. If major shortcomings are identified, the institutions will be informed accordingly. If discrepancies between ideal and reality persist, notably in the field of quality, the government has the option – with due regard to the proper procedures – of using coercive powers backed up by sanctions.

15.2   Accreditation and Evaluation Schemes in the Netherlands

The year 2003 marks the transition for the quality assurance systems of higher education in the Netherlands. A new accreditation system is being introduced. It builds upon (and will in part replace) the existing national systems of quality assurance.

First, we shall briefly describe briefly the previous quality assurance system and the system used until now to introduce new programmes. Then, we shall describe the design and outcomes of a pilot accreditation carried out by the Dutch HBO Council, prior to the introduction of the new accreditation system. Finally, we shall describe the new accreditation system as it has been developed so far.

15.2.1   The Quality Assurance System in the Netherlands

The Netherlands was among the first European countries to develop a formal system to assess the quality of teaching and research (van Vught & Westerheijden, 1993). In the 1980s a new steering philosophy replaced the detailed control of all kinds of input; the government would only check afterwards whether the *self-regulation* of the higher education system led to outputs in an acceptable range. In other words, the higher education institutions would be given more institutional autonomy if they proved that they 'delivered' quality education. True to a historical process, this 'new steering philosophy' was implemented before it was formulated. That happened in a policy initiative launched in the Dutch universities in 1983 concerning research, the 'Conditional Funding' (CF) policy.

This policy was intended to 'promote both quality and systematic discussion of priorities and the use of resources' in research in Dutch universities – accountability regarding government funding can be seen as an ulterior goal. The Conditional Funding policy was the first effort to assess how governmental funding for higher education was being used, changing the funding of fundamental university research from a 'give away model', included in the general grant to universities, to an 'exchange model'. A successful and satisfying exchange presupposes that the receiving party can assess whether it is getting 'value for money'.

The procedure chosen for the CF model was to have external committees of peers assess the research submitted by the universities and to guarantee the funding of the research group that was carrying it out for the next five years if the research was assessed positively. The information about research aims, activities and outputs (mainly publications) was to be supplied to the peers by the faculties. The external committees were appointed by the Royal Academy of Arts & Sciences, the most distinguished academic body in the country, which covered all areas of science. By using the principle of peer review, which is well-known in academia, and through the involvement of the Royal Academy, legitimacy of the procedure in the eyes of the academics was sought.

The research funding was allocated to the universities, not to the faculties or research programmes. It was up to the universities, therefore, to re-allocate funds from 'unprotected' to 'protected' research as they saw fit. However, there were very few re-allocations. The universities' decision-makers did not use the outcomes of the CF assessments for re-allocations, mostly because the assessments were very uniformly distributed. Very few research programmes were judged 'insufficient', and the peers declined to indicate 'excellent' research. The CF failed as a policy instrument for the re-allocation of funding.

What proved to be a much more influential aspect of the CF was that all research submitted for assessment was grouped into *research programmes*. Grouping together the research activities of several individuals started to become the main policy level in higher education research policy. The 'CF research programmes' became a lasting characteristic of research in the universities in the Netherlands, covering, at first, a significant percentage of all their fundamental research, and later practically all university-based fundamental research. Even when after two five-year rounds the CF faded away at the national level, most universities kept these research groupings for their internal administration, and they were at the basis of other research policies developed by the Ministry of Education & Science.

One of the main national policy initiatives that should be mentioned here is the training of post-graduate research assistants. Networks of researchers, often at an inter-university or even national level, were developed for that purpose. Later, these networks were institutionalised into 'research schools'. To have a research school recognised (for a five-year period) by the Royal Academy of Arts & Sciences is considered to be prestigious by universities. The CF research programmes may not always be recognisable in the themes of these research schools anymore, but for university decision-makers across all disciplines the CF procedure popularised the idea that research could be managed at a collective level.

Introduction of Quality Assessment of Teaching

A policy paper 'Higher Education: Autonomy and Quality' (HOAK) was published two years after the introduction of the CF. The idea of quality assessment was to be extended from research only to all major primary activities of higher education institutions – meaning, in fact, that quality assessment of teaching had to be developed.

In their negotiations about the implementation of HOAK in 1986, the Minister of Education & Science and the umbrella bodies of the universities, the Association of Universities in the Netherlands (VSNU) and the Association of *hogescholen* (HBO Council), reached the compromise that the umbrella bodies would co-ordinate the procedures to assure the government that they 'produced' quality teaching without too much waste of students and time, i.e. accountability with a special emphasis on dropout ratios and time to degree. In a spirit of self-regulation, the government would not use the outcomes of the quality assessments to further change funding of higher education after the cut-backs of the period before 1985. However, if a study programme was shown to be of low quality, and there were no improvements over a number of years (after a ministerial warning popularly called 'yellow card'), the government reserved the right to strike this study programme off the official register ('red card'), meaning that its diploma would no longer be recognised officially and that it would no longer be funded by the government, nor would students have a right to the study grant every student of a recognised programme is given.

In the hands of the umbrella bodies, the governmental goals of accountability and quality improvement changed to quality improvement and accountability – the change in order indicates a small but significant difference in emphasis.

The Principles, and their Implementation in Universities

For the design of the quality assessment procedure, the VSNU borrowed from the CF assessment procedure and from the decades-long US experience with programme review and specialised accreditation. Accordingly, the entity to be evaluated through the new procedure is the *programme*, i.e. the collection of courses leading to a specific *doctorandus* degree. Ad hoc *visiting committees* of external peers judge all programmes of study in an area of knowledge in the country, basing themselves on the information contained in the faculties' *self-evaluation reports* and on their own observations during two-day *site visits* to each of these faculties (see also Figure 1). At the end of each visit, preliminary comments and judgements about the study programme are given by the chair of the visiting committee. The final version of this text, following comments by the study programme, is included in the national, public *report of the visiting committee*.

The requirements for the self-evaluation report structure the self-evaluation process in the faculty. The VSNU guidelines for the report specify which topics should be addressed, e.g. programme aims, programme structure and content, student and staff information, data on graduates, issues of internationalisation and internal quality management. The structure of the report and the data to be used are prescribed in detail to ensure comparability across the country, but the faculty can emphasise issues it considers to be important.

Figure 1. Self-evaluation and visiting committees in assessment of teaching

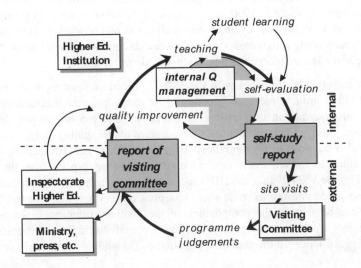

The self-evaluation reports are also the cornerstone of quality improvement: through the self-evaluation process, faculties ought to become aware of their strengths and weaknesses and begin to ameliorate the weaknesses, even if no external committee were involved – this is of course a normative, perhaps even idealistic picture, as sketched by proponents of self-evaluation processes.

The peer committee's judgements are collected in a national, public report, which includes the committee's frame of reference for judging the faculties, a chapter on the general state of affairs of teaching in the discipline in the country, and chapters on each of the programmes of study, with its strengths and weaknesses and the committee's recommendations for improvement. The visiting committees do emphatically not give a single, summary judgement of a study programme's quality. To do so would be contradictory to the multi-dimensional nature of the concept of quality.

This procedure has been in operation since the academic year 1987/88, the first year as a pilot project. Every year the VSNU appoints a number of ad hoc visiting committees to evaluate all programmes of study in their respective disciplines, thus covering all[2] programmes of study in a six-year cycle.

The Same Principles Implemented Slightly Differently in HBO Institutions

The HBO Council, the umbrella organisation of the HBO institutions, started assessing programmes of study in 1990, and because of the larger number of programmes it operates on an eight-year cycle to cover all areas of knowledge. In some areas with very many study programmes, two or more sub-committees visit them. Also, as a rule, the visits last no more than one day per study programme.

The most important differences with the VSNU procedure stem from the fact that the HBO study programmes are intended to be more 'practice oriented' than the academic programmes in universities. Applicability and job orientation therefore have higher priority. This influences the character of the quality judgements, and therefore also the ways of forming those judgements. Thus, the HBO Council issues its own guidelines for self-evaluation, which differ in some respects from the guidelines used by the VSNU; also, the HBO sector still being in the first round of evaluations, these guidelines are in some ways less prescriptive than those of the VSNU. And this can be seen in the composition of the visiting committees: whereas the VSNU mainly uses academic peers, the HBO Council visiting committees consist mainly of practitioners in the area of application of the study programme.

VSNU Quality Assessments of Research

After the demise of the CF procedure, the government wanted a new procedure for quality assessment of research in the universities. The procedure that the VSNU designed can briefly be characterised as an extension of experiences: of the CF experience on the one hand, and of the VSNU experience with quality assessment of teaching on the other.

From 1993 until 2003,[3] *external peer committees* judged fundamental university research according to four dimensions of quality: productivity, quality of output, relevance and long-term viability. *All* of a faculty's fundamental research was to be submitted, organised into *research programmes* as in the CF. The faculties provided the information again; bibliometric analyses of publication data were carried out by an independent bureau in a number of cases – this was new and not always part of the procedure. The committees might judge on the basis of this written information

---

2   With very few exceptions, mostly consisting of programmes that are unique in the country. Tailor-made solutions are developed for these 'orchid programmes'.

3   In 2003, all major research evaluation procedures were merged into a single one in co-operation of VSNU, KNAW and NWO.

only, but they also could interview research programme leaders or visit the faculties and laboratories. National, public reports were the main output of this procedure. In contrast to the teaching assessments, the research evaluations were given in summary figures for each research programme on the four dimensions of research quality. Productivity, quality of (key) publications, relevance of the programme and long-term viability of the research group were judged separately on five-point scales ranging from (1) insufficient to (5) excellent. As with the quality assessment of teaching, there was no direct connection between quality judgements and the government's (funding) policy for higher education. How the universities and faculties used the outcomes of the quality assessment procedures is the subject of the next section.

15.2.2   Effects

There is no direct connection between the quality assessments and government higher education policy. Specifically, there are no financial rewards or sanctions for the faculties concerned. The most important, but still marginal, financial consequence would ensue if students 'voted with their feet' (taking their tuition fees with them) by evading study programmes that are judged to be weak in many respects – but there is as yet no empirical evidence that they do. To ensure that the considerable amount of effort that goes into the quality assessments is not a 'paper tiger', but that these assessments are serious and that recommendations are acted upon, the government, through the Inspectorate for Higher Education, closely follows the visiting committees' reports and the follow-up by the universities. In the jargon of Dutch politics, this is called 'meta-evaluation'.

Since 1993 when the institutional arrangement concerning follow-up was renegotiated between the government and the higher education institutions, the Inspectorate has checked whether the universities react adequately to the visiting committee's observations (Scheele, Maassen, & Westerheijden, 1998). Note that the Inspectorate did not prescribe a certain method of follow-up. To decide on its own method of follow-up was part of the university's autonomy. The Inspectorate only required that some follow-up was planned and was put in writing in an 'Action Plan'. If no adequate Action Plan ensued, the Minister of Education issued a 'yellow card', i.e. a warning that unless thorough improvements were made quickly, the programme would be stricken off the register (CROHO) the following year. Such warnings were also given when study programmes were judged to be very weak in crucial aspects. If the Inspectorate discovered such 'worrisome cases', the Minister of Education asked the university to make rapid improvements. Warnings were issued in a small minority of cases – fewer in the university sector than in the HBO sector. This threat of sanctions has always been sufficient to induce improvements. Finally, the Inspectorate checked the follow-up in a mid-term review, three years after a visiting committee report is published. This was to ensure that quality improvement plans were implemented and did not remain paper plans until the next visiting committee six or seven years later.

The proof of the pudding was, of course, in what happened with these evaluations. They were not 'ritual dances' – the Inspectorate for Higher Education made sure of that. It has been established independently that non-utilisation by the higher education institution (usually, the faculty) was a relatively rare (Frederiks, 1996; Frederiks, Westerheijden, & Weusthof, 1994; Weusthof, 1994). This did not mean that all faculties slavishly followed all recommendations of the visiting committees. Frederiks (1996) estimated that about half of the visiting committees' recommendations were followed up. This was confirmed in 1999; it was found that virtually all recommendations endorsed by the visited programmes were followed up in the short or long term (Jeliazkova & Westerheijden, 2000). Even more important, there is no doubt that the visitation system has become part of mainstream university and higher professional education (Westerheijden, 1997).

15.2.3   The Programme Registration System

According to the 1993 Law on Higher Education and Academic Research (WHW), the following procedure was employed for the regulation of new programmes in higher education. The reason for introducing the system was Parliament's concern that there was too great a proliferation of study programmes in the second half of the 1980s. The outcome was the establishing of the Advisory Committee for Educational Programmes (ACO). Five of its members were appointed by the minister. Its task was to assess the plans for new educational programmes submitted by the institutions. Also, when changes were proposed in the educational and examination plans, the committee decided whether these were significant enough to represent a new programme. This kind of change mainly occurred in different types of specialisations within one programme. The conclusions of ACO were presented as an advice to the institution's management. The institution then decided whether to establish the new programme and to ask the minister to register it in the Central Registry of Higher Education Programmes (CROHO). Registration in CROHO meant that the institute might receive regular financing and that the students enrolled in the programme were eligible for student financing. If the minister decided not to follow ACO's advice, he notified Parliament. In assessing the new programmes, the ACO took into consideration the needs for higher education in terms of total number of programmes available and of national distribution ('macro efficiency').

This description left leeway for interpretation. However, the ACO informed the institutions regularly by detail on the specific procedures and the information to be submitted. For example, in the 2002 round, the institution had to demonstrate that it was indeed a new programme and that it did not diminish the transparency of the choice of programmes; that the programme met the quality requirements of the respective comparable programmes and that it was appropriate in terms of availability and geographical distribution of similar programmes.

In the first four years of the existence of the ACO, almost three-quarters of the programme proposals in the HBO-sector were rejected.

With the introduction of the accreditation scheme in 2003, the task of checking and approving new programmes is the responsibility of the NAO. This takes place on the institution's demand. The institution submits a profile description, a financial overview and a staff description of the programme. The submitted documents also indicate whether the programme is totally new or whether it already exists in other Dutch institutions. In making a decision, the NAO takes into account not only the quality of the programme, but also some financial aspects. Programmes that are totally new are in principle tested in more detail. The NAO recruits experts when necessary.

15.2.4   The Pilot Accreditation in the HBO-Sector

Already before the Ministry of Education, Culture and Science officially published the 'HOOP 2000' policy planning paper, the discussion around the Bologna process incited the HBO Council to explore accreditation, not only as an addition to the existing visitation model, but also as a possible substitute for it. An important issue for the HBO Council was whether it was possible to arrive at a more objective judgement of higher education quality. The HBO Council was mainly concerned with overcoming what it saw as the greatest shortcoming of the existing visitation system – that it produces a list of remarks and recommendations rather than an integrated overall assessment. The HBO Council took the initiative to carry out a pilot accreditation, which was to serve as the basis for a future discussion on the feasibility of introducing an accreditation system in the Netherlands. However, in practice, the pilot accreditation became one of several inputs to the discussion: not whether accreditation was feasible, but what were the right methods to perform it.

19 programmes in Social Work and 22 programmes in Commercial Economics took part in the pilot accreditation. A protocol was created, with a detailed description of the actors' tasks and of the rules for evaluation and accreditation decisions (*Protocol Proefaccreditering; Richtlijnen voor het accrediteringsproces*, 1999). The procedure was designed as follows:

First, a programme would carry out a self-evaluation study. Sufficient information was to be presented as well as an assessment based upon it concerning two distinct aspects: a) according to the guidelines for quality assessment of the programme according to the HBO standard requirements and b) according to the guidelines for assessment of management capacity.

Based on this self-study, the programme writes a three-part self-evaluation report. In the first part, general information on the institution and the programme is presented. The second part is an assessment of the programme according to the framework of the Accreditation Protocol. The framework consists of six standard criteria, further split into sub-criteria. Each of these is operationalised in a total of 80 verification points. The programme applies special calculation rules to reach an overall score of 'good', 'sufficient', 'average' and 'insufficient'. In the third part of the report, 'additional' information is presented which is to be used for a side letter with recommendations by the external visiting panel. This information is organised around 50 diagnostic questions. For each question, the programme also gives itself a score, without calculation rules.

An accreditation committee is in charge of setting up external review panels. The candidates undergo special training. After a two-day visit, the external panel writes an assessment report and gives an overall advice: positive, negative or conditional. Also, a confidential side letter with recommendations for improvement is presented to the programme after the final accreditation decision.

The pilot accreditation was monitored and evaluated by CHEPS at the request of the HBO Council (Goedegebuure, Jeliazkova, Pothof, & Weusthof, 2002). The independent monitoring and evaluation of the pilot accreditation led to two main conclusions: first, there seemed to be a general acceptance of an instrument that would demonstrate the quality of programmes in a more 'objective' way than the visitation system. On the other hand, however, the pilot accreditation exposed the problems created by too much detail and prescription of rules. It clearly showed that the balance between objectivity, legitimacy, and efficiency was not easy to find.

15.2.5 The New Accreditation Scheme

After Bologna, there was a serious discussion about the need to introduce accreditation in the Netherlands. The debate had already started around 1998. New dynamics and accountability, international transparency in Europe and beyond by positive statement of proven quality, openness of the higher education system, and the emergence of non-traditional suppliers were the key words behind the reform in the Netherlands. It became clear that the introduction of a bachelor-master system would mean adjustment of the binary system and therefore of the two-fold, though very similar, system of quality assurance. In addition, it was necessary to ensure the transparency of Dutch higher education for the international community, thereby improving its competitive position in the European knowledge market.

The Dutch Minister of Education, Culture and Science, after consulting the major stakeholders – the Association of Dutch Universities (VSNU) and the HBO Council, as well as the student organisations, decided to implement the Bologna decisions rapidly. In November 2000, the minister appointed a 'trailblazer' group to prepare the introduction of accreditation in the Netherlands and to develop the assessment frameworks for the new bachelor and master programmes. The committee developed recommendations on the basis of a study of international experience and intensive consultations with all the major stakeholders (Committee Accreditation of Dutch Higher Education, 2001). It was recommended to establish an independent Netherlands Accreditation Organisation (NAO). The new accreditation system began to be introduced as from late 2002. Thus, after introducing external quality assurance in the 1980s, the Netherlands was once again amongst the first in Europe to introduce a national accreditation system for all higher education programmes, both in the university and the higher professional education sectors.

All universities and higher professional schools are subject to the scheme, whether they are public or private, if they want to award bachelor's or master's degrees. The basic unit of the new accreditation scheme is the programme. There is a distinction between two types of programmes – academically oriented and professionally oriented. Both types may be offered by universities or higher vocational institutions (HBO) alike. Master's programmes and bachelor's programmes are accredited separately. Unlike the existing practice with visitations, similar programmes do not need to be visited at the same time and evaluated in clusters, although institutions may choose to do so.

The academically oriented bachelor's programmes are broader and are orientated towards a general background in science and acquiring basic research skills. The academically oriented master's programmes are of two types – for professional researchers with a sufficient specialisation and for academic professionals (doctors, lawyers, engineers, etc.). The professionally oriented bachelor's programmes target a particular profession, including practical experience. The professional master's programmes seek to build upon these programmes in two directions – in more depth with specific competences, or in broader types of multidisciplinary programmes.

Under the newly introduced accreditation system, an independent accreditation body, the Netherlands Accreditation Organisation (NAO) is established by law (www.nao-ho.nl). The NAO has independent members with expertise in the fields of higher education, professional practice and quality assessment. They are appointed by the minister. The accreditation system is based on the same principles of self-evaluation and peer review as the existing quality assessment system. The external assessment is carried out by quality agencies, in Dutch called Visiting and Assessing Bodies (VBI) and the accreditation is given by NAO. The formal consequences of (non-)accreditation are (loss of) study grants for students, funding of the programme (in public higher education institutions only) and awarding degrees with a legal status. Accreditation is granted for a period of six years, and new programmes need to be pre-tested. A programme is accredited either as academic or professional.

Bachelor and master programmes are accredited separately. The law specifies that accreditation must take into account the following aspects of quality: level of the programme, content of the programme, educational process, returns of education, sufficient facilities and an adequate quality assessment method.

In addition to accrediting existing programmes and licensing new programmes, the tasks of the NAO are: to check existing programmes for specific quality features on their demand, to strengthen the European and international dimension of Dutch accreditation and to maintain contacts in this area.

The development of the accreditation frameworks for existing and new programmes was one of the immediate tasks of the NAO. NAO discussed the new system intensively with the institutions, experts, trade unions, students and professional organisations. The accreditation frameworks were submitted for approval to the Minister of Education, Culture and Science. The accreditation framework was officially published in early 2003.

The accreditation framework for existing programmes consists of:

- An assessment framework, including aspects, facets and criteria,
- Rules for decision-making,
- Criteria to assess the procedure and the quality of the report produced by the quality agency,
- A description of the way existing programmes will be evaluated.

The following six aspects are subject to assessment: goals of the programme, contents of the programme, staff, facilities, internal quality assessment, outcomes. The different facets of these topics are to be assessed with the respective criteria.

Facets of the topic 'programme goals' are subject-specific requirements, level, orientation (professional or academic). Facets of the topic 'programme content' are orientation (professional or academic), relationship between programme goals and programme contents, coherence of the programme, student workload, entrance qualifications, duration, matching of form and contents, assessment and testing. Facets of 'staff' are professional or academic qualifications, adequate quantity, adequate quality of staff. Facets of the 'facilities' are adequacy, student supervision. Facets of the 'internal quality assessment' are evaluation of results, measures for improvement, involvement of staff, students, alumni and professional organisations. Facets of 'results' are level achieved, returns of education.

The institution can ask the external reviewers to assess exceptional quality features of the programme, which will be noted in the report, but will not influence the accreditation decision.

The assessment implies the use of a four-point scale (excellent, good, sufficient and insufficient) and decision-making rules based on specific weights of the criteria. The rules imply that, in order to obtain accreditation, a programme must score at least sufficient on each aspect. The score per aspect is a weighed sum of the facet scores.

One of the system's proclaimed aims is to preserve the diversity and the specific character of existing programmes. Hence, it was defined as broadly as possible. According to the NAO, it has consciously chosen a broader, flexible approach. This allows for input by the institutions and leaves room for the professional insight of the external reviewers.

Higher professional schools and universities take the initiative for accreditation. They invite a quality agency to assess the quality of a programme. The quality agencies are independent bodies that are registered with the NAO; the VSNU and HBO Council will lose their virtual monopoly. This does not mean that the quality agencies are certified by the NAO. The NAO produces an annual list of quality agencies that satisfy the requirements of expertise and quality. Therefore, the NAO does not assess itself, but gives the quality seal to programmes after reviewing the quality agency's conclusions. The aspects that should be looked at by the quality agency in order to qualify for accreditation are determined by the NAO. The NAO expects the quality agency to specify discipline-relevant criteria and requirements. The quality of work and the quality of the report produced by the quality agency are tested by the NAO. Quality agencies that produce weak reports may be deleted from the list of approved organisations.

Formal Stages of the Procedure

1. The institution applies for external assessment at a quality agency. This assessment covers the topics, facets and criteria presented in the accreditation framework.
2. The institution conducts a self-evaluation and produces a report.
3. The institution asks the quality agency to assess the quality of the programme based on the self-evaluation report. The quality agency visits the programmes and verifies the conclusions of the self-evaluation report. In addition, the quality agency assesses the quality of the self-evaluation. The quality agency establishes whether the programme satisfies the minimum requirements and formulates a conclusion which is presented in the report and supported by evidence.
4. The institution applies to the NAO for accreditation and submits a quality agency report, which should not be older than one year at the moment of submission.
5. The NAO assesses the quality agency report and may ask for additional information. The accreditation decision is taken within three months. In case of a

positive decision, the programme receives accreditation for six years. If the quality agency information is not sufficient, the NAO postpones the decision.

6. The institution may appeal.
7. The decision is made public.

The accreditation decision is seen by the NAO as the logical conclusion of a system of self-evaluations and peer review that functions well. The institutions produce a self-study report, which is verified by the visiting organisation, the NAO validates it and comes out with a clear 'yes' or 'no'. No conditional accreditation is allowed. However, this would not be the Netherlands if there were no room for ambiguity. One possibility for a second chance is the scenario in which the NAO, after requesting additional information and/or a second opinion, may just withhold a decision if not satisfied. The other possibility is the period of two years given to the programme to improve after receiving a negative decision. Given the serious consequences for students (no right to governmental support, no recognised diploma), this is a necessary condition to prevent damage caused by an abrupt closure of the programmes.

Since the new system is not functioning yet, only some parallels can be drawn with the existing visitation system. Since the accreditation scheme builds upon the existing routine of self-evaluations and visitation, it is logical to ask to what extent they are fit for accreditation.

What are the main differences? In the first place, the clear 'yes' or 'no' decision about the programme's minimum quality standard. This requires a more explicit definition of the reference framework and fewer ad hoc comparisons of the programmes during the assessment. The emphasis moves inevitably from process to output. Whether this new frame of assessment will lead to more differentiated judgements on the quality of Dutch programmes remains to be seen.

It is certain, however, that there will be consequences for the traditional separation between the academic and professional sector. Until now, any university programme was automatically considered academic. Under the new system, this is no longer the case. To what extent will this lead to a shift in the type and character of programmes offered by universities and professional schools? At master's or also at bachelor's level? These are questions awaiting an answer.

The choice for quality agencies is inspired by the idea to promote diversity in the system and to make it more open to international actors. However, given the scale of Dutch higher education, only the future will show how realistic this expectation has been.

15.2.6   Other Accreditation Bodies in the Netherlands

Dutch Validation Council. In the early 1990s, a proposal was made to establish a validation system for separate Master's programmes. The independent Dutch Validation Council (DVC) was established in 1997 at the request of the HBO Council. The HBO Council, universities and a number of employers' organisations are part of its Board. The task of the DVC is to promote national and international recognition of post-initial higher education programmes. This is done by establishing the quality and the required master's level. The council is concerned with recognising civil effect to positively validated programmes.

The Dutch Validation Council executes validation at request of the programme by means of a specific system. Independent expert panels establish the level and quality of the programme through specially developed procedures and instruments. If the result is positive, the Dutch Validation Council grants the programme the right to confer master's titles for a maximum period of four years. In future, DVC's activities will be integrated in the NAO system.

Certiked (Stichting Certificatie Kennisintensieve Dienstverlening). This organisation is specialised in quality management for knowledge-intensive service-oriented organisations and institutions. It issues certificates for covering international recognised standards such as ISO-9000, or other models such as EFQM, as well as specific professional requirements. *Certiked* is one of the candidates for a quality agency.

15.3   System Dynamics

15.3.1   Driving Forces and Social Problems

There have been some continuous themes behind decision-making in Dutch higher education regarding quality. One has been the balance between accountability and autonomy: reduction of ex ante regulation if higher education institutions showed they made good use of their greater autonomy. This has been part of government rhetoric since the early 1980s and a prime driver for the introduction of quality assessment.

This was accompanied by some doubt as to the suitability of higher education graduates (especially from universities) for the labour market. This is also linked to the efforts of the government to tighten the links between universities and their (economic) environment. In these efforts, quality assessment has been only one of the policy instruments next to funding for projects, incubators, etc. For the HBO colleges, this linking has been part of their mission from the outset.

Another major underlying driver for quality-related policies in the Netherlands – although in contrast with the previous element – has been what we would like to call a 'small country complex'. By that, we mean the conviction on the part of decision-makers that the high quality of Dutch higher education was not sufficiently recognised abroad because of our 'minority' language and our degree structure, which was not easily comparable with the degrees of other countries. This led to the readiness of the Dutch government to adopt innovative policy instruments that could show the Dutch quality standards to the outside world, and more especially its readiness to engage in international projects. It was the Dutch government, when it presided over the European Union in 1992, that introduced the issue of quality assurance on the European agenda. And it has been a pioneer in initiating or joining European projects ever since, including the recent 'Joint Quality Initiative', together with the Flemish government. Yet the major example of this driver is, of course, the way in which the Netherlands responded to the Bologna Declaration: it was among the first countries to restructure its degree and its well-established quality assurance systems.

The 'bottom-line' of policy is of course the costs of higher education. Cost containment has been a major concern for Dutch governments since 1977, when it was a major issue in the national elections. In relation to higher education, major budget cuts were made *before* quality assessment was introduced, as mentioned above. There was a conscious attempt in the mid-1980s to disassociate quality judgements and budget cuts, unlike the developments in the UK at the time. Nevertheless, continuous 'rationalisations' and per student budget reductions (taking inflation and the growing number of students into account) have created a threatening environment for Dutch higher education over the last two decades. Because of this financial context and stimuli from the ministry of education to engage in entrepreneurial activities, international trade in higher education (i.e. attracting foreign, non-EU students) has become one of the ways in which higher education institutions have tried to supplement their budget. Better international recognition was therefore of interest to the entrepreneurial higher education institutions as well: accreditation and well-known degree names could mean USPs (Unique Selling Points) for them.

15.3.2   Relationships among Schemes

The policy instrument 'landscape' in the Netherlands is becoming very simple: all major evaluation and approval schemes are now integrated under the NAO.

15.3.3   Consequences for the Higher Education System

We shall have to wait to see the consequences of moving to an accreditation system; yet it is clear that in the transition period there is much uncertainty at all levels. Who will be accredited, who will not? There has been talk during the preparation of NAO that 5 to 10 % of the requests must lead to non-accreditation to show that the danger was real: will this – if it comes true – affect the private sector only, or also public higher education institutions? What will the Minister of Education do if programmes that are vital for other policy goals are not accredited? (For instance: there is a severe shortage of teachers; would non-accredited teacher training programmes really be closed down?) Furthermore, how will the general standards framework of NAO be elaborated into quality agencies' checklists? Will the quality agencies be able to pay some attention to quality improvement – as promised in all policy statements – faced with the consequences of non-accreditation?

Students too are uncertain. In their talks with the NAO, they stressed control, especially control of quality of delivery. For them, as mentioned before, consequences will include eligibility for government student support. Students' options will be enlarged by the new accreditation system, as private higher education providers will be included in it on an equal footing, giving the same rights to government support. Whether this will lead to more quality-related choice of study programmes for students entering the higher education system (or re-entering it, e.g., at the master's level) is another issue worth studying in years to come.

For external stakeholders, the change to an accreditation system promises greater transparency of quality judgements, which until now were written for an audience of insiders – hence the market for magazines ranking the higher education institutions. In fact, employers' demands for more transparency were one of the drivers behind the HBO Council's pilot accreditation project.

Quite a different matter – which will have to be discovered in practice too – is whether the system of accrediting each programme separately will be sustainable. There are already some signs that reduction of effort is aimed at, e.g., some aspects common to a number of programmes in a single higher education institution could be checked through a 'lighter' mechanism.

15.4   Influence of Bologna and European Models

As mentioned in the previous section, the Bologna process has been taken up in the Netherlands as a major driver for higher education system change. The Bologna aims of international transparency and mobility within Europe and across the world were welcomed by Dutch policy-makers. The former has been mentioned as a first main driver of quality policy in the last two decades in the Netherlands. The latter was also mentioned, not so much in the 'friendly', 'co-operative' conception of student mobility or even graduate mobility in the European labour market, but more especially in the 'competitive' framework of attracting foreign, fee-paying students.

With respect to European models, the Netherlands has played the role of a model for other countries since the late 1980s through conscious 'promotional' activities by representatives of the Dutch quality assessment agencies. With the change to accreditation, the German case was used as a model for the development of the NAO (the example certainly was not followed slavishly, but discussions took place between representatives of NAO and the German Accreditation Council bureau).

The example of NAO and other elements of Dutch conceptions of quality (such as the preference for output quality, i.e. competences of graduates) were used in the wider European debate to set examples for other European countries, e.g., in the Joint Quality Initiative (JQI).

15.5 Individual Level Assessments

With the deregulation and privatisation movement of the 1980s and 1990s, the higher education institutions became independent employers in some respects (for more information see the parallel Enders & De Weert report). For the academic staff, this implied a move away from prescribed amounts of teaching or research hours per year, but also a move away from the seniority principle, i.e. automatic annual salary increases. Instead, individual performance was given some importance in higher education institutions' human research management (although that term was not used until recently). A main element here was the 'individual functioning talks' in the framework of staff appraisal schemes, which were to take place annually between teaching staff and their immediate superiors: in universities, lower-level teachers with their professor, professors with their dean, etc. These talks were not only meant to influence salary increases, but also to introduce career development into the higher education institutions, e.g. through teaching and research portfolios. However, these changes are still in their infancy; as De Weert reported in the parallel project report just referred to, committees have been at work and proposals have been made, but the old rules and regulations still apply. But with a new round of central negotiations coming up, the situation may change soon.

References

Committee Accreditation of Dutch Higher Education (2001). *Activate, Achieve and Advance: Final Report*. Amsterdam: Van de Bunt.

Frederiks, M. M. H. (1996). *Beslissen over kwaliteit*. Utrecht: De tijdstroom.

Frederiks, M. M. H., Westerheijden, D. F., & Weusthof, P. J. M. (1994). Effects of Quality Assessment in Dutch Higher Education. *European Journal of Education, 29*, 181-200.

Goedegebuure, L. C. J., Jeliazkova, M., Pothof, F., & Weusthof, P. J. M. (2002). *Alle begin is moeilijk: Evaluatie van de proefaccreditering HBO*. Enschede: CHEPS, Universiteit Twente.

Jeliazkova, M., & Westerheijden, D. F. (2000). *Het zichtbare eindresultaat*. Den Haag: Algemene Rekenkamer.

Protocol Proefaccreditering; Richtlijnen voor het accrediteringsproces (1999). Den Haag: HBO-raad.

Scheele, J. P. , Maassen, P. A. M., & Westerheijden, D. F. (Eds.). (1998). *To be Continued ...: Follow-Up of Quality Assurance in Higher Education*. Maarssen: Elsevier/De Tijdstroom.

van Vught, F. A., & Westerheijden, D. F. (1993). *Quality Management and Quality Assurance in European Higher Education: Methods and Mechanisms*. Luxembourg: Office for Official Publications of the Commission of the European Communities.

Westerheijden, D. F. (1997). A solid base for decisions: Use of the VSNU research evaluations in Dutch universities. *Higher Education, 33*(4), 397-413.

Weusthof, P. J. M. (1994). *De interne kwaliteitszorg in het wetenschappelijk onderwijs*. Utrecht: Lemma.

16 The Blurring Boundaries Between Accreditation and Audit: The Case of Norway

BJØRN STENSAKER

16.1 Introduction

Norwegian higher education has expanded significantly in student numbers during the last ten to 15 years. In the late 1980s, about 105,000 students were registered in higher education, while a decade later approximately 180,000 students were undertaking various forms of higher education (NFR, 2001, p. 95). The growth is complex. Universities experienced a decrease in the number of students after 1996, while the college sector increased the intake of new students. Some disciplinary differences are also noticeable. At universities, law and humanities seem less attractive to students in the late 1990s, while numbers have been fairly constant in pedagogy, social science and in the sciences. At colleges especially within health and social work an increase in student numbers is most visible (NFR, 2001, p. 96).

In Norway, the higher education system is divided into a university sector and a college sector. There are four universities. Established in 1811, and with over 30,000 students, the University of Oslo is the oldest and largest of the four. The other three, in Bergen, Trondheim and Tromsø, were all established at a much later stage. Six specialised university colleges in e.g. physical education, music, agriculture, also belong to the university sector, but with a much smaller number of students. The college sector comprises of 26 state colleges. This sector was reorganised in 1994, reducing the number of institutions from over 100 to the current number. The two sectors are approximately of equal size when it comes to the number of students – with the college sector on top, which implies that Norway has a larger college sector than many other European countries (Kyvik, 2002). There are also a substantial number of private higher education institutions in the country, but with the exception of the Norwegian School of Management (BI) with more than 10,000 students, most of the private institutions are quite small (in total there are approximately 21,000 students in the private higher education sector). In addition, over 20,000 students study abroad, while only around 4,000 foreign students study at Norwegian higher education institutions.

Traditionally, university degree types have been inspired by the continental university model, with a four-year first degree (cand.mag.), and a two-year second degree (cand.polit. etc.) to follow. Professional degrees in medicine, business administration, civic engineering etc., differ from this structure, even if the time frame for the

347

S. Schwarz and D.F. Westerheijden (eds.),
Accreditation and Evaluation in the European Higher Education Area, 347–369.
© 2004 Kluwer Academic Publishers. Printed in the Netherlands.

studies often is set to four or six years. In the college sector, the first degree has traditionally varied between two and four years. Normally, a second degree was not offered in the college sector. During the last decade, however, a few colleges have been granted the right to offer second-degree programmes and even doctorate studies in given subjects. Due to a major reform initiative in 2001, the degree system in Norway changed from the 1st of January 2003, introducing the Anglo-American bachelor–master system in higher education and the ECTS credit transfer system (St.Meld.Nr. 27, 2000-2001). This means that in the university and college sector, the first degree lasts for three years (bachelor), while the second degree lasts for two years (master). In addition, a Ph.D. is introduced, scheduled for three years. During the introduction of the new degree system, some of the professional degrees were adjusted to fit into the new system. Exceptions can be found in Theology, Psychology, Medicine and Veterinary studies. Teacher training will also keep its four-year time-schedule. However, as before, it will be possible for students to switch between studying at university and college, building their degree from various combinations at different levels of the two sectors.

If one looks at the programmes offered in Norwegian higher education, science, technical studies and social science programmes dominate, as these fields produce almost two-thirds of the degrees given annually in Norway (NFR, 2001, p. 100). A look at the number of doctorate degrees shows that most degrees are obtained in the sciences (26 %), in medicine (21 %), technology (19 %) and social science (18 %) (NFR, 2001, p. 103). As in many other countries, higher education in Norway has also become a more important arena for women. At present, almost 60 % of the students in higher education are women (NFR, 2001, p. 101), and the number of female doctoral students increased during the 1990s.

The labour market for graduates of higher education was fairly good during the 1990s. On average, only between 2 and 3 % of graduates with a university degree have experienced unemployment during the decade. However, some disciplinary differences do occur. In 2000, six months after leaving higher education, out of the candidates from the social sciences, humanities, law and the sciences, between 5 and 7 % were unable to find a job. For candidates in psychology, business studies, health the unemployment ratio is only between 1 and 2 % (NFR, 2001, p. 106). This picture is not very surprising. A high unemployment ratio for social science graduates could be explained, e.g., by the sheer number of candidates from these disciplines. Candidates with a university degree have normally found their job in the public sector, but this is gradually changing due to public sector cutbacks and the growing number of graduates from universities. Thus, the private sector will most likely become more important for graduates in the coming years.

As indicated earlier, most of the Norwegian higher education system is public with only one private higher education provider of some size. In 2000, the state-owned higher education institutions in the country accommodated 92 % of the total student population, and received 98 % of the public expenditure on higher education (Hämäläinen, 2001, p. 26). No student fees are paid to study in a public higher education institution. This situation indicates that the state is an important actor for the whole system, both as the resource provider and as the actor that regulates and steers the system. Traditionally the higher education system could be said to belong to the continental mode of steering with emphasis on input based factors (e.g. number of students) instead of output factors (number of graduates produced). However, during the 1990s the state steering of the sector changed. Signs of more autonomy for the institutions could be seen already in the early 1990s with some authority being transferred from the state (Stensaker, 1997), culminating in recent changes affecting the principles of funding in the sector (St.Meld.Nr. 27, 2000-2001). In this latest white paper on higher education it is proposed that an increasing share of the funding should be related to output based factors (number of credits, number of graduates). For institutions, the change means that they will be more responsible for their own economy, making institutional leadership more important. The challenge for institutions could be related to the fact that institutional leadership in Norwegian higher education has been rather weak, and that much power is located in the basic units at universities and colleges. However, signs that the institutional leadership was strengthened during the 1990s are becoming increasingly visible, along with more autonomous institutions (Stensaker, 1997, Bleiklie, 2000).

The changes in governmental steering until recently have not affected the procedures for approval of curricula, new study programmes or new higher education entities. Traditionally curricula in some areas (teacher training etc.) have been determined at the national level by the Ministry of Education. Approval of new study programmes and the establishment of new higher education entities have also been a responsibility of the Ministry of Education, but in a rather unsystematic way (Haakstad, 2001). This old system of 'authorisation' and 'recognition' changed on 1 January 2003, when a system of accreditation of Norwegian higher education was introduced as a part of a major reform effort to change the degree structure in Norway and further stimulate to more autonomous institutions (St.Meld.Nr. 27, 2000-2001).

16.2   Accreditation and Evaluation Schemes in Norway

Traditionally, Norway has been a typical representative for countries that put limited resources into the authorisation of new institutions and higher education programmes. The authorisation process has usually been taken care of by the Ministry of Education, and could be characterised as an administrative procedure. Even if a small expert panel usually has been consulted about a given authorisation, no study visits and other more in-depth evaluations were conducted. During the 1990s, Norway has also been quite modest when it comes to implementing other national systems for quality assurance, even if various pilot projects in the field of evaluation were initiated (see Stensaker, 1997). Thus, the political attention for quality assurance of higher education must be characterised as limited. Recent political initiatives in Norway, however, may contribute to change this picture considerably.

First, a new independent accreditation body the *Norwegian Agency for Quality Assurance in Education* (NOKUT) was created in January 2003. This body was established by a separate Act with its activities rather clearly specified in the text (UFD, 2002). NOKUT replaced the former Norway Network Council. This latter body had rather close ties with the Ministry, i.e., it was instructed by the Ministry, and had multiple tasks, including giving the Ministry of Education advice on strategic issues and taking care of various evaluations in Norwegian higher education. By law, the new body is secured a more independent status. The Ministry of Education cannot instruct NOKUT nor influence its activities in other ways than by law. Still, the Ministry has a final say on certain issues (creating new universities, change the status of current institutions from college to university, etc.). NOKUT has a staff of around 30, and is organised in three departments: one department for evaluation of institutional quality assurance systems, one department for accreditation of higher education institutions and programmes, and one department for recognition of foreign education and for giving advice to institutions regarding international credit transfer (ENIC/NARIC).

Second, formal accreditation schemes have been introduced along with NOKUT: Accreditation of universities and colleges according to institutional status and of study programmes at different levels has been established. Since the degree structure changed at the same time as the new system of accreditation was introduced, a consequence is that many studies are in a rather urgent need for a formal accreditation.

Third, an important premise for the accreditation schemes, introduced at the same time, is the requirement that every higher education institution, public as well as private, should have a functioning quality assurance system covering all higher education programmes offered. Every Norwegian higher education institution was expected to have a system implemented before the end of 2003 (UFD, 2002). The consequence of not having such a system, or that the existing system did not cover the minimum standards set, is not that an institution will lose it institutional status, or the accreditation for established studies, but that the institution will not be allowed to establish new programmes of study. In other words, not having an institutional quality assurance system restricts the institution's possibilities to expand and move into new fields of study. However, formally the need for an institutional quality assurance system is not subject to an accreditation process. Thus, the evaluative criteria developed related to validate the quality assurance systems will be presented after a more detailed description of the new major accreditation schemes.

16.2.1 Major Accreditation Schemes in Norway

Two major accreditation schemes exists in Norway, one related to determining the institutional status of higher education institutions, and one related to the accreditation of higher education programmes at various levels. In this section, each scheme will be presented separately.

Institutional Accreditation

The Ministry of Education has specified by law that there are formally three types of higher education institutions in Norway; Universities, university colleges (specialised universities), and colleges (either public or private). The institutions can opt for the preferred status themselves, but must be accredited by NOKUT to be allowed to use the title in their name. Institutions can also apply for a change of status, e.g. to go from being a college to a university, but must again go through an accreditation procedure, and obtain final approval from the Ministry of Education before such a change of status can occur. The relationship between the Ministry and NOKUT is in these matters such that NOKUT must approve a change of status before the Ministry gives the permission. The Ministry of Education cannot change the status of a given institution without the institution being formally recognised as having the quality to do so by NOKUT. However, NOKUT may provide institutions with such a quality label without the Ministry accepting the decision. Thus, the Ministry may for economic reasons reject institutional status changes.

To be accredited as either a state college or a *private college*, the following main criteria have been developed by NOKUT (2003):

- The institution must have a recognised quality assurance system (see above).
- The primary purpose of the institution must be related to higher education and research.
- The institution must have the right to award a bachelor-degree in one subject/discipline, and must have graduated students for at least two years.
- The institution must have R&D activities in relation to the higher education programmes offered, mainly carried out by its own academic staff, and where the staff as a main rule must have R&D tasks as part of their regular work plan.
- The institution must have an academic staff with formal scientific and pedagogic qualifications related to every higher education programme offered.
- The institution must have a library with competent staff, a collection of literature in the areas where higher education programmes are offered, and be connected to an electronic system for literature exchange and copying.
- The institution must have a board where academic staff and students are represented.

- The institution must have an infrastructure supporting higher education and research. This includes facilities for a relevant management and organisational structure, social welfare for students, adequate conditions for the academic and the administrative staff, available ICT-equipment for students and staff, an adequate number of lecture rooms, space for self-studies, project work, etc.

To be accredited as a *university college (specialised university)*, the institution must fulfil all criteria necessary to obtain status as either a state college or a private college. In addition, the following criteria apply (NOKUT, 2003):

- The institution must have the right to award a Ph.D. degree in at least one area, and must have successfully graduated students from the Ph.D. programme.
- The institution must demonstrate, in academic areas/disciplines where a Ph.D. degree is awarded, that accreditation standards specified by NOKUT for such degrees are met.
- The institutions must have the right to award a master's degree in minimally one academic area/discipline, and must have graduated students in at least two years.
- The institution must demonstrate, in academic areas/disciplines where a master's degree is awarded, that accreditation standards specified by NOKUT for such degrees are met.
- The institution must demonstrate, in other academic areas/disciplines, that it produces R&D of high quality and that it has a scientific staff with formal qualifications.
- The institution must have an infrastructure that is relevant for the research activities conducted, i.e. with an up-to-date research library that covers the Ph.D.-awarding areas of research, and with a sufficient collection of books and journals, with modern ICT-facilities, laboratories, with separate budget and plans for research, and with a management structure that ensures the quality of research activities.
- The institution must have a well established academic network both nationally and internationally.

To be accredited as a *university*, the institution must fulfil all criteria necessary to obtain status as either a state college or a private college and a university college. In addition, the following criteria apply (NOKUT, 2003):

- The institution must have the right to award master's degree programmes in at least five academic areas/disciplines, and must have bachelor's programmes in more academic areas/disciplines than those covered by the master's programmes.

- The institution must have the right to award Ph.D. degrees in at least four academic areas/disciplines, and where two of these must be related to regional needs and be of national importance. The institution must demonstrate a stable and continuing production of Ph.D. graduates in at least two of the four areas.

As shown, the institutional accreditation scheme initiated in Norway intends to cover all higher education institutions in the country, both in the public and in the private sector. As illustrated by the criteria sets, the institutional accreditation is partly a result of a prior accreditation of higher education programmes at various levels (see below). In other words, both teaching and research activities are included in the accreditation process.

NOKUT has a central position in this accreditation scheme in that all applications for obtaining a given status must be directed exclusively to this body. It is also NOKUT that receives all the data and the information needed in the accreditation process, and that organises the accreditation process, e.g. it appoints the external committee that is to analyse the application from the institution. It has been a tradition in Norway to appoint experts from other Nordic countries, representatives from business and society and students in external review committees (Stensaker, 1997). Most likely this practice will continue in the new accreditation schemes. Accreditation reports produced by NOKUT are public documents, available for any interested stakeholder.

No detailed timeframe for an institutional accreditation up to the point where the external review process is finalised is provided by the Ministry of Education or NOKUT. However, it is expected that such a timeframe will be developed, not least due to earlier complaints from private higher education institutions that the procedures in former 'approval' system took too long. The procedures for what happens after the external report is produced are more formalised. After the external report is finalised, it is sent to the institution without a formalised decision whether a given institutional status is given. The institution then is given five weeks to respond. Based on the reply from the institution, the Board of NOKUT decides whether accreditation is given. If rejected, the institution has to wait two years before a new application can be sent NOKUT. If accepted, NOKUT informs the Ministry of Education of its decision. It is then the Ministry that has the final say whether the accredited status is given. Students of accredited institutions have the right to obtain financial support from the state-controlled student support system.

There are other institutional accreditation schemes than those handled by NOKUT in Norway. However, contrary to the NOKUT schemes, these are voluntary for institutions. In the late 1990s, two business education institutions in Norway have obtained an EQUIS accreditation offered by the European Foundation for Management Development (EFMD). Institutions interested in this type of accreditation seem to have chosen EQUIS because of its international profile and recognition, and out of an interest to compete on the international student market, especially in the MBA-segment.

Accreditation of Higher Education Programmes

Along with the accreditation scheme for assigning institutional status, the Ministry of Education has also instructed NOKUT to develop standards and criteria for the accreditation of higher education programmes at all levels from introductory studies scheduled for 30 credits (ECTS) to Ph.D. programmes. However, when accrediting higher education programmes, differences between the public and the private higher education sector becomes visible. At present, the two sectors are regulated by separate acts, where the universities and university colleges (they are all public) in the new accreditation scheme developed for higher education programmes automatically receive an accreditation for all existing higher education programmes that they have the right to offer according to the Universities and College Act. In this act, these institutions have the right to establish new higher education programmes at all levels, including Ph.D. programmes (University colleges may not establish new Ph.D. programmes outside their 'core' academic area/discipline). For state colleges, the Universities and College Act provides the institutions with the right to establish new programmes up to the bachelor's degree level, and they can establish master's programmes in the academic areas/disciplines where they offer a Ph.D. degree.

For private higher education institutions, the situation is slightly different. The Private Colleges Act states that private higher education institutions must apply for accreditation of higher education programmes at all levels (bachelor, master and Ph.D.). As a transition arrangement, all existing programmes in private higher education institutions automatically receive an accreditation, but these institutions must apply for accreditation for any new programmes established. At present, political discussions is taking place with the intention to establish a common act for the public and private higher education sectors in Norway, which would erase the current differences in accreditation procedures. However, now already private higher education institutions can apply for an institutional accreditation either as a private college, a university college or a university, and may, if accredited as such, obtain the same right as public institutions have at present.

The main criteria developed by the NOKUT (2003) for accreditation of higher education programmes up to 30 credits (ECTS) are as follows:

• The institution offering the programme must have a managerial structure and follow the regulatory framework specified in the Private Colleges Act.

- In the curriculum, the name of the programme must be specified together with information on whether parallel programmes exist in the public higher education sector. The curriculum must also specify admission rules, objectives of the programme, skills required from students, teaching and learning methods, examination rules and regulations and syllabus.
- The academic staff must demonstrate scientific and pedagogic qualifications at the same level as for teaching in accredited institutions.
- The higher education programme must have an adequate infrastructure i.e., access to lecture rooms, sufficient level of ICT-support etc.

The main criteria developed by the NOKUT (2003) for accreditation of higher education programmes between 60 and 120 credits (ECTS) are as follows:

- All criteria specified for higher education programmes up to 30 credits must be fulfilled.
- The higher education programme must be characterised by academic progression, internal cohesion and societal relevance.

The main criteria developed by the NOKUT (2003) for accreditation of higher education programmes qualifying for a bachelor's degree (180 credits ECTS), are as follows:

- All criteria specified for higher education programmes up to 120 credits must be fulfilled.
- The programme must be based on a formal description of rights and obligations of students, staff and the institution.
- The curriculum must specify the academic areas/disciplines the programme builds upon, the work load of students, the scientific and pedagogic qualifications of the staff, and must ensure that the programme qualify as a basis for master's degree applications.
- The programme must be organised in a way that academic quality is secured and improved, i.e. the academic staff must be of a sufficient number and be stable, national and international relations must be documented and the academic staff must be actively involved in and have formal possibilities to be involved in R&D.

The main criteria developed by the NOKUT (2003) for accreditation of higher education programmes qualifying for the master's degree (300 credits ECTS), are as follows:

- The programme must be based on a formal description of rights and obligations of students, staff and the institution.

- The programme must have an adequate name and be specific on the master's degree awarded (Master of Arts, Master of Science, etc.).
- The curriculum must specify the academic areas/disciplines the programme builds upon, the work load of students, and the expected competences after graduation.
- The programme must provide students with experience of scientific work.
- The programme must have a sufficient infrastructure (ICT-support, library, laboratories, etc.).
- The programme must contain a thesis by students, either as an individual work or as teamwork. In discipline-based, vocational and experience-based master's degrees, the thesis must count for at 30 to 60 credits (ECTS).
- The programme must have a scientific and pedagogic qualified staff, with senior qualifications in the staff in core areas of the master's degree. The scientific qualifications of the staff must match the profile of the programme, and external examiners must document the same qualifications as the scientific staff.
- The scientific staff must have an active research profile, and must have formal arrangements that ensures time for research.

The main criteria developed by the NOKUT (2003) for accreditation of higher education programmes qualifying for the Ph.D. degree, are as follows:

- The programme must be based on a formal description of rights and obligations of students, staff and the institution.
- The programme must have an adequate name and be specific on the Ph.D. degree awarded.
- The programme must have a formal plan including a description of courses that secure students formal training in methodology and history of science.
- The institution awarding the Ph.D. degree must have a solid academic basis, including an active and stable research oriented staff. The research conducted must be relevant for the core areas of the Ph.D., and be both theoretically and empirically oriented. At least eight people with at least associate professor qualifications must have formal full-time positions in connection with the programme. Most of the teaching and tutoring must be done by the full-time staff.
- The programme must document the scientific qualifications of the staff through their international publications (in journals, etc.).
- The bachelor's and master's degree programmes supporting the programme must be of a quality and extension to function as a solid basis for a Ph.D. programme (e.g. graduate a sufficient number of candidates).
- The institution awarding the Ph.D. must document its national and international networks through participation in scientific conferences, research networks, exchange arrangements of students and staff, etc.

- The programme must have a sufficient infrastructure (ICT-support, libraries, laboratories, support staff, locations, lecture rooms, etc.).
- The programme must have formal routines for assuring the quality of teaching and tutoring, specifying how quality is improved over time.
- The institution must document the regional and national importance of the Ph.D. programme.

As illustrated by the accreditation criteria for each programme, research activities, research qualifications held by the staff and research networks increase in importance as one moves from lower degree programmes to higher degree programmes. The described criteria sets also cover all disciplines and academic areas except for some professional programmes where specific criteria are not yet developed.

NOKUT is the main player also for the accreditation of academic programmes. It specifies when and how accreditation of a certain programme will take place. Thus, the body can itself decide on the reasons for initiating a re-accreditation process of programmes at any level. In addition, NOKUT decides on the methods used for accreditation. The standard method used will be a mix of self-evaluation and external review, with publication of a report afterwards. As with the institutional accreditation, reviewers will most likely be a mix of domestic and Nordic experts in various disciplines. Some student representatives and some societal and industry representatives will in most instances be selected to serve on the committees.

No time schedule for the accreditation process from application to completion of the external review process has been specified yet. However, after the external report is finalised, it is sent to the institution that then is given five weeks to respond to the claims and findings made. The board of NOKUT then decide whether accreditation is given, and the decision is sent to the Ministry for final approval. If the application is rejected by the board of NOKUT, the institution must wait up to two years before a new application may be sent (NOKUT may allow the institution to send a new application before that time if only minor details lack before accreditation can be given).

Concerning re-accreditation of programmes, no criteria are yet specified for this procedure. Due to an ambition of keeping 'bureaucratic' procedures to a minimum in NOKUT, there is some hesitation about adopting a cyclic model of re-accreditation. Thus, at present, there are no procedures concerning when re-accreditation is to take place, only how it should be carried out. When going through a re-accreditation process, the institution have between three and six months to initiate actions if re-accreditation is not given. If accreditation is withdrawn, the decision is sent to the institution with a copy to the Ministry of Education. The institution must immediately close the programme, i.e., examination and graduation of students cannot take place, and new students are not allowed into the programme. The institution must also make sure that its students can take their exams at another higher education institution. Students of accredited programmes have the right to obtain financial support by the state-controlled student support system.

There are other programme accreditation schemes in Norway than those handled by NOKUT. However, these are voluntary systems, most often designed for vocational or professional programmes (e.g. engineering), research laboratories or for the accreditation of a single department. The ISO-standard is a typical representative of these systems, where the accreditation is conducted by organisations with a licence to perform such tasks from the ISO. Only a limited number of programmes have been accredited by such systems.

16.2.2   Complaints and Legal Handling of NOKUT's Accreditation Decisions

The Ministry of Education has appointed a special complaints committee consisting of five members to deal with institutional disagreements regarding NOKUT's possible negative decisions on institutional accreditation or accreditation of programmes. One of the committee's members is a student, and the chairman of the committee must fulfil the formal criteria to function as a judge in a civil court.

The committee has the right to make a formal decision when four out of five members are present. The decisions made by the committee cannot be taken further in the legal system.

16.3   Major Approval Schemes in Norway

Even if the new accreditation schemes developed could be interpreted as a shift from an informal 'approval' system to a more formalised system, this does not mean that approval schemes have lost their significance in Norwegian higher education. On the contrary, a new approval scheme has been introduced linking the control functions of the accreditation schemes with more improvement-oriented procedures (see below).

16.3.1   Evaluation of Institutional Quality Assurance Systems

Both institutional accreditation and accreditation of academic programmes rely on the existence of an institutional quality assurance system. By law, all Norwegian higher education institutions, public and private, are mandated to implement such a system by the end of 2003. These systems of quality assurance will be evaluated by NOKUT. Contrary to the accreditation schemes described above, this process is not labelled as an accreditation process, but as a process of approval. The consequence of not having an approved quality assurance system is that the right to establish new programmes is withdrawn. The institution loses neither the right to its institutional status (university, state college, etc.) nor its existing accreditation of programmes. It is in other words a limitation in the institutional autonomy that is proposed. Below are the ten criteria specified for the evaluation of the institutional quality assurance systems listed (NOKUT, 2003):

- How the quality system is linked to and is a part of the strategic ambitions and work of the institution.
- The specified objectives for the institutional work on quality.
- How the quality system is embedded in the leadership at all levels in the organisation.
- That the quality system is organised in such a way that it ensures extended participation in the organisation, with clearly specified responsibilities and duties.
- The collection and analysis aggregated to the institutional level of data and information from internal assessments that are necessary to establish a satisfactory overview of the quality of every programme.
- That analysis is conducted concerning how the defined objectives are met.
- How and in what way information and results from the quality system are used as a basis for decision-making and further improvement of the quality of the institution.
- Clarify how the quality system contributes to better management of financial, human and organisational resources.
- That students take an active part in the work to improve quality.
- That an annual report is delivered to the board of the institution, in which an overview and an assessment of quality of the institutions are given, along with an inventory of measures and processes initiated to further improve the quality of programmes.

In the criteria developed by NOKUT, it is emphasised that the quality assurance system is the responsibility of the board and the leadership of the institution. No formal requests concerning how an institutional quality assurance system should look like are specified by NOKUT. The size, objectives and profile of the individual institution must, according to NOKUT, be allowed to influence on what a quality assurance system should look like. Also when it comes to documentation (quantitative) the institutions are given much discretion. No such quantitative information is required to be reported to NOKUT even if NOKUT may demand certain information when a quality assurance system is evaluated.

The Ministry of Education (UFD, 2002) has ordered that an evaluation of the institutional quality assurance system must take place at least every sixth year, but that the prime objective with the evaluation of the quality assurance systems is not control but to develop well-functioning systems where dialogue and frequent communication between the external experts and the institution is considered to be a vital characteristic. The external experts must specify in what area the system is adequate and where the system needs improvement. The Ministry has also made it clear that it is expected of the institutions to establish routines that secure continuous improvements of the quality system (UFD, 2002).

16.3.2   Recognition of Internationally Obtained Education and Credits

NOKUT has a special section that deals with recognition of international obtained education and credits. This is the Norwegian ENIC/NARIC equivalent, which also includes the Lisbon Recognition Convention unit. Normally, recognition is provided by the individual institution in Norway after individual application, but NOKUT has been mandated to develop general recognition criteria, i.e., a framework that Norwegian institutions may use when dealing with individual applications. In this way, it is hoped that students will experience equal treatment from different institutions. To be recognised as higher education in Norway, a given programme or a course must be recognised as belonging to the category higher education also in the 'exporting' country. Both private and public higher education institutions may handle applications for recognition within areas in which they have the accredited rights to do so.

16.4   Other Supra-Institutional Evaluation Schemes

The Research Council of Norway (NFR) has the responsibility to conduct research assessments, and NOKUT and NFR have been ordered to try to co-ordinate their evaluation activities to minimise the administrative burden and the work-load of the institutions. Traditionally such co-ordination was rare, something that has triggered institutional complaints. Research assessments are conducted regularly by the NFR, and the signals are that this activity will increase in scale and scope in the coming years (NFR, 2001, p. 11).

A typical research assessment in Norway is built up in much the same way as the accreditation process. A self-evaluation is followed by an external peer review, which subsequently produces a public report on its findings and recommendations. Normally, external peer review committees consist of international experts in the field. Contrary to many evaluation activities in education, research assessments usually bring in experts also from outside the Nordic countries. Research assessments are conducted each year and often have a national and disciplinary scope, i.e., in mathematics, in political science and so forth. However, the outcomes of such assessments usually have not been very dramatic. Few rewards or sanctions are attached directly to the assessments.

At present, there is some overlap between the research assessments conducted and the up-coming accreditation schemes. As shown above, research activities are normally a part of the accreditation criteria, at least in higher degree programmes and in institutional accreditation processes. Thus, it may be expected that the two processes will collect and analyse some of the same data. How institutions will respond to this, and whether the new accreditation regime will 'occupy' some of the territory of the NFR remains to be seen.

As in many other OECD-countries, there are also stakeholders in higher education that perform their own 'evaluations' of higher education. In Norway, four newspapers in the last four years have interviewed a substantial number of students of higher education in order to find out what they think about the programme they are enrolled at, and the institution at which they are affiliated. The study, known as 'Stud.mag' or the student satisfaction survey, covers all higher education institutions and programmes offered in Norway, although a limited number of programmes are selected each year. The questionnaire used for the interviews is developed by NIFU, an independent research institute specialised in higher education issues that also performs the quantitative analysis of the data. The result is published each year in the newspapers. The study is likely to continue and is met with an increasing interest, also among higher education institutions. In addition, the data from the study have been used to analyse a range of issues in higher education and represent a valuable source of information for higher education researchers (see e.g., Wiers-Jenssen & Aamodt, 2002, Wiers-Jenssen, Stensaker & Grøgaard, 2002).

16.5   Potentials and Problems of the Accreditation System

It is not easy to pinpoint any specific reason why an accreditation system was introduced in Norway. In the 1990s, a growing interest in evaluation and performance of the higher education system can be detected. Not least, a pilot project of national evaluations in various disciplines was tested out, leading to conclusions that a special body for putting quality issues on the agenda should be established, along with a more systematic approach for evaluating the higher education system (see e.g., Stensaker, 1996, p. 80). Other conclusions from the pilot project were that the higher education institutions should take a more systematic approach in assuring the quality of their programmes, and that the leadership of the institutions needed more information on the work conducted at lower levels.

In 1998, the Norway Network Council was established with the multiple purposes of giving the Ministry of Education advice on strategic issues in higher education and having the responsibility of developing a national system for evaluating higher education. The Council initiated several projects to stimulate institutional interest for quality, among them several institutional evaluations with the intention of both checking quality of teaching and learning directly, and the work conducted to secure and improve the quality of programmes offered (NNR, 1999). However, the council struggled with its legitimacy, especially in the university sector, which accused the council of not having the skills and competencies to evaluate all types of higher education institutions. One of the reasons for this scepticism can be traced back to the establishment of the body, which mainly was a result of a re-organisation of several other councils related to the college sector. The consequence was that the new body had a staff not specialised in or recruited for evaluative tasks.

In the late 1990s, a separate commission for higher education was established, the so-called Mjøs-Commission (NOU, 2000). This Commission had the task to study the consequences of the increase in student numbers in higher education and how to adjust the system to the new situation. The Commission argued among others that to handle the growth in student numbers and to increase the efficiency of the system, more emphasis should be placed on competition among institutions and that more weight should be given to output rewards (NOU, 2000, p. 43).

One of the suggestions of the committee was to propose a new accreditation body with an independent status and a staff specialised in quality evaluations and assessments, which could act as a rigid quality controller of such a new system. An underlying premise for this proposal may be related to a wish to treat public and private higher education more equally. In the 1990s, private higher education institutions needed to apply to the Ministry of Education for every new programme offered, and such approval could often take up to two years to obtain. Private higher education institutions complained that this situation represented a huge advantage for the public sector (Stensaker, 2000, p. 98). The new accreditation system may indeed contribute to change this situation, since both public and private higher education institutions are scrutinised using many of the same criteria.

The institutional accreditation scheme may seem to be a rather dominating one if one compares it to accreditation schemes in other European countries, which focus more on programme accreditation (Westerheijden, 2001, p. 68). The reason is related to the fact that at present there is a strong 'institutional drift' in Norway. Several of the existing state colleges are in the process of opting for university status. This process can be found in several other countries as well (Kyvik, 2002), but in Norway it will have to be handled by the new institutional accreditation system. By defining the criteria for university status (most important: five master's degrees and four Ph.D. degrees where two must have at least regional relevance), it is up to NOKUT to decide whether university standards are met in the future. However, it is still the Ministry that decides whether university status is formally given, and this is likely to be a decision where economy will matter much.

The establishment of an accreditation system in higher education cannot be said to rest on research in the field. The decision in Parliament to establish the accreditation system neglected research suggesting that the big challenge related to quality in Norwegian higher education perhaps was not to control it more but to develop it further due to weak institutional systems for and attention related to quality issues

(Stensaker, 1996, Handal et al., 1999, Stensaker & Maassen, 2001). The social-democratic government that received the report from the commission seemed to agree with such views and proposed in the white paper that followed that the existing Norway Network Council should continue its work with an emphasis on quality improvement. However, in Parliament this proposal was voted down and the suggestion for the establishment of an accreditation system was raised again. The conservative majority in the Parliament voted in favour and thus succeeded in establishing such a system and an independent body (NOKUT) conducting the accreditation. This was one of the few issues from the social-democratic government that caused disagreement in the Parliament. Other reform proposals such as changing the degree structure and increasing the efficiency of higher education were supported by a large majority in the Parliament. Later in 2001, the social-democratic government resigned and a conservative government took over with a new Minister in charge of implementing the substantial number of reform proposals made.

However, whether NOKUT really represents a big change in Norwegian higher education can be questioned for a number of reasons. First, when it comes to personnel, NOKUT is staffed with many of the same persons that worked for the former Norway Network Council. The director general is the same and several others holding key positions in the staff also worked in the former council. Second, if one takes a closer look at the procedures proposed by NOKUT, striking similarities appear between suggestions made by the former council and the institutional quality systems suggested by NOKUT (see NNR, 1999). The improvement-oriented focus of the institutional quality system is kept, and the audit approach suggested by the old council seems to be continued by NOKUT. This seems like a deliberate strategy by NOKUT (Haakstad, 2001).

The potentials of the new system are that it seems to combine elements of reporting, evaluation and accreditation in a somewhat joint system. The basis of all the accreditation activities lies in the existence of an institutional quality assurance system that also has some built-in reporting activities that can be used for accreditation purposes. There also seems to be some cohesion between the different accreditation schemes. For example a rejected institutional accreditation may force institutions to apply for programme accreditation in areas, where before they had rights to establish programmes. There also seems to be huge overlaps between the criteria used for accrediting Ph.D. programmes and the criteria used for institutional accreditation of universities and university colleges. The fact that many of the accreditation standards also seem to be quite 'soft', emphasising the existence of processes rather than checking of explicit and quantifiable standards, point in the same direction. One of the fears of a full-scale accreditation system proposed was that it could cause heavy administrative burdens for the institutions and contribute to an increased bureaucratisation of Norwegian higher education (see NOU, 2000, Stensaker & Maassen, 2001). This is still a possible unintended outcome of the new system, especially since not only institutions, but also programmes at all levels must undertake an accreditation process.

For higher education institutions, the new accreditation procedures will most likely contribute to further strengthen institutional leadership. The fact that institutional leadership is made formally responsible for the institutional quality assurance system, and that institutional developments can be severely restricted by not obtaining programme accreditation support this assertion. A strengthened institutional leadership, on the other hand, may limit the power that departments traditionally have had in Norwegian higher education. The criteria describing the institutional quality system make it clear that departments to a much larger degree than before must report to the institution about 'quality failures', and also open up for increased institutional 'interference' in departmental decision-making.

Whether NOKUT represents a shift in the power structure at national level is more difficult to project. Formally, the establishment with its independent status and based on the fact that the Ministry cannot instruct the body in other ways than through legal acts, suggests that power has been transferred from the Ministry to NOKUT. In this perspective, the establishment of NOKUT represents a decentralisation in Norwegian higher education. Procedures that traditionally belonged to the Ministry have been taken over by NOKUT, and the new system makes it easier to differentiate between decisions made on expert criteria and decisions based on political considerations. On the other hand, it is still the Ministry that has the final say when it comes to granting institutions a certain status (e.g., to become a university). Thus, one may also claim that it is only the 'unimportant procedural' aspects that have been moved out of the Ministry, making it more of a political secretariat for the political leadership. In this perspective, the changes are not so much about decentralisation but a rearrangement of the dominant position the state has in Norwegian higher education. How the board of NOKUT will function is, however, of great significance in the latter perspective. Giving accreditation to institutions and programmes that the Ministry at a later stage turn down, may create tensions that over time may weaken the legitimacy of the system, something which can trigger a 'softer' Ministry. The fact that governments in Norway usually have not been based on a majority of members of the Parliament can contribute to weaken the Ministry. Norwegian higher education history suggests that when questions about new higher education institutions are on the agenda, the interest of the Parliament usually increases. The establishment of the regional colleges in the 1960s, and the establishments of several Norwegian universities show that issues that have both a national and regional interest trigger processes where political rather than expert criteria matter most.

The interest organisations of students in Norway supported the reform initiatives and seem to look forward to the establishment of institutional quality systems where student assessment of teaching and learning are to have a central place. To the degree that such systems actually contribute to improve the programmes offered, students may be served better by the new approaches. Whether the accreditation system, especially of programmes, will have the same effect, is more difficult to project. The old approval system where the Ministry regulated the establishment of new programmes and the traditional external examiner system, which have been turned into a voluntary system for institutions, seemed to have kept quality at a reasonably high level in the country in the past. After the reform initiatives with the introduction of new bachelor's and master's degrees, it is expected that students will receive more guidance from teachers and will be followed up more closely than in the past. Whether such follow up will take place is, first and foremost, an economic question, and may have more influence on programme quality than the new accreditation system per se. The *Stud.mag* study, mentioned before, also show that most Norwegian students are relatively satisfied with the quality of education they receive (Wiers-Jenssen & Aamodt, 2002), a fact that could diminish the effect of a system focused on minimum standards. If only very few programmes lose their accreditation, a consequence would be that the majority of the students will not notice much of the accreditation system. If however, a programme stands in danger of losing accreditation, the consequences for students may be dramatic since, in the worst case, they must transfer to another institution. In this case, the new accreditation system may represent a severe treat to students who have been identified to programmes of weak quality.

The latter situation also brings us to the possibility that the new accreditation may increase the 'juridification' of higher education. This tendency may occur also due to other elements in the changes proposed, not least as a consequence of the new contracts that are to be established between the institutions and individual students. In these contracts, rights and obligations of the two parties are specified in a detailed way, and students may take legal actions against violations of the agreed contract. In the accreditation system, in the complaints committee the legal influence perhaps is most visible. This committee, consisting of five persons, of whom the chairman must have qualifications to act as a judge in a civil court, will decide all complaints from the institutions. The rather 'soft' criteria suggested by NOKUT imply that much discretion is left to this committee when deciding how certain criteria should be interpreted. A possible consequence is that the committee may pay more attention to legal rather than to expert views when dealing with the complaints.

16.6   The International Dimension of Norwegian Higher Education

It is tempting to interpret the recent reform initiatives in Norway as a direct response to the Bologna process. The changes in the degree structure, the new grading system and the new accreditation system ring some familiar bells for students of the Bologna Declaration. Nevertheless, one should be careful to argue that the new accreditation system in Norway is directly derived from the Bologna process. The interest for quality assurance has a broader foundation than 'just' to adapt to international policy developments, as indicated above.

That being said, the international dimension has played a role in developing the new quality assurance system. Looking into the established procedures, three sources of inspiration are in particular noticeable: Sweden, Europe (Bologna Declaration) and to some extent the current GATS negotiations. Sweden seems to have been the role model when developing the institutional quality assurance system, but also some of the procedures the new accreditation schemes will use, bear great resemblance to the audit system that was implemented in Sweden in the mid-1990s. The former Norway Network Council may be an important player leading to this result. Not least, the former council published in the late 1990s a report specifying how Norwegian higher education should be evaluated in the future (NNR, 1999). In this report, it was recommended that future Norwegian evaluation systems should be based on an audit-procedure due to its 'flexibility and open approach' (NNR, 1999, p. 81). The fact that a Swedish expert participated in the pilot project in addition may have led to this strong focus on the Swedish experiences.

This does not mean that the Bologna Declaration and the present GATS negotiations are unimportant in the Norwegian context. For politicians and for the Ministry of Education, these processes are of great importance. A closer analysis of political documents paving the way for the recent reforms in Norwegian higher education shows many references to the Bologna Declaration, to the need to internationalise Norwegian higher education and to attract foreigners into the domestic higher education system (see e.g., St.Meld.nr. 27, p. 16 and 38-41). The interest in the internationalisation of higher education is not new in Norway. Norwegian students for decades have travelled abroad and at present about 10 % of the total student population are enrolled at various foreign higher education institutions. Due to a rather generous student support scheme that makes Norwegian students very attractive to fee-based programmes abroad, the Ministry of Education follows the GATS negotiations closely. When it comes to the new accreditation schemes, both the Bologna process and the GATS negotiations seem to have been important sources of inspiration for Norwegian policy-makers, at least when it comes to introducing the term accreditation in Norwegian higher education (see e.g., the NOU, 2000, chapter 15).

However, even if the term accreditation may stem from these processes, and even if several countries have implemented accreditation schemes during the latter years, it still seems rather difficult to find a common 'European model' for accreditation. Fierce discussion on how a transparent European system for quality assurance should look like and on what 'platforms' it should be based, have complicated any policy adaptation attempt. Except for the term accreditation, there seems to have been much insecurity among Norwegian policy-makers on the content of such a system. In the Mjøs-report that laid the foundation for the latest reforms in Norwegian higher education, accreditation systems are only discussed on a couple of pages in the almost 700-page report (NOU, 2000, p. 357-359). In other words, there was little clarification concerning the substance of the accreditation schemes.

Thus, for implementers of the new accreditation system the challenges have been to 'operationalise' these schemes and to provide them with substance. A look at the accreditation schemes as they appear today point to the tendency that the new schemes are a re-built (Swedish) audit model that builds on the past experiences and on pilot projects carried out by the former Norway Network Council. One might claim that the accreditation schemes have been somewhat 'transformed' during implementation and that the implementers in this respect may have learned from the experiences of 'the first generation' of accreditation schemes developed in Central and Eastern European countries (see Westerheijden, 2001 for a more detailed description). In this way, some of the shortcomings of existing accreditation systems, i.e., the conservative nature of judgements reached and the lack of an improvement orientation, may be addressed. In a recent article by one of the staff members of NOKUT, this seems to be one of the central intentions of the new body (Haakstad, 2001, p. 82). An additional advantage with such a combined accreditation/audit approach may be found in its potentially efficient way of integrating various processes in a joint system. Whether the accreditation schemes in fact will trigger such effects remains yet to be seen.

16.7   An Integrated Approach for Improvement and Control?

One conclusion that may be reached from this chapter is that what seems to be an accreditation system adapted to future expectations about deregulated higher education markets and the ongoing European and global integration processes, is geared heavily to pressing domestic needs at the same time. (The public/private dimension and the need to deal with 'institutional drift'.) During implementation the somewhat 'solution-driven' changes related to the Bologna process also show signs of being adjusted to prior experiences in evaluation and shortcoming in the quality of Norwegian higher education provision. The result seems to be a hybrid between (solution-driven) international developments and domestic needs.

The interesting questions for the future include how the new accreditation system in Norway matches the developments in other countries. For instance, in the Nordic countries a system for exchange of students and staff exists that may be affected by the new accreditation system. Will the other Nordic countries accept the accreditation given by NOKUT, or will Nordic and/or international developments put pressure on the Norwegian accreditation schemes to adjust to emerging 'standards' in this field? In relation to this, it is also interesting to see whether the monopoly

NOKUT has in the accreditation area at present will continue in the future. Even if other accreditation agencies are allowed to accredit Norwegian higher education also in the new system, it is only the 'stamp' provided by NOKUT that at present provides students with access to the state supported student financing system. At present, the new accreditation system seems to represent a desire for national control over higher education. This is, however, not unusual in a European perspective (Westerheijden, 2001, p. 73).

Also domestically, the new accreditation schemes represent a challenge, not least in terms of integrating the new accreditation schemes with other quality assessment activities in the sector. Not least are Norwegian higher education institutions mandated to have systems that secure the staff a good working environment ('HMS', which stands for health, environment, security). At present, these HMS systems are not a part of the accreditation schemes developed even if in some areas they overlap considerably, e.g., when it comes to staffing and infrastructure. Furthermore, the reform and the new legislation also guarantee the students a physical learning environment (not regulated before), where it is currently suggested that the existing Labour Inspection Authority (*Arbeidstilsynet*) should monitor the learning environment. In these areas, a potential exists for integration and rationalisation.

Traditionally, the Ministry demanded several annual (quantitative) reports about the activity and 'production' of the higher education institutions. In the new system, these reports are supposed to be part of the institutional quality system upon which that all accreditation activities should be based. This 'performance indicator' system has provided the Ministry with important information about the quality and efficiency of the higher education system, and the intention with the integration in the institutional quality system seems to be that the institutions themselves must take independent actions on the basis of these data to a larger extent than before. In the new system, the quantitative indicators will also be sent to the Ministry where they will be an important element in the new and more output-based financing system.[1] In other words, improvement and control, and quality and funding will become more tightly coupled both at the institutional and at the national levels. In the discussions about the new accreditation system in Norway, the problematic relation to the new funding systems has been raised frequently. The fear is that quality standards may suffer due to possible institutional budgetary gains. This is a question that also needs to be investigated closely in the coming years.

---

1   The new funding system for higher education in Norway was introduced as of the budget year 2002. In it, grants to higher education institutions consist of three main components: a) a basic component (approximately 60 % of the total allocation), b) an education component (approximately 25 %) based on the number of completed student credits, the number of graduates (scheduled to begin in 2005), and the number of exchange students (in + out), c) a research component (approximately 15 %) which consists of result-based allocation (competitive), and a strategic allocation.

References

Bleiklie, I., R. Høstaker & A. Vabø (2000). *Policy and practise in higher education: reforming Norwegian universities*.London: Jessica Kingsley Publishers.

Haakstad, J. (2001). Accreditation: the new quality assurance formula? Some reflections as Norway is about to reform its quality assurance system. *Quality in Higher Education*, 7, 77-82.

Handal, G., K. Lycke & I. Hatlevik (1999). *Studiekvalitet i praksis*. Oslo: Pedagogisk forskningsinstitutt, Universitetet i Oslo.

Hämäläinen, K., J. Haakstad, J. Kangasniemi, T. Lindeberg, M. Sjölund (2001). *Quality assurance in the Nordic higher education – accreditation-like practices*. (ENQA occasional papers 2) Helsinki: European Network for Quality Assurance in Higher Education.

Kyvik, S. (2002). *Changing relationship between university and non-university higher education sectors*. Paper presented at the 24th EAIR-Forum in Prague 2002.

NFR (2001). *Det norske forsknings- og innovasjonssystemet – statistikk og indikatorer*. Oslo: Norges forskningsråd.

NNR (1999). *'Basert på det fremste...'? Om evaluering, kvalitetssikring og kvalitetsutvikling av norsk høgre utdanning*. Oslo: Norgesnettrådet rapport 2/1999.

NNR (2002). *Norgesnettrådets pilotprosjekt med utvikling av et kvalitetssystem. Rapport fra pilotprosjektgruppa*. Oslo: Norgesnettrådet.

NOKUT (2003). *Forskrift om standarder og kriterier for evaluering og akkreditering av høgre utdanning* (Høringsutkast). Oslo: NOKUT.

NOU (2000). *Frihet med ansvar. Om høgre utdanning i Norge*. Norges offentlige utredninger (2000: 14). Oslo: Statens forvaltningstjeneste.

St.Meld.Nr. 27 (2000-2001). *Gjør din plikt – krev din rett. Kvalitetsreform av høyere utdanning*. Oslo: Kirke-, utdannings- og forskningsdepartementet.

Stensaker, B. (1996). *Organisasjonsutvikling og ledelse. Bruk og effekter av evalueringer på universiteter og høgskoler*. Oslo: NIFU rapport 8/1996.

Stensaker, B. (1997). From accountability to opportunity: the role of quality assessments in Norway. *Quality in Higher Education*, 3, 277-284.

Stensaker, B. (2000). *Høyere utdanning i endring. Dokumentasjon og drøfting av kvalitetsutviklingstiltak ved seks norske universiteter og høgskoler 1989-1999*. Oslo: NIFU-rapport 6/2000.

Stensaker, B. & P. Maassen (2001). *Strategier og metoder for kvalitetsutvikling. En drøfting av noen sentrale forslag og synspunkter hos Mjøsutvalget*. Oslo: NIFU skriftserie 10/2001.

Trondal, J., B. Stensaker, Å. Gornitzka & P. Maassen (2001). *Internasjonalisering av høyere utdanning. Trender og utfordringer*. Oslo: NIFU skriftserie 28/2001.

Westerheijden, D. F. (2001). Ex Oriente Lux?: national and multiple accreditation in Europe after the fall of the wall and after Bologna. *Quality in Higher Education*, 7, 65-75.

Wiers-Jenssen, J. & P. Aamodt (2001). *Trivsel og innsats. Studenters tilfredshet med lærested og tid brukt til studier. Resultater fra 'Stud.Mag' undersøkelsene*. Oslo: NIFU rapport 1/2002.

Wiers-Jenssen, J. & B. Stensaker & J. B. Grøgaard (2002). Student satisfaction. Towards an empirical deconstruction of the concept. *Quality in Higher Education*, 8, 183-195.

UFD (2002). *Forskrift om akkreditering, evaluering og godkjenning etter lov om universiteter og høgskoler og lov om private høyskoler (Foreløpig versjon)* Oslo: Utdannings- og forskningsdepartementet.

17 Accreditation and Evaluation in Poland: Concepts, Developments and Trends

EWA CHMIELECKA & MARCIN DĄBROWSKI

17.1 Introduction

The legal regulations adopted in Poland in 1990 and later (AHEd, 1990; ASTD, 1990; ASCSR, 1991; AHVE, 1997) were conducive to a quantitative expansion of higher education. The past decade saw the creation of over 250 non-state institutions and over 20 state vocational institutions of higher education, while the state academic institutions greatly increased their enrolment at all levels of study. During this period the total number of students increased approximately four-fold, which means that we are definitely witnessing mass higher education in Poland. The tables below illustrate the size and structure of the Polish higher education system (Chmielecka, 2000; Central Office of Statistics, 2002, www.stat.gov.pl).

Table 1. Student numbers

Academic year	2001/2002	2000/2001	1999/2000	1990/1991
Students	1,718,700	1,584,800	1,431,900	408,800
Percentage of age cohort	Net 32,7 Gross 43,6	Net 30,6 Gross 40,7	Net 28,0 Gross 36,9	Net 9,8 Gross 12,9

In the academic year 2001/02, 70 % of students were enrolled at public universities and the remaining 30 % at private ones; 62 % were charged fees and only 38 % were getting free education. The latter shows that Polish youth is strongly motivated to enter higher education.

Table 2. Numbers of institutions of higher education

Academic year	2001/2002	2000/2001	1999/2000	1990/1991
Public higher education institutions	123	115	113	106
Private higher education institutions	221	195	174	6
Total	344	310	287	112

S. Schwarz and D.F. Westerheijden (eds.),
Accreditation and Evaluation in the European Higher Education Area, 371–393.

The Polish higher education system has a complex structure. There are universities (in a traditional sense of the word), universities of technology, universities of economics, universities of agriculture, medical universities, pedagogical universities (or academies), academies of physical education, academies of fine arts, theological academies, state higher schools for vocational education and private higher schools (mainly for vocational education).

The professional titles awarded to graduates of higher education institutions in Poland are as follows:

- the professional (vocational) title of *licencjat* (BA) is awarded following the completion of 3 or 3.5 years of higher professional education;
- the professional title of *inżynier* is awarded following the completion of 3.5 or 4 years of higher professional education in technical areas, agriculture, economics and related areas;
- the title of *magister* (MA) is awarded following the completion of single-cycle 5 or 6 year *magister*-level courses in a given field of study.[1] Equivalent titles include *magister edukacji* (in Education), *magister sztuki* (in Fine Arts), *magister inżynier* (in Engineering), *magister inżynier architekt* (in Architecture), *lekarz medycyny* (in Medicine), *lekarz stomatolog* (in Dentistry) and *lekarz weterynarii* (in Veterinary Medicine). The title of *magister* may also be obtained following the completion of 2 or 2.5 year second-cycle *magister*-level courses, for which holders of the professional title of *licencjat* or *inżynier* are eligible.

To be awarded any of the above titles students must complete all subjects and internships or a practical placement included in the curriculum, submit and defend a diploma project or thesis and pass a diploma examination. Upon graduation, each student receives a diploma in a specific field of study, three copies of the diploma and, upon request, a diploma in a foreign language.

The list of fields of study (programmes) in which university-type institutions in Poland may award professional titles of *magister* contains 101 entries. The Central Council for Higher Education defines this list according to section 42.1.1 of the Act on Higher Education (AHE, 1990). The names of the fields of study (programmes) that are offered in schools of higher professional (vocational) education and lead to the title of *licencjat* or *inżynier* are in accordance with the list of fields of study defined by the Central Council of Higher Education for Higher Education Schools. The list of programmes includes names of more than 170 specialist options currently offered. Names of specialist options are not regulated, and this list is open.

---

1   For a brief explanation of this typically Polish organisational concept in higher education, see section 4 of this chapter.

In Poland, there is a strong tradition of respecting studies at *magister* or degree level, which are regarded as true 'higher studies'. The *licencjat* is rejected, as both students and employers aspire to the MA. Many professions require additional certificates awarded by professional associations.

The unemployment rate in Poland is very high and in September 2002 it reached the figure of 3,112,592 people (17.5 %). The number of registered unemployed higher education graduates in September 2002 was relatively small (26,415). That meant that the number of unemployed university graduates was at the level of 18.5 % of the unemployed among the graduates from all school types, while within the group of all registered unemployed it came to 0.85 %, which testifies to the low unemployment among the university graduates. In immediately preceding years it was at a lower level, whereas in the 1990s the demand for university graduates had even exceeded supply (http://www.mpips.gov.pl).

The influences of actors such as state institutions and political parties, trade unions and others are moderated by a very strong tradition of university autonomy. The most important factor which orientates the existence and the development of universities (public and non-public) is The Act on Higher Education of 1990. It supplies the collegiate bodies of public universities with great authority and allows non-public universities to form their decision-making structures independently. According to the Act, the main role of the Ministry of Education and Sport is to control the universities' performance in keeping with the requirements of the law. The Parliament of the Republic of Poland, by accepting the budget together with the funds for maintaining higher education, remains the only political body that has a significant influence on these funds. Political parties, trade unions and other organisations seem to be inconspicuous. They may, however, be more prominent at the local level, where the organs of the local government (and related political organisations) create and manage local universities.

17.2 The National System of Quality Assurance in Higher Education

17.2.1 Accreditation

There are two fundamental accreditation schemes in Poland. The first is national (state-owned), represented by the State Accreditation Committee (*Państwowa Komisja Akredytacyjna*, PKA) and has been in operation since January 2002. The second is called 'environmental' or private and is represented by accreditation committees formed by the academic communities who are willing to accredit certain groups of programmes (fields of study) delivered by higher education institutions (usually of a certain type). The 'environmental' committees of the universities represented in the Conference of Rectors of Polish Universities (KRASP) co-operate within the framework of its Accreditation Committee (KA KRASP). SEM F operates separately. These committees had been created before PKA came into existence.

Since these two schemes are of a very different character they will be described below separately (Wójcicka, 2001, 2002; Wójcicka & Chmielecka, 2001).

The State Accreditation Committee (*Panstwowa Komisja Akredytacyjna*, PKA)

As from 1 January 2002, the State Accreditation Committee (PKA) offered programme accreditation nationally. It is compulsory for all degree programmes for both levels (*licencjat* and *magister* degree) offered by any higher education institution, both public and private. The PKA accreditation covers teaching (in all of its aspects) as well as scientific research. These two subjects constitute the main part of the PKA accreditation standards.

The academic community, the Central Council for Higher Education and the Ministry of National Education, had requested the creation of a national accreditation organisation since 1994 (Kawecki, 1996; Chwirot, 1998; AKA, 1997; Wnuk-Lipińska & Wójcicka, 1995). The PKA is a state institution. It was established through an amendment of The Act on Higher Education (of July 2001), which defined the PKA's fundamental obligations, competences and procedures. The law also gives PKA the right to co-operate with other accrediting institutions in Poland and abroad.

The PKA consists of 65 members, appointed by the Minister of National Education and Sport (MENiS). The Minister's decisions are based on a candidates' list, which he receives from the PKA. Candidates are entered on the list following a survey that the PKA organises amongst the university Senates. The Committee sets its own statute regulating its basic activities and the competences of its bodies and organs. The Committee has sub-committees for humanities, natural sciences (mathematics, physics and chemistry), agriculture, forestry and veterinary sciences, medical sciences, physical education, technical sciences, economics, and social studies and law (AAHEd, 2001; KRASP, 1998).

The PKA's Office is part of the Ministry of the National Education and Sport. The projects of the Office are supervised by the Director of the Office, who has the rank of a Vice-Director of the department of the Ministry. The minister appoints and dismisses the Chairman and the Secretary of the PKA from among the Committee members. The Committee is controlled and reviewed by the Ministry.

The PKA submits opinions to the Ministry on the:

1) creation of universities,
2) universities' right to conduct higher studies in defined fields and at certain levels of education,

3) creation by a university of a subsidiary or an exterior faculty,

4) evaluation of quality of a given field of study (programme). The evaluation of a field of study is carried out if a programme is newly created (within three years of its launch or being promoted from licence or engineer to master's degree), if an application is made to be upgraded to a master's level degree programme, if the PKA's Presidium chooses so, or at the Minister's request.

5) evaluation of teachers' educational quality,

6) respecting the requirements for delivery of higher education.

Probably the prime stakeholder is the Ministry of National Education and Sport (MENiS). Positive evaluations by the PKA are the basis for MENiS' approval and decision-making concerning the establishment or continuation of universities and/or fields of studies. Negative evaluations could lead to its decision to terminate or suspend teaching in a certain field.

Amongst the most important stakeholders and institutions engaged in the scheme are, second, academic teachers and higher education institutions and their units. For them, obtaining feedback on schools that comply with the basic education quality standards will give additional motivation to enhance the quality of their work. Gaining accreditation means their stabilisation on the education market and public confirmation of the basic quality of studies. They also hope to remove the worst units from the higher education system and thus increase competition on the educational service market.

A third category of stakeholders is the other accrediting institutions (especially 'environmental' ones). The accreditations they offer gain additional value, with the fundamental accreditation of the PKA as a background.

Outside academia, students, parents, and employers are affected by the scheme. They receive basic information about the credibility of schools and their achievement of fundamental quality standards. For students, for instance, this will enable better-informed choices of the place to study, and for employers it will help them for the recruitment of employees.

The PKA accreditation is free of charge. The Committee's activity is financed from the state budget. The Minister defines (through an order) the way the projects of the Committee are administrated and financed, the remuneration of its members and the conditions of reimbursements of travel costs etc. associated with meetings and reviews. The remuneration of the Council and the Committee members will be evaluated in relation to the minimal basic wage of an ordinary professor.

The formal stages of the procedure are as follows: an evaluation team is appointed to carry out an educational evaluation at a certain university unit. The Secretary of the Commission, in accordance with the Chairman of the Team, appoints the evaluation team, which consists of five persons. The chairman of the Team must be a Committee member. The evaluation proceedings cover: the self-evaluation, the visit by the evaluation team, the preparation of the report, the consideration of the application for accreditation, and the resolution of the PKA Presidium which can be graded as follows: distinguished, positive, conditional, negative. The grades: 'distinguished' and 'positive' are granted for a period of five years. The resolution concerning the conditional grade includes the recommendations and the terms of their realisation. The Committee's resolution is passed on to the Minister and to the university. If the evaluation is negative, the Minister (having considered the type and range of the stated violations) withdraws or suspends the approval to run a given field of study at a given level of education.

The formal duration of the stages of the procedures is about four to six months. In case of disagreement with the PKA Presidium's resolution, the university may apply for reconsideration of the case. The application should be submitted to the Committee within 14 days from delivery of the initial resolution. The application is considered during a common session of the evaluation team and the Committee Presidium within thirty days.

Generally speaking, the PKA's activity is transparent and the resolutions of the PKA Presidium are published on the PKA's website. It lists the fields of education (universities) evaluated during a given period, as well as the results of the accreditation.

The first accreditation proceedings began in 2002. Until January 2003, approximately 150 procedures were initiated, and 13 have been completed. Accordingly, at the time of writing it was too early to summarise the experiences. But one can notice that the procedures are being implemented in accordance with the official assumptions. The results have been published. Of the thirteen completed proceedings, two had a negative grade. One of the two universities that received a negative decision announced in public that it would bring the decision before the Supreme Administrative Court. It is not known yet how MENiS will regard the negative evaluations. It might decide to close or suspend certain fields of education. As these are the first cases, the academic community is awaiting the MENiS decision. It is commonly expected that, due to the heavy workload of the PKA, its tight budget could cause difficulties in their implementation.

The 'Environmental' Accreditation Scheme

The 'environmental' accreditation scheme includes a number of accreditation agencies:

- The Association of Management Education 'Forum' (SEM F)
- KRASP Accreditation Committee, including amongst others:
  - University Accreditation Committee (UKA)
  - Accreditation Committee for Medical Universities (KAUM)

- Accreditation Committee for Technical Universities (KAUT)
- Foundation for Promotion and Accreditation of Economic Studies (FPAKE).

All the 'environmental' accreditation schemes listed above offer accreditation for fields of study in their discipline at both *licencjat* and *magister* levels. Their accreditation standards cover both teaching in its all aspects and scientific research. Their standards of teaching quality are set at a higher level than the requirements of the PKA.

In 1993, the Association of Management Education 'Forum' (SEM F) was founded mainly by private business schools. Since most of them had a 'vocational' rather than an 'academic' status, they were not involved in the framework of KRASP. Nevertheless, the SEM F's institutional character, accreditation standards and procedures are typical of 'environmental' accreditation schemes. In 1994, twelve SEM F members signed the Agreement of Business Schools on Quality of Education and implemented – for the first time in Poland – an accreditation system for educational programmes and managerial staff training. At the end of 2002, SEM F conducted accreditation for the following fields of study (only full-time): Management and Marketing, Finance and Banking, Economics, Informatics and Econometrics, Informatics, as well as for the Master of Business Administration (MBA) programmes and one-year Managerial Study (Bielski, 2002; Kwiatkowski, 2001; SEMF, 2002; www.semforum.com.pl).

The Rectors' Conference of Academic Schools of Poland (KRASP) considers ensuring the quality of higher education to be a core activity. In August 2000, KRASP made it known that it would support the activities of the 'environmental' accreditation committees. Therefore, an Accreditation Committee was established by the Resolution of the KRASP Plenary Assembly on 7 June 2001. According to the Resolution, the KRASP Accreditation Committee is a forum of co-operation of the accreditation committees appointed by the conferences of rectors of particular university types, which are members of KRASP. The Committee itself does not undertake accreditations. These activities remain in the competence of the 'environmental' committees. The Committee's tasks include (Woźnicki, 2001; Kraśniewski, 2001):

- verifying the correctness of accreditation standards and procedures applied by the 'environmental' committees;
- co-ordinating the activities of the 'environmental' accreditation committees; especially adjusting the accreditation principles and proceedings to the fields of study in different types of universities;
- representing the accreditation committees operating within the KRASP framework internationally;
- inspiring the activities of the KRASP organs in education quality;

- conducting information and educational activities in the field of accreditation.

The Committee is financed by the KRASP. However, this does not apply to accreditation procedures; since their costs are borne by the 'environmental' committees.

The Accreditation Committees were established by the Conferences of Rectors of the respective universities (KAUM in 1997, UKA in 1998, FPAKE in 2000 and KAUT in 2001). The Committees represent all state universities in their fields in Poland. The disciplines accredited in the scheme are as follows:

- UKA: all fields of study in the universities, in accordance with the MENiS listing. The Guidebook of UKA, published annually, contains the list of these fields and names of the university units that offer them (UKA, 2002; Chwirot, 2001, 2002; http://main.amu.edu.pl/ects/uka/uka.html).
- KAUM: Medical studies (the faculties of Medicine), Medical analysis, Pharmacy, Dentistry (Gembicki, 2002; Mirecka & Gembicki, 2001).
- KAUT: all fields of study offered by the technical universities. In 2002 KAUT launched its first accreditations for selected fields of study (Konczakowska, 2002; KAUT 2002).
- FPAKE by the end of 2002 prepared accreditation standards and launched accreditation for the following fields of study: Management and Marketing, Finance and Banking, Economics, International Relations, Informatics, and Econometrics. Work on standards for 'Commodities science' and MBA has begun. FPAKE's accreditation procedure covers the field of study offered full-time and all other forms, e.g. extra-mural or part-time (Chmielecka, 2001; Strahl, 2002; www.fundacja.edu.pl).

In addition to the KRASP member accreditation agencies mentioned in the list above, the Accreditation Committee for Agricultural Universities (KAUR), the Accreditation Committee for Pedagogical Universities (KAUP), the Accreditation Committees for Physical Education Academies (KAAWF), the Accreditation Committee for Universities of Fine Arts (KAUM) are also formally included in the Accreditation Committee of KRASP. Each was established by the appropriate Conferences of Rectors. However, their activity remained at the pilot stage of accreditation procedures until early 2003. They do not have websites or other official information sources, therefore they are not treated in more detail in this chapter. Nevertheless, it can be expected that they will soon become more active. When that is the case, all Polish universities will be covered by the 'environmental' accreditation network (Borecki, 2002; Król, 2002; Socha, 2001, 2002).

The main group stakeholders and engaged institutions are as follows:

- Academic teachers and universities and their units: accreditation confirms the high quality of education of schools (faculties) and employed teachers. Obtaining the 'environmental' accreditation gives a distinguished position in the educational market, as it confirms a high (above-average) quality of the educational service. Lack of 'environmental' accreditation may suggest lower education quality.
- State Accreditation Committee (PKA); as the 'environmental' accreditation applies higher standards than the PKA, the results could point to interesting areas for PKA accreditation.
- For KAUM, we can add as an interested party the federal Department of Education of The United States, which suspended in 1996 recognition of physicians' diplomas issued in Poland for lack of an external quality control system in Poland. As half the faculties of medicine in Poland conducted programmes in English for foreign students, it became urgent to appoint an Accreditation Committee. Its activity was well received and the US Department of Education restored the diploma recognition, stating that the Committee's procedures corresponded to the American standards of accreditation.
- Sponsors and supporting institutions.
- Organisations making ranking lists of higher education institutions and of programmes: in the majority of them, accreditation gives additional points to units.

As for ownership, we find three main models. First, UKA, KAUM, KAUT are institutions established by the Conference of Rectors. As neither Conferences nor Committees are legal entities, they cannot be regarded as the 'owners' according to the law. It could be maintained that these accreditation agencies are 'propriety' (initiative) of the university communities in Poland and are managed and controlled through the bodies appointed by them.

The second model is that of the FPAKE. The FPAKE is a foundation that 'belongs' to the founders, e.g. to the Foundation Board, as the founders can decide about its liquidation. The composition of the Board changes with the regular elections of rectors, since only acting rectors may be Board members.

Third, the SEM F is an association, which therefore 'belongs' to its members. In 2002 SEM F was composed of 62 members, mainly teachers of managerial education, and representatives of the corporate world; while amongst the supporting members there were 26 higher education institutions and other institutions related to managerial education, mainly private business schools.

The activities of UKA, KAUT and KAUM are under the control of their Rectors' Conferences. The Committees send them annual reports each year, together with a financial settlement. The FPAKE is subject to the legal regulations on foundations. This obliges it to submit annual reports to the internal organs and to MENiS. The report must deal with substantial parts, as well as the finances, prepared by an accounting company. SEM F has a Revising Committee, which is in charge of controlling the Association's activities within the time limits given by law. As for the accreditation standards, they are reviewed permanently by the committees' experts according to the regulations given by their statutes.

Students, parents and employers receive reliable feedback concerning the high (above-average) quality of education, which enables better grounded choices of where to enrol, and helps employers to recruit. Information about the accreditation will be disseminated more particularly to these groups of stakeholders.

The 'environmental' accreditation agencies were created in order to balance the standards of education quality at the Polish universities, to contribute to the upgrading of the quality and to create a system of accreditation in accordance with the agreed evaluation systems applied in the European Union. To fulfil these objectives they:

- determine, on the basis of recommendations from expert groups, the standards for the quality of education in specific fields of studies; (the KAUM accreditation is based on procedures and standards of American accreditation adapted to the Polish context; the SEM F and FPAKE are strongly influenced by the EQUIS accreditation scheme).
- determine what documentation is necessary in the accreditation process;
- decide about the commencement of the accreditation procedure for the study area at a school which asks for it;
- oversee the process of each accreditation;
- nominate expert groups and their chairmen, and members of evaluation teams;
- receive reports of evaluation teams;
- award, refuse or defer accreditation for specific fields of study at given schools (KAUM, FPAKE, SEM F) or prepare requests for the Rectors' Conferences (UKA, KAUT) to do so;
- perform all other activities necessary to fulfil their mission.

Their accreditation is voluntary, given for three to five years and payable (approximately € 2,500 to € 4,000).

UKA, KAUM and KAUT conduct their activities in keeping with the common law. There are no specific legal regulations. FPAKE runs its activities according to the legal regulations on foundations, and SEM F on the basis of the law on associations.

The founders of UKA and KAUT finance the costs of their functioning. The Medical Universities finance the costs of KAUM by paying annual fees, the amount of which depends on the number of students and the Commission's needs (including the number of completed accreditations). The Medical Universities do not bear any other accreditation costs. According to its statutes, FPAKE obtains funds for its activities through donations, endowments of its sponsors ('benefactors') and the income of the company operated by the Foundation. The SEM F obtains funds for its activities through entrance fees and membership premiums, donations, inheritances, endowments, the incomes through its statutory and economic activity, and incomes from the public.

The accreditation procedures adopted by all committees are very similar, differing only in some details, and consist in the following steps:

- Forming experts groups to define specific standards for the quality of education in specific fields of study, based on the general standards adopted earlier.
- Application by a university unit for a field of study to be accredited.
- Self-assessment by the school (in case of KAUM, these documents may be 1,500 pages!).
- Establishing an evaluation team to:
  - conduct a comprehensive review and assessment. The evaluation is to be conducted according to the general and specific standards defined, and includes a mandatory site visit;
  - prepare a written report on the review and assessment conducted and to present it to the committee, together with the recommendation to award the accreditation, to defer it until specified conditions are met, or to refuse accreditation.
- The committee discusses the report during a plenary session and makes a decision as to whether to award, defer or refuse accreditation.

The preconditions that must be met before an accreditation procedure may begin are the following:

- The unit of the institution (a faculty, an institute, a chair) which applies for accreditation for a given area of studies applies internal methods of stimulating and evaluating the quality of the education that is offered;
- This area applies a system of credit points that is congruent with the European system (ECTS);
- The area of studies and the quality of education meet the staff quality requirements set by the committee.

The formal duration of the procedure is about six to ten months. Key and specific criteria of the committees' accreditation can differ, but they usually include: mission and strategy, students, teaching staff, facilities and administration, teaching process, scientific research, social and corporate environment.

All committees adopted rules concerning objections regarding the procedures, for instance UKA nominates an appeals team and the accredited university has the right to appeal to the Rectors' Conference.

The documentation, the process and the conclusions of the accreditation procedures are generally confidential. The decision about awarding the accreditation to an area of study is made public usually on the websites and by publishing annual reports that show that the accreditation procedures were completed successfully.

So far, there has been no formal link between the committees' accreditation and approval of other decision-making processes (for instance by PKA or the Ministry).

By January 2003, UKA had conducted some 250 accreditation proceedings covering approximately 30 fields of education in 17 universities and over ten other types of higher education institutions. In the five years of KAUM's activity, all medical faculties of all Medical Universities have undergone the accreditation process. Until the end of 2002, 19 programmes obtained SEM F's accreditation and a few re-accreditations were completed. In 2001/02, KAUT elaborated the procedure and the general standards of accreditation and started accreditation procedures for 26 fields of study. In January 2003 the first – over ten – accreditation proceedings were expected to have been completed. In 2001/02, FPAKE elaborated its accreditation procedures and standards. By January 2003, 16 accreditation proceedings in five fields of study were in progress. None had been completed when the present report was written.

17.2.2   Approval Scheme

Approval is not based on accreditation. In Poland it refers only to newly created universities, fields of study, subsidiaries and external faculties of already existing universities. Periodical approval (i.e. prolonging the permission for the existing universities) is based on the accreditation procedure of the State Accreditation Committee.

In order to understand better the basic forms of approval in Poland, one must say a few words about the recent history of higher education in Poland. According to the Act on Higher Education of 1990, public universities were established in virtue of a law by Parliament. The statute of the university was issued by the Minister, together with the opinion of the Central Council of Higher Education (which also issued an opinion about the application for creating the university). The Minister also appointed the first rector. According to the same Act, non-public universities were established in virtue of an authorisation issued by the Minister of National Education (together with the opinion of the Central Council of Higher Education. New fields of study were created through a similar procedure).

The Act on Higher Vocational Education was adopted in 1997. It regulated the control of quality of education in the entire vocational sector of higher education (public and non-public). Since then, all vocational schools (leading to the *licencjat* or the *inżynier* degree) operate under the authorisation of the Minister of National Education, after receiving the opinion of the newly created KAWSZ, the Accreditation Committee for Higher Vocational Education (Witkowski, 2001). The Central Council kept its competences with regard to academic institutions (non-vocational higher education). The legal task of the Accreditation Committee for Vocational Education was to issue opinions about creating new institutions and fields of study and conducting periodical accreditation in vocational institutions of all types. Decisions were made by the Minister of National Education. The Committee existed until the end of 2001.

The Amendment of the Act on Higher Education of July 2001 created the State Accreditation Committee (PKA), described above. It took over the role of issuing opinions about creating new universities, subsidiaries and fields of study from the Central Council and from KAWSZ and passing them on to the Minister. This procedure refers to launching fields of study which are already on the list accepted by the Ministry. But applications for creating new types of study programmes (as yet unlisted) and their education standards are subject to the Central Council of Higher Education's opinion.

The Minister, following the Act regulations and the opinions of the Central Council for Higher Education, sets the fundamental standards, which are later used by PKA to evaluate the field of studies:

- the conditions which should be fulfilled by the university that wants to launch and maintain a field of studies at a certain level (in particular the number of academic teachers holding a scientific or academic degree, included in the staff's minimum requirements; the type of employment and the ratio of employees to the number of students),
- the names of the fields of study,
- the standards of teaching within each field of study and at each level of education; concerning the graduates' profile, overall content of studies of certain subjects, both within the group of general, basic subjects and those connected with each field,
- the teachers' education standards, considering the graduate's profile, the teachers' education subjects, internships, curriculum content and required skills,
- the detailed conditions for establishing a subsidiary or an exterior faculty of the university; taking into consideration the obligation to comply with the field of studies' training requirements (as far as its creation and running at a certain level is concerned).

The university must immediately advise the minister about the loss of capacity to conduct higher studies (including changes in staff employment that influence the permission to conduct higher learning). If the university does not comply with these regulations within six months, the minister decides whether to suspend the university's rights to conduct higher learning in the given field at this level.

If the assessment by the State Accreditation Committee is negative, the minister withdraws or suspends the authorisation to conduct higher education in the field of study at that level of education, depending on the type and range of the stated violations.

17.2.3   Evaluation Scheme

There is no separate evaluation scheme of a supra-institutional nature in Poland. Elements of evaluation are included in the accreditation procedures, especially in the 'environmental' accreditation. The self-assessments and *peer reviews* may take the form of a weakness and strength analysis of the institution or programme. It offers recommendations for the improvement of the weaknesses. However, none of the 'environmental' accreditation committees has yet appointed an expert body to carry out evaluations at the request of higher education units without comparing the standards and that have not ended in accreditation.

17.3   System Dynamics

17.3.1   Driving Forces: Quality

The basic reason for creating and developing the accreditation system in Poland was concern about the quality of education, which was threatened by the fact that higher education in Poland had become 'mass education'. The quantitative growth had become necessary (the population with a university degree still remains below 10 %) and is the justified pride and achievement of Polish society. However, the growth was not followed by appropriate funding from the state budget. The grant per student decreased dramatically. But the law authorised charging students for studies in non-public higher schools and for studies (other than full-time) in public universities. These two factors helped to develop fee-based studies (extramural in public universities and in the private sector). Unfortunately, the state organs did not control these studies effectively as far as their quality was concerned. The growth caused additional threats to quality because of:

- insufficient teaching staff: whereas the number of students quadrupled, the number of academic teachers increased only 20 to 25 %;

- teaching staff hold several regular posts simultaneously, which worsens the quality of teaching and research. This is partly due to the low salaries of academic teachers, which are regulated nationally for public universities.

This went hand in hand with insufficient quality control, which consisted exclusively of approval based on the Act on Higher Education and the activities of the Central Council and the Ministry of National Education. This caused anxiety in (part of) the academic environment and led to the following:

- since the mid-1990s, with the continuous demands for a state system of accreditation; there was no excuse for the ten-year delay of the law's amendment (the first post-communist law on higher education was promulgated in 1990);
- creation of the agencies of 'environmental' accreditation;
- focusing on the most significant threats to quality (among the accreditation standards): students' attitude towards the staff, minimal programme requirements, etc.;
- creating accreditation schemes directed to fields of study, as these are the basic higher education units.

17.3.2   Driving Forces: Political and Social Factors

The political factors include the preparation of the Polish higher education system for the forthcoming accession to the European Union, greater competition of universities on the European education market, and stimulating international co-operation and student and staff mobility.

As far as the social problems are concerned, the accreditation scheme leads to:

- Ensuring minimum quality by removing low-quality units. This accompanies the advent of mass higher education and adjusts the higher education market in Poland to these new contexts.
- Publishing PKA's results in the media should draw public attention to the threats to higher education and to the reasons for this, including the need to increase the state's higher education budget.
- Marking the institutions with distinctive quality of education, thus setting competition mechanisms.
- Implementing quality-enhancing mechanisms in universities.
- Changing teaching staff's attitude towards quality education.

It is far too early to say whether these goals have been achieved, as the state accreditation system is only in its infancy. In the case of UKA and SEM F (which have been in operation for a few years) we can confirm their positive influence.

17.3.3   Why Not Evaluate?

As mentioned above, there is no separate scheme of supra-institutional evaluation. This mechanism is included in the 'environmental' accreditation schemes. Their review reports end with advice for accreditation and with a summary of the weaknesses and strengths of the accredited field of study. Why does it happen this way? It is very difficult to answer this question. It could be said that uncontrolled commercialisation, massification and the 'pathologies' threatening the quality mentioned above made the universities more sensitive to quality assurance mechanisms which would provide them with certified quality (i.e. accreditation) and make them more credible. Accreditation was more urgent and socially important than quality improvement per se. Maybe evaluation can be a next step. For example: FPAKE is planning to launch an advising system for quality assurance, but still as an initial step towards accreditation.

17.3.4   Relationships Between Schemes

As mentioned, the approval of existing institutions is based on the accreditation conducted by PKA. It consists in verifying the conformity of universities' activities with the teaching standards for the fields of study. PKA passes the result on to ME-NiS, which makes the decision about continuing them or not. Concerning the approval of the creation of new universities, subsidiaries, fields of study, or authorisation to confer the master's degree, the evaluation is also being carried out by PKA, whereas MENiS makes the decisions. Here there is full co-operation between PKA and MENiS. In case of a negative opinion of PKA, the Minister must take the steps defined in the Act, e.g. suspend the field of study.

The relations between approval and accreditation are exiguous. In some cases the 'environmental' accreditation standards for a field of study and the teaching standards elaborated by the Central Council are similar and were worked out by the same team of experts (e.g. for the field of psychology, accredited by UKA).

We have two typical accreditation models in Poland. One is 'top-down', constituted by law and involving state authorities (PKA). The other is 'bottom-up', constituted by the academic community (the committees of the KA KRASP and SEM F). Their reciprocal relations and emerging co-operation together form a constantly evolving system of external quality assurance. What is rather unusual is that the academic movement appeared first, followed by that of the state. The interdependence of PKA and the 'environmental' institutions is a fundamental problem. The discussion over a model of their co-operation had preceded the Act amendment and the creation of PKA and has been continued since. However, no decisions were reached.

The institutions that are members of KA KRASP suggested the following arrangements. As the accreditation conducted by committees within KRASP is voluntary and is closely linked to the required quality of education, and as PKA's task, in accordance with the Act, consists in verifying whether the university fulfils the minimum requirements advising on applications for approval, it seems clear that both schemes complement each other. The question then is whether, as the 'environmental' committees proposed, a field of study that has already obtained 'environmental' accreditation should be awarded PKA accreditation easily (after a lighter procedure)? PKA has not reacted positively on this so far. The 'environmental' committees are afraid that the creation of PKA, with its compulsory accreditation at a basic level and its possibility to grant a 'distinguished' grade, will decrease the demand of the academic community for the voluntary 'environmental' accreditation. This could imply that their activities will be wasted. However, they wish to convince PKA to take advantage of the 'environmental' committees' attainments, since PKA's projects are vast and its budget is limited. PKA acts under very strong pressure. Its resistance to the offered co-operation is justified: taking advantage of the 'environmental' accreditations must be confirmed by total credibility of their evaluations. That is why there is a need for a 'cap' institution (like KA KRASP), which enables the rectors' conferences to confirm the integrity of the 'environmental' accreditation.

The second important type of relation is co-operation between the 'environmental' institutions. These institutions are formed 'bottom-up'. They have institutional independence and substantial autonomy. They have in common:

- self-regulative accrediting institutions;
- voluntary, paid, periodical accreditations;
- self-regulative standards (always for the 'fields of study');
- almost identical procedures of accreditation: application submitting, appointing the peer review team, self-evaluation, peer review team visit, the report, the decision about the accreditation issued by the Accreditation Committee.

What separates them, apart from some organisational differences, is the nature and level of accreditation criteria requirements. Yet these institutions are willing to co-operate and clearly strive for a 'common currency' for their accreditations and, maybe later, mutual acceptance of their accreditations or common accreditations for related fields of study offered by universities of different types. So far, their co-operation has taken the following forms:

- common sessions of the chairmen of the 'environmental' committees in KA KRASP to exchange information and sound out possibilities of co-operation;
- joint conferences, training, seminars, publications;
- mutual consultations on standards and accreditation criteria;

- forming mixed peer review teams (i.e. with members from universities of different types), e.g. FPAKE and UKA in the case of programmes in economics;
- joint accreditation for some fields of study: e.g. UKA and KAUT accredited together chemistry and some other fields of study;
- participation of representatives of various university types in the activities of accreditation committees: thus, the FPAKE committee consists of representatives of universities, technical universities and agricultural universities, which all offer economics.

There is now a variety of accreditation leading to a 'common currency'. For example: fields concerning management may obtain (apart from PKA's accreditation) SEM F, FPAKE and UKA accreditation. Each is of a slightly different nature. It is being discussed whether we should strive for unification of standards and criteria or keep the variety, which allows the universities to have several separate evaluations. So far, variety has more supporters. However, KA KRASP represents committees that are under its auspices, e.g. in the negotiations with PKA and in international forums, so the committees must give importance to the high and comparable standard of their accreditations.

In sum, we should remember that the external system of quality evaluation which was created and developed in 2002 is still in its infancy and will certainly evolve and change. It is difficult to predict the directions of its evolution. Discussions are in progress; and there is a will to maintain the variety of evaluations.

17.3.5 Consequences of Accreditation

The consequences of the creation of the accreditation scheme are different. The PKA controls the basic quality level, enforcing minimal requirements. There were cases where universities, having been informed about PKA accreditation procedures for one of their fields of study, replied that they had just stopped the recruitment or closed the field, which, in practice, means that they did not fulfil the minimal requirements and that the forthcoming PKA evaluation would end these fields of study. Hence, a positive influence of the common and compulsory PKA accreditation can be seen: the universities expecting PKA accreditation verify their own functioning.

The main consequences of 'environmental' accreditation include:

- Growing awareness concerning quality. Within the few years of their operation, it became obvious that quality assurance systems are necessary in higher education institutions; opposition and scepticism to accreditation, which previously existed in the academic environment, have almost vanished.

- Creating a large group of persons who are competent in matters of quality assurance mechanisms and engaged in their implementation. It is difficult to estimate the exact figure, but considering the number of peer review teams and expert group members, those who are in charge of self-evaluations at universities; and people who participate in programmes such as TEMPUS and the others devoted to the quality of higher education, it would represent a few thousand (mainly connected with UKA)
- Spreading practices linked to accreditation standards; e.g. ECTS, transparency of the teaching processes, student surveys, etc.
- Establishing offices or rectors' plenipotentiaries responsible for quality assurance in many universities.
- Ensuring fair competition on the market between higher education institutions, making clear which of them are better than others.

For students, at present, the most important changes are the following:

- better information about the quality of studies, and hence a better possibility of choosing their institution;
- greater influence of students on the teaching processes (through feedback e.g. in surveys, greater transparency of the teaching procedures, and larger choice of courses);
- greater mobility through the ECTS system.

As the accreditation enhances quality of education, and is expected to continue to do so in future, we can expect:

- better educated graduates, who will make up the social and professional elites;
- better use of public funds for higher education;
- information for parents and students about where it is best to study, which means better use of private funds for education;
- better recognition of graduates by employers;
- introducing this sector of Polish public life into the European higher education area – which brings us to the topic of the next section.

17.4   Drivers from Abroad

All accrediting institutions quote in their documentation that their fundamental targets are their will to introduce Polish higher education into the European education area and to create procedures and standards in accordance with those of European Union accreditation schemes (e.g. the ECTS system). The oldest 'environmental' committees (SEM F, UKA) took advantage of assistance funds (TEMPUS, PHARE, and others). These funds enabled them to co-operate with Western accreditation institutions and experts to draft their own procedures (study visits, seminars and training, in Poland and abroad). The committees that were established later (KAUT, FPAKE) often based their approaches on the example of the older Polish accreditation committees. All were greatly influenced in their standards and approaches by this exposure to European and – especially in the case of KAUM – American accreditation.

The appointment of the State Accreditation Committee fulfils the postulate requiring each education system in Europe to possess a central accreditation and approval system, which would cover all higher education institutions in the country (*Furthering the Bologna Process*, 2001; *From Prague to Berlin*, 2002; Kraśniewski, & Macukow, 2002).

Some of the accrediting institutions are members of European and international accreditation organisations and/or their networks, or they intend to apply for membership after they have developed their activity. Thus, PKA and UKA are members of the Network of Central and Eastern European Quality Assurance Agencies in Higher Education (http://www.ceenetwork.hu/index.html), and SEM F is a member of EQUIS; and is also deeply involved in CEEMAN's activities.

The basic difference and source of the most significant problems faced by Polish accreditation institutions that are willing to adopt the European pattern of accreditation is the *'field of study'*. The entire higher education system in Poland is based on 'fields of study'. 'Fields of study' are neither pure programmes nor institutions, although they must be conducted by university faculties. The list of recognised fields of study is given by MENiS. The basic or minimal curriculum requirements for each field of study are also centrally set. The recruitment of students is conducted collectively within a given 'field of study'. This system was reinforced by the State Accreditation Committee, which created its accreditation model according to fields of study. The universities applying for accreditation are therefore interested in the accreditation for a field of study. That is why 'environmental' accreditation committees also adopted a field-of-study structure of assessment. But the Polish higher education system also requires accreditation of institutions, because the most important threats to education quality are not the programme content but the functioning of universities. This is why the accreditation standards combine institutional assessment requirements and curriculum requirements, which are very often separated (SEM F, KAUM) into two individual issues (which does not conform with the patterns that are common in Europe).

The second problem and reproach reported by Western reviewers concerning 'environmental' accreditations is that they are established by the rectors' conferences, i.e. by the authorities of universities, and not by the 'scientific community itself' (Westerheijden, 2001; Wójcicka, 2001a). However, rectors are elected by the communities of their universities, and the Accreditation Committees' projects, such as the expert teams' elaborations of standards and, above all, the assessment teams' tasks are carried out by representatives of the academic community (which do not represent the decision-making structures in the university).

It is also reproached that *all* accreditation systems in Poland focus on the 'input' of the education process and not on the graduates' competences and added value achieved within the education process, i.e. output. (By the way, an 'output' accreditation model would minimise the discrepancies between the accreditation for the field of study and that of the institution, mentioned above). There is a question then whether the Polish accreditation scheme is capable of adopting the above quality assessment model and whether it could be applied if the main problems of the quality of education were strictly related to the university's 'input'. Such solutions are the outcome of a long-lasting evolution and preparation of the academic environment of the EU countries and the much higher funds that they have available, e.g. to follow their graduates' careers. Nothing similar has existed in Poland as yet.

17.5 Other Forms of Assessment

We could mention the following elements of assessment, covering all universities:

- An obligatory assessment of academic teachers' achievements in public universities. Article 104 of the Act on Higher Education states that all academic teachers should be subject to evaluation at least every four years, at the request of their superiors, or before the termination of their appointment. The rules of this assessment are set by the university, but it was regulated nationally that the university can dismiss an employee who had negative grades twice. If the employee does not obtain the doctor's degree within eight years of employment, or the *doctor habilitatus* degree within nine years after obtaining the doctorate (unless the statute of the university states otherwise), this also leads to dismissal (the so-called employee 'rotation').
- An assessment of the State Committee for Scientific Research (KBN) of all units (in universities as well as in research institutions) leading to the award of one of four categories with regard to their research standing.
- An assessment of the Central Commission for Scientific Title and Degrees of how an individual obtained the *doctor habilitatus* degree or the title of professor. The assessment focuses on the candidates' achievements to obtain the degree or the title; and indirectly evaluates the activities of the scientific councils (faculty councils) that apply for awarding the degree or title.

The relations between accreditation proceedings and the assessments above are not very explicit. However, the evaluation criteria of certain 'environmental' institutions (e.g. FPAKE) include questions about systematic staff review and the ways of using of outcomes, similarly for the number of *habilitation* professor procedures. In addition, the KBN research category is taken into consideration in the assessment standards of an academic institution, which considers a high KBN category as a confirmation of a high level of scientific research.

References

AAHEd (2001). Amendment of the Act on Higher Education of July 2001.

AHEd (1990). Act on Higher Education of 1990.

AHVE (1997). Act on Higher Vocational Education of 1997.

ASCSR (1991). Act on the State Committee for Scientific Research of 1991.

ASTD (1990). Act on Scientific Title and Degrees of 1990.

Akademicka Komisja Akredytacyjna (1997). Instytut Problemów Współczesnej Cywilizacji, Warszawa

Bielski, M. (2002). Komisja Akredytacyjna Stowarzyszenia Edukacji Menedżerskiej Forum. In Chmielecka, E. (ed.), Akredytacja–krajobraz polski. Łódź, FEP, p. 21-25.

Borecki, T. (2002). Komisja Akredytacyjna Uczelni Rolniczych. In Chmielecka, E. (ed.), Akredytacja–krajobraz polski. Łódź, FEP, p. 31-35.

Central Office of Statistics (2002). Higher Schools and their Financing in Academic Year of 2000/2001. Warsaw, Central Office of Statistics.

Chmielecka, E. (2000). Changes in Higher Education. In Kolarska-Bobińska, L. (ed.) The Second Wave of Polish Reforms. Warsaw, Institute of Public Affairs, p. 61-80.

Chmielecka, E. (2001). Komisja Akredytacyjna FPAKE, In Wójcicka, M. (ed.) Jakość kształcenia w szkolnictwie wyższym. Słownik tematyczny Warszawa. p. 54-55.

Chwirot, S. (1998). I AKA, i UKA, Forum Akademickie nr. 3/98, p. 22-23.

Chwirot, S. (2002). Uniwersytecka Komisja Akredytacyjna. In Chmielecka, E. (ed.), Akredytacja–krajobraz polski. Łódź, FEP, p. 13-17.

Chwirot, S. (2001). Uniwersytecka Komisja Akredytacyjna. In Wójcicka, M. (ed.) Jakość kształcenia w szkolnictwie wyższym. Słownik tematyczny Warszawa. p. 122-125.

FPAKE (2002). Informator FPAKE.

From Prague to Berlin. The EU Contribution - progress report (2002).

Furthering the Bologna Process. Report to the Ministers of Education (2001). Prague.

Gembicki, M. (2002). Komisja Akredytacyjna Uczelni Medycznych. In Chmielecka, E. (ed.), Akredytacja–krajobraz polski. Łódź, FEP.

KAUT (2002). Informator KAUT na rok akademicki 2001/2002.

Kawecki, J. (1996). System oceny jakości kształcenia w szkołach wyższych. Warszawa, Rada Główna Szkolnictwa Wyższego.

Konczakowska, A. (2002). Komisja Akredytacyjna Uczelni Technicznych In Chmielecka, E. (ed.), Akredytacja–krajobraz polski. Łódź, FEP.

Kraśniewski, A., & Macukow, B. (2002). 'Deklaracja bolońska i co dalej?', Miesięcznik Politechniki Warszawskiej, nr. 6.

Kraśniewski, A. (2001). Komisja Akredytacyjna Konferencji Rektorów Akademickich Szkół Polskich. In Wójcicka, M. (ed.) Jakość kształcenia w szkolnictwie wyższym. Słownik tematyczny Warszawa. p. 55-57.

KRASP (1998). Model Publicznej Szkoły Wyższej i jej otoczenia systemowego. Zasadnicze kierunki nowelizacji prawa o szkolnictwie wyższym (ed. J. Woźnicki), Warszawa: KRASP.

Król, J. (2002). Komisja Akredytacyjna Uczelni Pedagogicznych. In Chmielecka, E. (ed.), Akredytacja–krajobraz polski. Łódź, FEP, p. 29-31.

Kwiatkowski, S. (2001). Komisja Akredytacyjna Stowarzyszenia Edukacji Menedżerskiej Forum. In Wójcicka, M. (ed.) Jakość kształcenia w szkolnictwie wyższym. Słownik tematyczny Warszawa. p. 58-61.

Mirecka, J., & Gembicki, M. (2001). Komisja Akredytacyjna Uczelni Medycznych. In Wójcicka, M. (ed.) *Jakość kształcenia w szkolnictwie wyższym. Słownik tematyczny* Warszawa. p. 61-65.

SEM F (2002). System akredytacji programów kształcenia menedżerskiego SEM F. Warszawa, SEM F.

Socha, S. (2001). Komisja Akredytacyjna Akademii Wychowania Fizycznego. In Wójcicka, M. (ed.) *Jakość kształcenia w szkolnictwie wyższym. Słownik tematyczny.* Warszawa. p. 51-52.

Socha, S. (2002). Komisja Akredytacyjna Akademii Wychowani Fizycznego. In Chmielecka, E. (ed.), *Akredytacja–krajobraz polski.* Łódź, FEP, p. 35-39.

Strahl, D. (2002). Komisja Akredytacyjna FPAKE. In Chmielecka E. (ed.), *Akredytacja–krajobraz polski.* Łódź, FEP, p. 39-43.

UKA (2002). *Jak zdobyć znak jakości? - Informator UKA na rok 2002.*

Westerheijden, D. (2001). Opinion on the project of accreditation standards of FPAKE. Unpublished working paper for FPAKE.

Witkowski, M. (2001). Komisja Akredytacyjna Wyższego Szkolnictwa Zawodowego. In Wójcicka, M. (ed.) *Jakość kształcenia w szkolnictwie wyższym. Słownik tematyczny.* Warszawa. p. 65-68.

Wnuk-Lipińska, E., & Wójcicka, M. (eds.) (1995). *Jakość w szkolnictwie wyższym,* Warszawa, Uniwersytet Warszawski.

Wójcicka, M., & Chmielecka, E. (2001). The Polish System of Quality Assurance: Results of Top-Down and Bottom-Up Initiatives (research findings). In *Quality Assurance in Higher Education: quality, standards, recognition*proceedings of the 6th Biennial Conference of International Network for Quality Assurance Agencies in Higher Education, Bangalore, India 19-22 March 2001, p. 181-184.

Wójcicka, M. (2001a). Recenzja dotycząca projektu 'Procedur i standardów akredytacji FPAKE'. Unpublished working paper for FPAKE.

Wójcicka, M. (2001). Kłopotliwe rozdwojenie. *Forum Akademickie,* nr. 6, p. 34-38.

Wójcicka, M. (2002). Krajowy system jakości - rocznik 2002. In Chmielecka, E. (ed.), *Akredytacja–krajobraz polski.* Łódź, FEP, p. 9-13.

Woźnicki, J. (2001). Komisja Akredytacyjna KRASP. *Perspektywy,* nr. 6, p. 25.

http://forumakad.pl/archiwum/2001/02/artykuły/05-z_prac_krasp. htm
http://main.amu.edu.pl/ects/uka/uka.html
http://www.buwiwm.edu.pl
http://www.ceeman.org/about/index.html
http://www.ceenetwork.hu/index.html
http://www.fundacja.edu.pl
http://www.kaut@uci.agh.edu.pl
http://www.mpips.gov.pl
http://www.semforum.com.pl
http://www.stat.gov.pl

18 Portugal: Professional and Academic Accreditation – The Impossible Marriage?

ALBERTO AMARAL & MARIA JOÃO ROSA

18.1 The Higher Education System[1]

18.1.1 Main Components

The Portuguese higher education system is binary. It includes both private and public universities and polytechnics. In the public sector there are 13 universities, one Open University *(Universidade Aberta)* and an independent institute, ISCTE (*Instituto Superior de Ciências do Trabalho*); there are also 16 polytechnics – the University of the Algarve and the University of Aveiro include some polytechnic schools – and 32 non-integrated schools. This subsystem also includes a network of nursing institutes, three institutes for training technicians for health services (Lisbon, Porto and Coimbra), a school of hostelry and tourism, and a school of art restoration. Some public higher education is dependent on the Armed Forces and Police Forces (Military Academy, Air Force Academy, Naval School and the Higher School of Police).

In the private sector, there are nine universities and 72 polytechnics (including non-integrated polytechnic schools).[2] There is also a Catholic University which was established under a concordat between the Portuguese State and the Holy See.

In sum, polytechnics are vocationally-orientated and do not carry out fundamental research. Only applied research was conceived for the sector. On the other hand, the mission of the institutions in the university sector includes both fundamental and applied research.

18.1.2 Degrees Awarded

The main degrees awarded by the different types of higher education institutions are summarised in Table 1.

---

1   We are grateful to all who contributed to this report with their comments, information and advice. We are especially indebted to Professor Fernando Ramos, Professor Machado dos Santos and our colleagues from *Cipes*. We are also grateful to Dr. Stefanie Schwarz for her very pertinent comments.

2   Some institutions have more than one regional campus. If they are counted separately, the number of universities increases to 14 and the number of other institutions to 98.

S. Schwarz and D.F. Westerheijden (eds.),
Accreditation and Evaluation in the European Higher Education Area, 395–419.

Table 1. Degrees awarded by types of higher education institutions

Degree	Institution/Sector	Length
Bacharelato	Polytechnics	3 years
Licenciatura	Universities/Polytechnics	4/6 years
Mestrado	Universities	+ 2
Doutoramento	Universities	+ 3 (+)

18.1.3   Size of the Different Components

The number of students per type and sector is given in Table 2 for the academic year 2001/02. The public sector served over 70 % of all students. Most students (54 %) attend universities, either public or private.

Table 2. Student numbers by type and ownership

Public			Private		
Universities	Polytechnics	Army/Police	Universities	Polytechnics	Catholic U.
171,014	108,136	1,456	41,331	60,186	10,136

18.1.4   Transition to the Labour Market

The Portuguese higher education system expanded rapidly in the 1980s and early 1990s, with a major contribution from the private sector. Expansion of higher education and diversification, as well as the increase in student enrolment in fields that were of economic importance have been explicit government policy goals for more than a decade. However, these policy goals have not been fully attained, both because of the mushrooming of the private sector in a direction that goes against the aims of the diversification policy (geographical distortions and insufficient supply of technical degrees) and because of the academic drift of the polytechnics.

The new private institutions were not sound academic and financial projects, but rather short-term, profit-making attempts. This is confirmed by the type of courses provided, by the extremely rapid expansion of these institutions, by the lack of research activities, by reliance on the moonlighting of the teaching staff of public institutions, and by the lack of enthusiasm for quality assessment issues. If this provided good business for some, it compromised the future credibility of an important part of the system.

The uncontrolled expansion of the private sector, the public polytechnics' academic drift and excessive pedagogical autonomy of public universities led to a great mismatch between the outputs of higher education and the needs of the labour market. This increased graduate unemployment rates and paved the way for professional accreditation. More recently, due to a combined effect of a drop in the total number of candidates and an increase of new places in the public sector, many places in higher education are now left without candidates, especially in private institutions. Hence, private institutions are entering a difficult fight for economic survival. At the same time, candidates are more aware of the labour market situation and avoid study programmes with negative employment prospects. This will affect the offer of study programmes. This was already visible in the enrolments of new students for the academic year 2002/03, as some of the less popular study programmes were confronted with a drop in the number of candidates – in some cases, there were none!

18.1.5 Steering of the System

In Portugal, the most visible actors involved in higher education are the government (represented by the Ministry of Science and Higher Education[3]), the CRUP (Portuguese Council of Rectors), the CCISP (the co-ordinating structure of public polytechnics) and the CNE (National Council for Education). The private sector also has a strong influence, but it prefers to use a well-established network of political and economic interests, rather than visible institutional structures.

The most important actor is the Ministry of Science and Higher Education. In Parliament, all political parties emphasise the strategic role of education in the context of Portuguese economic, social and political development, but, in general, political activity is reduced to generic political statements, while high technical quality is conspicuously absent from political debates. According to the Portuguese sociologist Boaventura de Sousa Santos this is the result of what he calls the 'parallel state'.[4] The General Directorate of Higher Education of the Ministry is responsible for all administrative processes related to higher education, but, regarding public universities, its role was greatly reduced by the 1988 University Autonomy Act.

---

3   Before the present government, there was a Ministry of Education (all levels of education, including higher education) and a Ministry of Science and Technology (responsible for research). Now, higher education is merged with research in a new ministry for Science and Higher Education.

4   The new Constitution approved in 1976, after the 1974 revolution, was very left-wing. But none of the governments elected after the Constitution was approved could be considered as Marxist or extreme left. This led to a gap between the objectives and intentions of legislation and the social and political tissue that they intend to regulate. Over the years, many laws have fallen into oblivion. The Constitution was progressively amended to eliminate the more obvious ornaments of a socialist ideology. This is what Santos calls the 'parallel state'.

The Council of Rectors of Portuguese Universities (CRUP) and the Polytechnic's Co-ordinator Council (CCISP) are two of the main actors in the national higher education policy, but social and cultural traditions have so far maintained CCISP as a weaker political stakeholder than its university partner.

According to the University Autonomy Act (article 4), CRUP's mission is 'to co-operate with the State in the making of national policies for education, science, and culture'. Co-operation, at this formal level, is expressed in compulsory advising functions on all legislative projects concerning higher education. However CRUP's political weight has been more important than this formal role could suggest. This was probably due to the fact that the rectors of most Portuguese universities were elected for more than one term, and were thus able to create strong personal ties that enabled them to define a common set of academic values which were expressed in clear strategic choices in the relationships with other political actors.

CRUP was created by Decree Law 107/79 of the 2nd of May 1979, but it became active with the discussion and implementation of the Law of Autonomy and its structure was modified by the Decree Law 283/93 of the 18th of August 1993. The conduct of CRUP has been in harmony with the characteristics of Portuguese society, namely a low public profile, avoidance of unnecessary conflicts, and a strong negotiating capacity. In general, CRUP does not publicly criticise the government's actions, avoids political partisan influence and prefers to negotiate with the help of sound technical documents produced by its members and approved by the Council.

However, CRUP has taken a very critical stance regarding the uncontrolled expansion of private higher education and the government's role in facilitating the accumulation of teaching activities in both public and private institutions, as it became immediately apparent that the development of the private sector would also downgrade some areas of the public sector. One of the reasons why CRUP decided to lead the implementation of the quality assessment system was the public universities' opinion that the evaluation system guaranteed their quality vis-à-vis the private sector and had a moral effect on the behaviour of the academic staff. CRUP also produced policy papers about the higher education system, which addressed amongst others the problems of diversity and the relationship of universities with polytechnics[5] and stressed the importance of life-long learning. Public discussions of these policy papers were organised to shape the future changes of the system.

Another important actor is the students' unions. Following the 1974 revolution, students participated at all levels of institutional governance. For a long time after the revolution, because many of their leaders were more concerned with political

---

5   CRUP favours the diversity of the higher education system, with additional short cycle vocational diplomas that could help to solve the problem of dropouts, but is critical of the polytechnic's academic drift.

party warfare than with academic policies, students' unions were not very visible in the definition of higher education policies. However, a governmental decision to increase the level of tuition fees (previously kept frozen for decades) acted as a catalyst of student discontent, thus propelling students' organisations into a much more active role in the definition of political regulation instruments such as fees, grants, students' social welfare or *numerus clausus*.

The most absent actors are employers' organisations. Paradoxically, whilst governments initiated a new discourse which gave the market a more important role in the regulation of higher education and emphasised the importance of higher education as a factor for the development of economic activities, Portuguese employers and their organisations were far from assuming the statute of effective political actors, thus confirming what Santos calls the heterogeneity[6] of the Portuguese state.

18.2   Accreditation Mechanisms

18.2.1   Control by the State

At present, there is no national accreditation system that is run or controlled by the state (see section 18.3.5 for some very recent changes). At the level of study programmes, state control is exercised through their bureaucratic approval, but the situation is different for the various segments of the higher education system.

For instance, Article 7 of the University Autonomy Act (Law 108/88 of 24 September 1988) grants public universities full pedagogic autonomy – meaning that they have almost complete freedom to start, suspend or cancel study programmes – and they have used this extensively. At present, there is even a feeling that they have too much pedagogical autonomy. This makes effective co-ordination of the sector almost impossible. It is true that the Ministry must register new degrees,[7] but it cannot refuse registration unless the degrees are illegal (e.g., because of the length of the programme or the total number of credits needed to obtain the degree). If that is not the case, then the Ministry's only option to dissuade the institution from launching

---

6   After the 1974 revolution, Portugal emerged from decades of isolation. In a few years, 'the Portuguese corporative state went through a transition to socialism, a fordist regulation and a Welfare State regulation, and even a neo-liberal regulation. The structure of the state presents, in each moment, a geological composition with several layers, sedimented in different forms, some old, some recent, each one with its own internal logic and its own strategical orientation. This is the meaning of the heterogeneous state.'

7   The General Directorate for Higher Education of the Ministry of Science and Higher Education is responsible for the registration of all teaching programmes of public universities and for the preparation of all the requests for the establishment, modification or closure of courses of public polytechnics. It is also responsible, for the preparation of the legal procedures of the requests for recognition and authorisation of the courses of public polytechnics and private higher education institutions.

the new study programme is to determine that the students who are enrolled in that programme will not be counted for funding purposes. But this has never occurred.[8]

In contrast, public polytechnics are not allowed to create, suspend or cancel study programmes: they have to submit all proposals to the Ministry for approval. It is also important to remember that, in principle, private institutions are also subject to strong control by the Ministry: They must ask for permission before starting or modifying any study programme and must apply for state recognition of all their degrees and diplomas for them to command the same status and recognition for academic and professional purposes as those conferred by public institutions.

At the level of the institutions, the Ministry has full power of approval. The establishment of a new public institution is an act of the government that in general takes the form of a Decree-Law approved by the cabinet. The establishment of a new organic unit in an already existing public institution (e.g., a new school or faculty in an existing university) starts with the approval of a proposal by the Senate, but this proposal must also be approved by the Ministry. As for private institutions, they cannot start operating without previous approval by the Ministry.

The Special Case of Medicine and Dental Medicine

The government decided (Council of Ministers deliberation of November 1998) to implement a special programme for health sciences. One of the main reasons for this was the present lack of physicians as a result of the *numerus clausus* in the schools of Medicine during the 1980s – a World Bank recommendation. Concerning Medicine and Dentistry, the proposals for the establishment of new schools or study programmes are evaluated by International Review Teams that produce recommendations that follow the traditional quality assessment methodology: the institution that presents the proposal produces a self- evaluation report and the review team visits the institution and produces an evaluation report.

There are also plans to create an accreditation system for hospitals' clinics and health centres where physicians can be trained.

The Special Case of Teacher Training

Decree-Law 290/98 of 17 September established the National Institute for Accreditation of Teacher Training (INAFOP) which was under the orders of the Ministry of Education. INAFOP was responsible for accreditation and professional certification of teachers for nurseries and schools of basic and secondary education. This was the

---

8   The Ministry's funding formula is proportional to the students' enrolment. The only exception was the creation of a new study programme in Law by the Universidade do Minho. But after two years, this decision was reversed.

only case where the Portuguese state established an accreditation agency supported by the Ministry of Education. However, the new government that came into power in 2002 decided to close down the accreditation agency because of its interference with the pedagogic and scientific autonomy of higher education institutions.

18.2.2   The National System for Quality Assessment

Both because of the imposition of the Law of Autonomy and because of quality problems raised by the very rapid development of the private sector of higher education, there was a national consensus around the need to set up a national quality assessment system. Public universities regarded the quality assessment system as a guarantee of their quality vis-à-vis the private sector, as well as a means to moralise the behaviour of some academic staff.

A commission of the Portuguese Council of Rectors (CRUP) therefore decided to lead the implementation of the quality assessment system. In October 1992, a seminar on evaluation was organised at the University of Porto; under the presidency of the Minister of Education with the participation of experts from France, the Netherlands and the United Kingdom. The different evaluation systems already implemented in Europe were examined. Following this debate, the Council of Rectors decided to choose the Dutch system as a model because of its emphasis on quality improvement, the recognition that higher education institutions should be responsible for the quality assessment system and its compatibility with the University Autonomy Act.

To implement the system CRUP decided to launch an experimental phase by using the Dutch system in five disciplines: Physics, Computer Sciences, Electrical Engineering, Economy and French. This experiment was designed with technical assistance of the Dutch VSNU and the University of Twente. With their help, several seminars were organised for the rectors and the Faculty deans, the representatives of the institutions to be evaluated, the members of the visiting committees, etc. A Portuguese version of the Dutch *Guide for external program review* was prepared with the necessary adaptations. Later, CRUP created the Foundation of the Portuguese Universities, a private institution which was independent from the universities and resembled VSNU. It became responsible for the quality assessment system for public universities.

These initiatives were taken in agreement with the Ministry of Education and with its collaboration and support. At the same time, a draft version of the Law of Quality Assessment was prepared in consultation with the Ministry and CRUP. Because of the complexity of the Portuguese higher education system (universities and polytechnics, both public and private), it was decided that the law proposal which would be submitted to Parliament should only define the general characteristics of the quality assessment system, leaving the definition of its details to specific protocols to be negotiated between the Ministry of Education and each of the higher education subsectors. The final version of the law was passed by Parliament in 1994 as Law 38/94 of 21 November. It defines the items to be evaluated in Article 3:

a.   The teaching, in particular the curricular structure, the scientific level, the pedagogical processes and their innovative characteristics;
b.   The qualification of the teaching staff;
c.   The research carried out;
d.   The links with the community, in particular through service rendering and cultural activities;
e.   The facilities and the pedagogical and scientific equipment;
f.   The international co-operation projects;
g.   The students' demand, school achievement and the mechanisms of social support;
h.   The interdisciplinary, inter-service and inter-institutional collaboration;
i.   The insertion of the graduates into the labour market;
j.   The efficiency of organisation and management.

This assessment has the following objectives, according to Article 4 of the Law:

a.   To promote the quality of the activities;
b.   To inform the educational and Portuguese communities in general;
c.   To ensure more accurate knowledge and a more transparent dialogue between higher education institutions;
d.   To contribute to the regulation of the higher institutions network.

A close observation shows that the Portuguese law retains most characteristics of the Dutch methodology. The main objective of the quality assessment system is to improve the activities of the institutions; the results of evaluation will also be used for accountability purposes. The institutions of higher education will have main responsibility for the quality assessment system.

The most important document of the quality assessment activities is the self-study report that is submitted to the external visiting committee. The system is national (all institutions are involved), periodic (once a complete round of evaluations is completed, a new one is launched) and comprehensive (all the disciplines and study programmes will be examined). The students will participate in the quality assessment activities and the external visiting committees will take their opinions into account. The final evaluation reports will be made public and will contain the responses from the evaluated institutions.

There will be no direct relation between the results of evaluation and the level of funding of the institutions; the funding formula of higher education institutions does not depend on the results of quality assessment.

The results of the evaluation will have implications for the institutions. In the case of successive negative evaluations or when, upon a negative evaluation, the institution fails to implement the recommendations of the visiting committee, the Minister of Education can take one or more of the following actions:

a. To decrease or to suspend the funding given – public institutions.
b. To suspend the registration of the degrees conferred – public universities.
c. To suspend the degrees offered – public polytechnics.
d. To withdraw the permission to confer degrees – private institutions.
e. To suspend the accreditation of the degrees offered – private institutions.
f. To suspend the degrees conferred – private institutions.

The evaluation will be by discipline and will be implemented in successive phases, starting with quality assessment of education. Later, the system will be extended to research activities and to extension services offered to the outside community.

The Inspectorate has no direct action in the evaluation activities; its sole role will be to validate the data produced by the institutions for evaluation purposes if there is any doubt about their reliability.

The universities/polytechnics and public/private divide has led to three sub-systems of evaluation (public universities, public polytechnics, private sector), each with its own Evaluation Council. Decree-Law 205/98 of 11 July established the National Evaluation Council for Higher Education to co-ordinate these sub-systems, ensure the 'harmony, cohesion and credibility' of the overall system and carry-out the meta-evaluation of the system, if necessary with support from foreign experts.

Below, under 'international influences', we present a comparison of the Portuguese and the Dutch systems to elucidate further the organisation of the Portuguese national quality assessment system.

18.2.3 The Role of Professional Associations

Professional associations (*Ordens*) are professional public corporations in the traditional liberal professions (lawyers, doctors, engineers and pharmacists), public bodies with an associative basis, or in the English terminology 'statutory membership organisations', working within public law. Following the 1974 revolution the number of these professional associations trebled.

Table 3. Professional associations and labour market access

Profession	Initial year	Labour market access	First year	Accreditation of professional study programmes	First year
Lawyers	1926	Training + Examination		Wants to develop an accreditation system for Law study programmes	
Architects	1998	Examination and/or training	2002	Has an accreditation system (21 accredited study programmes)	2000
Biologists	1998	Degree		Wants to develop a certification system for Biology study programmes	
Economists	1998	Examination + training	1998	Has a system that is not a proper accreditation system and visits to institutions very rarely take place	1999
Nurses	1998	Degree		Wants to introduce examinations and to develop an accreditation system.	
Engineers	1936	Examination + training	1994	Has developed an accreditation system (88 accredited study programmes)	1994
Pharmacists	1972	Examination and/or training	2004	Wants to develop an accreditation system	2003–2004
Doctors	1938	Degree*			
Dentists	1998	Degree		Wants to introduce training periods and to develop an accreditation system	
Veterinary Doctors	1990	Degree		Wants to develop an accreditation system	
Official Copyholders of Accounts	1999	Examination + training	2000		
Solicitors	1944	Degree		The new statute allows for the introduction of examinations and/or training periods and the development of an accreditation system	

Table compiled by Professor Fernando Ramos. * Doctors generally follow training periods (internships) of up to six years.

Professional associations that can limit or condition access to professional exercise (in some relevant cases, professionals can only practise if they are members of the professional association) need to be established by an Act of Parliament or by a governmental Decree-Law duly authorised by Parliament.

Despite these precautions, there is a large number (some even say excessive) of professional associations (*Ordens*): for Pharmacists, Economists, Engineers, Lawyers, Nurses, Doctors, Veterinary Doctors, Dentists, Architects, Biologists, Official Copyholders of Accounts. There are also a Chamber of Solicitors, an Association of Nutritionists and an Association of Technical Engineers.

The requirements to become an effective member of a professional association vary substantially according to the profession (see Table 3). In some cases, holding the appropriate degree is sufficient. In other cases, admission is allowed following a training period and/or an examination. In 1994, the Engineers' Association (*Ordem dos Engenheiros*) established an accreditation system and apparently other professional associations are following suit. As a general rule, when an accreditation system exists, graduates from accredited higher education institutions have direct access to effective membership.

The Engineers' Association

Anyone who intends to work as an Engineer must become a full member of the Engineers' Association. And to become a full member of the association it is necessary but not sufficient to hold a recognised degree in Engineering. The Association must have accredited the study programme or candidates must pass an examination organised by the Association. This confers great power to the Engineers' Association: if the study programmes in Engineering at University A are not accredited, students are not sure to become chartered engineers because they need to pass the Association's examination, while students enrolled at University B where study programmes were given accreditation know that they will automatically become effective members of the association.

The system of accreditation uses a methodology that is quite similar to the national system of quality assessment. Accreditation is periodical and is supported by a self-evaluation report and a visit by a review team. The Association publishes a list of all accredited study programmes but not of those programmes that have been refused accreditation.

The accreditation process is voluntary but accredited study programmes have a competitive advantage. The accreditation is given to study programmes and not to Faculties or Departments, since different programmes offered by the same faculty can have varying levels of quality.

The accreditation process is quite complex, demands a lot of bureaucracy and takes 13 months on average. Any institution demanding accreditation for their study programmes must apply to the Association, and provide copies of the self-evaluation reports for each study programme to be accredited and copies of the institutional report. The self-evaluation reports must follow the guidelines set by the Association.

The study programmes' self-evaluation reports contain detailed information about the organisation of the study programme, duration, enrolment, core and optional courses (with the number of teaching hours and credits for each course,[9] as well as its contents), curricula vitae of all professors, pedagogical methods, details of the recommended bibliography, data on the employment of graduates, etc.

The institutional self-evaluation report contains general information about the institution, including the composition of the Executive Board, budget, total enrolments (in all study programmes), data on research activity and contracts with industries, research contracts, as well as information about general courses and professors (this refers to information about courses that are taught simultaneously to students of more than one study programme).

The review team visits the institution for one or two days and interviews members of the Executive Board, Professors, Students and Staff. After the visit, the review team drafts a preliminary report that includes the main findings, the team's opinion about the clarity, objectivity and completeness of the elements of the self-evaluation reports and an appreciation of strong and weak points. However, when drafting the report, the review team should try to avoid giving any impression about the final accreditation decision. This report is forwarded to the institution, which will check that there are no factual errors.

The review team then finalises the report, which includes recommendations for improvement of the study programme, and a recommendation for a positive or negative decision concerning the accreditation process. The report also contains a detailed explanation of the rationale that justifies the recommendations.

The report is submitted to the joint appreciation of the Council for Admission and Qualification (of new individual members of the Association) and of the Council for Accreditation. The final decision is forwarded to the Association's National Executive Board that ratifies it. The Faculty is then notified of the final decision in writing. The final decision can take one of three forms:

- Full accreditation for a period of six years, when renewal of the accreditation will be necessary.
- Conditional accreditation for a period of three years, with recommendations of improvements that need to be implemented over that period and must be confirmed by a review team, once the approbation period is over.
- Refusal of accreditation, with a list of the reasons that support this decision.

---

9 This only refers to courses that are specific to the study programmes. Details of other courses which are common to other study programmes (e.g., Mathematics or Physics) are presented in the institutional self-evaluation report.

The whole procedure is confidential and can only be made public with the permission of the institution. However, the Association publishes a list of the accredited study programmes (but not of those programmes that were denied accreditation).[10]

The Architects' Association

The statutes of the Architects' Association determine that to become a member a graduate must hold a degree in architecture that is recognised by the Association. Candidates may be asked to pass an examination that is organised by the Association to determine their professional aptitude and/or to be on probation for a period of one year under professional tutelage approved by the Association.

The National Executive Board of the Association has approved proposals put forward by the National Council for Admissions to define objective criteria for the exemption of the aptitude examination, which are renewed periodically and based on the curricula of the study programmes, the learning conditions and evaluations. This means that the Architects' Association has established a system for the accreditation of study programmes that is similar to that which is implemented by the Engineer's Association. This system has been in operation since the end of year 2000 and by 2003 when this chapter was written, 21 study programmes had been accredited, allowing their graduates to automatically become effective members of the association.

The objectives and methodology of the accreditation system of the Architects' Association follows very closely those that have already been in operation since 1994 for the accreditation of Engineering study programmes. As with engineering programmes, the architects' system is voluntary, periodical, based on institutional and study programmes self-evaluation reports, peer review visits and an external evaluation report. The results of the exercise can be full accreditation for six years, or accreditation for shorter periods (there is more flexibility than in the case of engineering, since a three year period is not imposed).

However, this system presents an important innovation: the Association accepts that the information for the accreditation process which is supplied by the institution may be collected from already available sources such as the internal and external reports of the National Quality Assessment System. This reduces the bureaucratic work impinging on institutions and may contribute to greater compatibility between the two parallel systems. It is important to emphasise that accreditation is based upon the fulfilment of an EU directive on the recognition of architects, as minimum conditions for accreditation are:

• Study programmes must be officially recognised.

---

10 More information can be obtained from FEANI's website: www.feani.org.

- Study programmes must be of the level of a university degree.
- The contents of study programmes must comply with article 3 of EU Directive 85/384/CCC of 10 of June.
- The minimum duration of study programmes is five years and about 4,000 hours of classes (full-time), or the part-time equivalent.
- There is a medium term objective of 4,500 hours of classes.

The Pharmacists' Association

The new statutes of the Pharmacists' Association were approved by Decree-Law 288/2001 of 10 November. They allow the Association to define objective criteria that enable candidates to be exempt from admission examinations. These criteria, which must be periodically revised, will be based upon the contents of study programmes, the educational resources and the methods of assessment.

Following the approval of the new statutes, the Pharmacists' Association decided to implement an accreditation system of study programmes that was discussed with its members and higher education institutions The objectives and procedures will follow fairly closely the system implemented by the Engineers' Association.

The Pharmacists' Association has an innovative system for the renewal of the professional membership card. The card needs to be renewed every five years. Renewal is subject to the accumulation of a minimum number of credits obtained through lifelong education activities. These include continuing education programmes, postgraduation programmes (including master's degrees, PhDs, and *agregações* – equivalent to the German *Habilitation*), scientific research activity, etc. In order to recognise the credits of continuing education programmes the Association is also creating an accreditation system for institutions and agencies that provide that kind of programmes.

The Economists' Association

The Economists' Association has not established a formal system of accreditation and only under very special circumstances will there be institutional visits by review teams. The Association will take into consideration the results of the National System of Quality Assessment and a training period is obligatory before candidates are admitted. The informal 'accreditation' criteria include:

- The programme has been officially recognised (registered) by the Ministry.
- The study programme was evaluated positively in the National System.
- A curriculum that guarantees the transmission of a minimum technical knowledge and a culture appropriate to professional exercise.
- A minimum number of credits in specific scientific areas.

The Dentists' Association

The statutes of the Dentists' Association do not allow for the establishment of an accreditation system for study programmes in Dental Medicine. However, the Association intends to launch an accreditation system and has submitted a new proposal of statutes to Parliament. So far, no decision has been taken.

The Veterinary Surgeons' Association

This Association intends to introduce an accreditation system with a clear European emphasis. The Commission's Directive 78/1027/CEE established the minimum criteria for Veterinary Surgeons to be allowed to practise in the Union. The Commission's Directive 89/98/CEE, while defining the conditions for recognition of three-year higher education diplomas, eliminates the automatic recognition of professional qualifications by allowing member states to control the quality of the professionals. This may be seen as a restriction compared to the former Commission's Directive 78/1026/CEE which conferred automatic accreditation to all three-year (and longer) European degrees.

The national representatives of the profession and their organisations launched a pilot project for international evaluation of European Schools of Veterinary Medicine in 1986. It has finally resulted in the approval by the Veterinary Surgeons Training Advisory Committee of an evaluation protocol. The Portuguese Association would like to restrict the accreditation of Portuguese Veterinary schools to those with a positive European evaluation.

The Biologists' Association, the Nurses' Association, the Chamber of Solicitors

So far, none of these organisations has implemented a system of accreditation. In general, the condition for membership is to hold a recognised Portuguese degree, or a foreign degree that is equivalent to a Portuguese degree, or a degree from a European country which comes under the laws of the European Union. None of these associations demands a training period under conditions they approve. However, all three would like to implement accreditation systems for those study programmes that entitle graduates to professional practice.

The Medical Association

The Medical Association does not have an accreditation role regarding undergraduate teaching of Medicine. However, it plays a very important role in the control of internships after the students leave university. A good critical analysis of the present situation was provided in a recent evaluation of the Portuguese medical schools by a review team of the Association of European Universities. It showed the lack of participation of the university in specialisation training that 'is managed by the professional specialised associations in the medical sector (practitioners), in co-operation with the Ministry of Health, and with very little influence from the academics'; there is one national 'college' for each specialisation.

The Lawyers' Association

The role of the Lawyers' Association is rather similar to that of the Medical Association. So far, the Lawyers' Association does not have a role in the accreditation of study programmes in Law but it is responsible for the professional training of future lawyers. Indeed, students after leaving the university must go through a training period in an established lawyers' office where they work as practitioners. The training period is, in principle, controlled by the professional association.

The new head of the Lawyers' Association recently declared his intention to establish a system for periodic accreditation of study programmes, but it has not been implemented so far.

The Association of Official Copyholders of Accounts

Membership is determined by appropriate academic qualifications, an examination and a training period. The introduction of an accreditation system is not foreseen.

Technical Engineers

Short-cycle three-year courses which lead to the academic degree of *Bacharel* are offered by the polytechnics.

In parallel with the *Ordem dos Engenheiros*, there is a similar Institution called the APET – *Associação Portuguesa dos Engenheiros Técnicos* – which has implemented its own accreditation procedures to grant the professional title of *Engenheiro Técnico* (Technical Engineer). APET has developed a similar accreditation system in co-operation with the Engineers' Association,. APET also has close links with FEANI and a substantial number of the short cycle courses are now registered in the EurIng index.

Recent changes in legislation allow Polytechnics to offer a two-tier degree programme that confers a *licenciado*, which has the same legal status as degrees conferred by university engineering schools. APET has been replaced by ANET (*Associação Nacional dos Engenheiros Técnicos*), an association under public law whose statutes are approved by Decree-Law 349/99 of 2nd September. The transition was not smooth and accreditation activities have been suspended.

18.3   Analysis of the Different Systems and their Relationship

18.3.1   Driving Forces for Accreditation

The main driving forces for accreditation are the rapid expansion of higher education, the recognition that some educational provision is of low quality and a serious mismatch between the outputs of higher education and the needs of the labour market. These driving forces gave rise to a movement headed by the engineers' association that led to the emergence of professional accreditation. Other professional associations are following the example of the engineers.

18.3.2   Other Approval Schemes

There are three main evaluation/approval schemes which are not based on accreditation: registration and/or approval of institutions and study programmes by the state, the national quality assessment system and various schemes run by professional organisations.

Registration and/or Approval by the State

In principle, the state controls both the quantity and the quality of educational provision. Quantity is controlled through the establishment of a system of *numerus clausus* for all study programmes of universities and polytechnics, both public and private. Every year, the higher education institutions make *numerus clausus* proposals for every available study programme, but the Minister takes the final decision.

The registration of study programmes by the Ministry has become a necessary condition for enrolments in a new study programme. This can be seen as an *a priori* system of control of both the quality and the adequacy of the new study programmes for the needs of society and the economy. However, it remains to be seen if this will be an effective system of regulation.

Repeating what we stated at the beginning of this chapter, expansion of higher education and diversification, as well as increase of student enrolment in fields that were considered of economic importance has been explicit government policy goals for more than a decade. However, these policy goals have not been fully attained, both because of mushrooming of the private sector in direction contrary to the aims of the diversification policy (geographical distortions and insufficient supply of technical degrees), and because of some academic drift of the polytechnics. In this process the State is very much to blame and it demonstrates that the system of registration was not a very effective regulation device. Only the characteristics of Portuguese society can explain why expansion and diversification have occurred in a direction that runs counter to explicit government policy goals when polytechnics and the private sector had to submit their study programme proposals to the approval of the Ministry of Education.

Some problems raised by this recent evolution are due to a paradoxical situation whereby the government has the power and the instruments to regulate the system, but frequently abstains from using them. Indeed, Portuguese society can be considered rather gentle and permissive. Conflicts seldom lead to violence, harsh measures are very seldom enforced and a lot of sympathy for the weak is frequently expressed. It is also true that there are many laws with a strong regulatory character, but they are not always taken very seriously. For the same reason, the state has difficulties in enforcing any credible system of *a posteriori* control and generally prefers to resort to *a priori* scrutiny of proposals submitted to the approval of the Ministry of Education. In practice, however, private institutions have a strong lobbying capacity, allowing them to obtain official recognition without close scrutiny of the legal demands or the quality of teaching. And it is true that the national practice of avoiding conflicts and not taking harsh decisions has often resulted in late approval of proposals. Indeed it is no surprise to see that the Ministry, instead of answering with a clear yes or no the demands of private institutions, sometimes decided to ignore all legal deadlines by choosing not to answer at all. And it is no surprise to observe that many private institutions have illegally initiated study programmes without the necessary governmental permission, being later absolved by retroactive governmental decisions that legalise the situation when problems could become serious.[11]

It is obvious that the state has important responsibilities in the present crisis, since it promoted the uncontrolled expansion of the private sector through negligence and lack of rigour in law enforcement, thus yielding to a private sector *veni, vedi, vici* approach. Moreover, we must remember that the state has kept the main regulation of the system. These omissions have had serious consequences. So it is no surprise that private institutions have been encouraged to develop without any effective state control neither of the offer of study programmes or quality in the illusion that there was an ever-growing market for higher education.

A new law (Law 1/2003 of the 6th of January) established a kind of buffer organisation, the Advisory Council on Higher Education. We write 'kind of', because, although its 17 members are appointed by institutions such as the Council of Rectors of the Portuguese Universities, the Council of the Presidents of the Portuguese Polytechnics or the Association of the Presidents of Private Higher Education, this Advisory Council is presided by the Minister or its representative. The Council will for-

---

11 Not long ago, the President of the Republic, faced with one of these retroactive decrees, refused its promulgation without the approval of a decree that clearly established that illegal higher education institutions would be closed down, if necessary with the help of the police.

mulate opinions about the development priorities of the higher education system and the establishment and recognition of new institutions. However, it is too early to determine whether the new system will be more effective than the previous one in regulating the higher education system.

National Quality Assessment System

The main objective of the national quality assessment system is to improve the quality of educational provision. The final reports are made public but they are in general rather cryptic and carefully written to avoid rankings, and as such have been a frustration for the national media. There is now some public feeling that the published results are rather useless as a source of information for the public and rather ineffective as instruments for quality improvement.

Schemes Run by Professional Organisations

In general, the aim of these schemes is to guarantee that new graduates are prepared for professional practice. These schemes are considered appropriate.

18.3.3 Relationship Between Accreditation and Other Schemes

There is no formal relationship between the existing accreditation systems and other quality assessment schemes. However, in the national quality assessment system, when evaluating study programmes that train for professions, it is common practice to invite in the peer review team at least one representative from the professional association. More recently, conversations were initiated between the national system and the Engineers' Association to see if the two systems could be combined in order to avoid 'evaluation fatigue' of the higher education institutions. In other cases, the Association (architects) allows institutions to use data from the national quality system self-evaluation report as elements for accreditation. In other cases, the Association (economists) does not have a formal system of accreditation and relies upon the results of the national quality assessment system.

The only formal relationship exists within the professional associations themselves: graduates from accredited study programmes automatically become members of the association without taking the examination that are organised by the association for the admission of new members.

18.3.4   Consequences of Accreditation

Consequences for Institutions and Scholars

The obvious consequence of refusal of accreditation of a study programme by a professional association will be a loss of prestige and capacity to enrol students in that study programme. This may be a serious threat now that the total number of candidates for higher education is substantially lower than the total number of vacancies. And lower enrolments mean lower budgets, both for public and private institutions. The budget may also become insufficient to support scholars' research activity, or even worse, their salaries.

Consequences for Students

Graduates from a study programme or institution that is not accredited by a professional association must pass an examination of the association in order to be able to register as full members and be entitled to practise their profession. The advantage for graduates from accredited study programmes is automatic registration as effective members of the association.

Consequences for Other Stakeholders

There are no dramatic consequences for other stakeholders. The most obvious is the loss of public prestige of non-accredited institutions and programmes. Employers may also avoid hiring graduates from the less prestigious institutions and/or study programmes.

18.3.5   Recent Developments and Projections for the Future

Law 1/2003 was passed by Parliament and published on the 6th of January. Its articles 36 and 37 are relevant for the present chapter, as they establish an 'academic accreditation' to be implemented by the same agencies responsible for the quality assessment system, and they define the consequences of refusal of accreditation both for study programmes and for institutions. The Law, however, does not clarify the relationship of this system with the accreditation schemes run by professional associations.

The full consequences of this new law are difficult to assess. It is not clear if the accreditation powers will be completely transferred to the quality assessment agency, thus depriving professional associations of their present powers of accreditation, or if the two systems will be allowed to run in parallel, with the obvious risk of contradictory decisions. A better alternative would be to combine the two systems, thus offsetting the danger of overburdening the institutions with an excessive number of quality exercises.[12]

Article 36. Accreditation

1.	Academic accreditation consists in the verification of the fulfilment of the requisites necessary for the establishment and functioning of higher education institutions and for the registration of study programmes.
2.	Accreditation is the responsibility of the quality assessment agency.
3.	The results of accreditation are 'accredited' and 'not accredited'.
4.	The decisions of accreditation or of non-accreditation of higher education institutions and of study programmes are forwarded to the Minister of Science and Higher Education for the purposes mentioned in the following paragraphs.
5.	The refusal to accredit a higher education institution may imply the suspension and cancellation of the authorisation to operate or of the recognition of its public utility, according to the case.
6.	The refusal to accredit a study programme may imply the cancellation of its registration, with the subsequent suspension of its operation.
7.	In the case of the two previous paragraphs the Ministry will establish the conditions allowing students to transfer to another higher education institution.

Article 37. Accreditation of study programmes

1.	The accreditation of a study programme also implies the accreditation of its curricula.
2.	The accreditation of curricula also implies the public recognition of all courses taken, thus allowing students to continue studies in a different higher education institution.

On the other hand, the consequences of accreditation (article 36, §§ 5 and 6) are not very different from those of a negative quality assessment (see below, Law 38/94 of 21 November).

It is true that the final reports of quality assessment exercises, because they are made public, are usually drafted with care. This means they very seldom offer clear bases for drastic decisions such as cancellation of study programmes. If the quality assessment agency is forced to produce an accreditation-type conclusion – a yes or no

---

12 It is not clear to what extent the two systems can run in parallel. A distinction between 'academic' and 'professional' accreditation does not seem to provide clear and non-overlapping boundaries for both systems. Professor Vital Moreira considers that, since higher education degrees are public or publicly validated – and this will be reinforced by a national system of accreditation – the re-accreditation by professional associations does not make sense (one may even have doubts about its constitutionality). Professional associations represent the interests of their associates, whereas the state represents the general interest, and as such the corporative interest cannot override the general public interest.

answer – this will give the Minister a much more sound basis for action. Indeed, the Minister has publicly complained on several occasions that the conclusions of the reports of quality assessment agencies were quite obscure, and this may explain the provisions for accreditation in the new Law.

Article 5. Evaluation results

1. The results of the evaluation shall be considered by the Ministry of Education to the effect of the application of measures adequate to the nature of the evaluated activities, in particular: a) Increase in public financing. b) Incentive to the create new courses or develop the already existent courses. c) Enhancement of the support to scientific research activities. d) Introduction of development contracts, aiming at the correction of the deficiencies and disparities found during the evaluation procedures. 2. If the results of the continuing evaluation of the higher education institutions are negative, they may determine the following measures: a) Reduction or suspension of the public financing whenever the institutions do not follow the reviewers' recommendations. b) Suspension from the register of the courses in the public higher education system. c) Cancellation of the authorisation for courses in the public higher education polytechnic system to function. d) Cancellation of the authorisation for the functioning of courses or the recognition of degrees in the private higher education system.

18.4   European and Global Influences

18.4.1   Europe and GATS

So far we cannot detect any great influence of ideas, concepts or perceptions regarding Europe, such as the Bologna process, on the accreditation and evaluation schemes. Cases of a more evident European influence are where the Commission has produced directives concerning the professions of nurse responsible for general care, dental practitioner, veterinary surgeon, midwife, architect, pharmacist and doctor. It is believed that the subsidiarity principle means that quality assessment or accreditation is a competence that is reserved for the member states and cannot be transferred to Brussels or to a European centralised accreditation agency.

No decisive measures have been taken to follow the orientations defined by the Bologna process: there are still four different degrees (see Table 1) and there is deep disagreement about the changes that are necessary to comply with Bologna. Most universities still offer five-year study programmes in Engineering, Economics, and Law, while Pharmacy and Architecture offer 5.5- and 5- or 6-year programmes respectively. A recent law (Law 1/2003 of 6 of January) determines that study programmes must be organised within a credits structure 'to comply with the orientations of the Bologna process, to promote internal and international mobility of students and to facilitate lifelong education activities through credit accumulation', but there is no visible action.[13]

Regarding globalisation, we can only detect that recent legislation contains provisions against franchising education activities. Following the 1997 Lisbon Declaration on mutual recognition of diplomas, there is a system for almost automatic recognition of foreign doctoral degrees., which however excludes degrees conferred under franchising. And a new law (Law 1/2003, article 16) explicitly forbids franchising activities.

18.4.2   Influence of Other International Models

There has been some international influence on the implementation of the Portuguese national quality assessment system. At the time when references to quality started to find their way into political discourses and legislation, the Ministers of Education of the EU, then under Dutch Presidency, agreed that the Commission should take the following steps to strengthen the evaluation of higher education in Europe:

1. Comparative study of the evaluation methods used by Member States.
2. Development of a limited number of co-operative pilot projects in this area.
3. Creation of mechanisms to strengthen European co-operation, taking into account the concrete previous evaluation experience.

The comparative study of the evaluation methods used in the Member States was published in October 1993. A European Pilot Project on quality assessment was carried out in 1995 using a methodology that included elements that were common to the existing national quality systems. Some members of the European academic community were afraid that this initiative may lead to a new European centralised bureaucracy and to a quality assessment model that followed the existing national quality systems. The vice-president of the Confederation of European Rectors Councils, Professor Michel Cousin, held a joint meeting with the Council of Rectors

---

13 Likewise, most German universities chose to postpone the implementation of the Bologna process, according to a recent survey by the Federal Statistical Office. The study shows that the new bachelor/master 'European-type' courses represent only 2 % of total student enrolment. The lack of enthusiasm for the conversion to the new European curriculum is mainly due to the professionals' strong attachment to the traditional *Magister* and *Diplom* degrees which usually take at least ten semesters to complete (see www.educationews.com/newsletter4/ Newsletterweb.htm).

of Portuguese Universities where he pointed to the dangers of the Ministers' decision and advised Portuguese universities to start a national system as soon as possible in order to avoid the imposition of one of the available models. This advice was taken seriously and the Portuguese national system was implemented soon afterwards with technical support from the Dutch VSNU and the University of Twente. However, there are some differences between the Portuguese system and the initial Dutch system:

1. In the Portuguese system there is no meta-evaluation by the Inspectorate.
2. As the external credibility of the evaluation system will be reinforced if the independent character of the external visiting committees is stressed, the members of the visiting committees will be appointed by the structures which represent the different sectors of higher education (e.g. the Foundation of the Portuguese Universities, in the case of the public universities) from lists of experts previously submitted to the approval of the Minister.
3. Once an evaluation report is completed, the institutions, if they so wish, can respond to the report, and the response will be included as an appendix. However, the institutions must report to the Minister the procedures to be followed by the institutions for the implementation of the recommendations of the visiting committee to eliminate the weak points of the degree programme.
4. Besides the normal evaluation by discipline, the possibility of evaluating an institution as a whole has also been considered for the future.
5. The law also considers the need to set up a national database on the higher education system to ensure that the data from the different institutions are uniform, thereby allowing for comparisons.

18.5   Other Activities

18.5.1   Research

In general, research money is allocated under a competitive system based upon an evaluation of research centres and groups by pools of reviewers with a majority of international experts. The level of funding is linked to the results of evaluation.

It is important to know that until quite recently (March 2002) the Ministry of Education was mainly responsible for the 'education' budget of higher education institutions, whereas the Ministry of Science and Technology was mainly responsible for funding research. Both ministries had their own quality assessment systems, which used different rules and regulations and different approaches to quality assessment.

The new government has a different structure: a Ministry of Education that is no longer responsible for higher education, and a new Ministry of Science and Higher Education, which is responsible for higher education and for the activities of the former Ministry of Science and Technology. This new organisational structure may lead to changes in evaluation mechanisms, but it is yet too early to know what the future developments will be.

18.5.2 Institutional Evaluation

The national legislation for quality assessment of higher education (Quality assessment Act no. 38/94, of 21st November) contains provisions for institutional evaluation. However, so far this system has only carried out discipline-based evaluations.

18.5.3 International Activities

The Portuguese universities have played an important role in the development of the system of Institutional Reviews offered by the EUA (former CRE) – European University Association – to its member institutions. The University of Porto, together with the Universities of Utrecht and Gothenburg, were responsible for the initial experimental exercise that led to the final design of the system. Later, the University of Lisbon, the Technical University of Lisbon, the New University of Lisbon, the University of Minho, the University of Aveiro, the University of Algarve and the Catholic University (i.e. 80 % of the total Portuguese membership of EUA) were all reviewed by EUA.

18.5.4 Other Activities

There were some dispersed evaluation activities. We can refer, for instance, to benchmarking exercises promoted by the Columbus Association (University of Lisbon) and experiments using TQM and ISO 9000 certification for higher education institutions (e.g., the Polytechnic Institute of Porto).

18.5.5 Open Questions

The autonomy laws transfer to individual higher education institutions decisions concerning the promotion of academic personnel, subject to some general rules such as filling the vacancies by means of a public (national or international) process and participation of outside peers in the decisions about the candidates. However, criticism has been voiced about the closed character of these job openings, as in general most candidates come from within the institution, and some people have suggested that promotions should be decided at a national level, following a more independent evaluation of the candidates' CVs. This is not very different from the old practice in France and Italy. So far, this has not been taken seriously.

19   A Decade of Quality Assurance in Spanish Universities

JOSÉ-GINÉS MORA

19.1   Introduction

The traditional Spanish higher education system, which was regulated by the State, was obviously not interested in accountability. However, it has now become more autonomous, and accountability is therefore necessary. In Spanish higher education, accountability and assessment are recent, but they are developing very rapidly. Generalised assessment of individuals and institutions began in the early 1990s. Now, academics' teaching and research activities are evaluated on a regular basis. Promotion and some salary increases depend on assessments (Mora, 2001). Moreover, in 1995, after several pilot projects, the Council of Universities established the National Programme for Assessment of Quality in Universities (Mora, 1997; Mora and Vidal, 1998) to introduce a systematic assessment of universities. Within a few years, Spanish universities set up new offices to support quality assurance programmes and thousands of people are now participating in self-assessment activities and external visits around the country. Regional governments are also involved in these programmes and have even created their own quality agencies. The final impact of these activities has been uneven: some universities and regions are very active in this matter (for instance, Catalan universities with the support of the dynamic Catalan Agency for Quality); in others, the impact has been less pronounced because neither the university leaders nor the regional governments have shown special interest in quality assurance.

After ten years' experience in quality assessment, a new law on higher education (LOU, see the next section) came into force recently. It established that syllabi must undergo assessment, certification and accreditation. These can be carried out by the newly created National Agency for Quality Assessment and Accreditation (ANECA) or by regional agencies in areas where they exist. The LOU also obliges degree programmes to undergo a process of accreditation in order for them to be considered official qualifications. This system of setting minimum accreditation standards has been established to ensure the quality of all study programmes. This represents an important innovation in Spanish higher education regulations. Prior requirements have always had to be met in order to obtain official approval, but no further checks were made after that. The accreditation of study programmes is currently at an experimental stage and it will be at least two years before it is introduced. In line with the most up-to-date accreditation criteria commonly used in other European countries, an accreditation system is being developed to find out whether

S. Schwarz and D.F. Westerheijden (eds.),
Accreditation and Evaluation in the European Higher Education Area, 421–443.
© 2004 *Kluwer Academic Publishers. Printed in the Netherlands.*

programmes provide students with the expertise (knowledge, skills and attitudes) required by the labour market.

We shall now present a detailed analysis and description of the activities undertaken in the field of quality assurance and those planned in the area of accreditation. Before that, we shall present a brief analysis of the structure of the Spanish university system.

19.2   The Spanish Higher Education System

19.2.1   Legal Framework

To understand the current quality assurance movement in Spain, one must study the recent history and structure of its universities. Spanish universities, the oldest of which were founded in the Middle Ages, remained relatively unchanged until the 18th century and were under the influence of the Catholic Church. At the beginning of the 19th century, liberalism stemming from the French Revolution changed the structure of the state. Under the 'Napoleonic' system of higher education adopted by Spain, the universities were agencies that were regulated by laws and norms issued by the state. Everything in the daily functioning of a higher education institution was a consequence of external rules that applied to all educational institutions. Until very recently, academic programmes in all institutions had the same curricula. Universities had no specific budgets and expenditure was regulated by the state to the minutest detail. Professors were appointed after a strict selection procedure as members of a national body of civil servants.

In this stifling atmosphere of state regulation, quality assurance as it is currently understood did not have its place. The higher education processes, from the financial issues to the number of teaching hours of a course, followed established state rules and there could be no deviation from these rules, at least in theory. The control of the processes was exclusively *ex-ante*, and criteria and standards were pre-established. The system relied on the integrity of appointed 'professor-officials' to ensure strict applications of the rules. Only in cases of glaring misbehaviour did the state intervene *ex-post* to remedy the problems.

This strictly regulated higher education system was also an elitist system whose main goal was to train the ruling class of the modern state, especially the civil servants. Spanish universities, like their French and Italian counterparts, had a strong professional orientation. The teaching process focused on the transmission of skills that were essential to the development of professions, many of which were part of the state structure. The strict system used in the selection of civil servants functioned as an *ex-post* system of quality control.

The situation described above began to change in the 1970s, when the system started to shift from an elite system to mass higher education. Legal changes also helped to trigger a complete renovation of the higher education system. The 1983 University Reform Act (LRU) formed the basis for the emancipation of higher education from the control of the state, as in other European countries during this decade (Neave and Van Vught, 1991). The main changes introduced by this Act were that:

- universities became autonomous entities which could establish their own programmes and curricula;
- institutions were conceived as independent and competitive units;
- professors were no longer part of a national body and began to 'belong' to each university;
- responsibility for universities was transferred to regional government; and
- institutions began to receive public appropriations as a lump sum and be able to allocate funds internally. There was not only a shift of formal control from the government to the institutions, as in other countries (Woodhouse, 1996), but also a movement from the national government to the regional governments.

The situation seems to have stabilised recently as a result of the drop in the birth-rate which has led to a slight drop in student numbers. The need for greater investment in buildings and academic staff has also begun to stabilise. However, two factors have led to a new situation in Spanish universities: a new legal framework which was drawn up by the government towards the end of 2001 (the *Ley Orgánica de Universidades* [Organic Law on Universities], hereafter referred to as *LOU*), and the Bologna Declaration, which affects all European higher education systems. Important curricular and organisational changes are required in order to adapt to the new situation, in addition to changes in the teaching methods. Once again, after a long period of flux, Spanish universities are now facing the need for radical change.

The new law made certain changes to the legal structure of higher education. Among the most noteworthy are:

- the incorporation of lay persons in the running of university (always a minority group);
- the election of the rector by direct vote (as opposed to being elected indirectly by the senate);
- greater academic staff representation, which implies a slight reduction in student representation;
- the requirement that academic staff have to obtain national habilitation before being appointed by universities; and
- the obligatory accreditation of degree programmes by the new National Agency for Quality Assessment and Accreditation (*Agencia Nacional de Evaluación de la Calidad y Acreditación*, ANECA).

In general, the law gives universities and autonomous regions more independence to organise themselves as they wish. This is a positive feature because it allows both universities and regions to rethink their legal regulations and adapt them to the new situation. This could perhaps have been done without the LOU, but it has created the need to introduce changes. Many university statutes may improve because they are better adapted to a situation which is very different from that of 25 years ago, at the end of the Franco dictatorship. Moreover, the autonomous regions are starting to draw up their own university laws with their own regulations and to set up their own agencies to assess the quality of teaching and institutions. This is interesting because it will allow for the differentiation and improvement of universities: their heads must be interested in promoting change and they must be located in an autonomous region whose governors are also concerned about the competitiveness of its universities. It is still too soon to see the first results, but it can already be seen that some regions are doing more than others on this front.

19.2.2 Basic Structure

Higher education in Spain consists almost exclusively of universities (50 public and 14 private). Most students enrol in public universities, although an increasing number of private universities enrol roughly 6 % of higher education students. There are three basic types of university programmes: short-cycle programmes, which are more vocationally oriented and last for three years; long-cycle programmes, which last for five or six years; and doctoral programmes, which add two years of course work and require the preparation of a research-oriented thesis after a long-cycle degree. Doctoral programmes are mainly followed by students who are interested in an academic career. Generally speaking, people with greater economic resources or intellectual capabilities have preferred long cycles university programmes.

The Spanish higher education system has become a mass system. The gross enrolment quota for the 18- to 23-year-old population is 41 %, and it is around 55 % for new entrants in higher education among the 18-year-old cohort (Mora et al., 2000). The increase in recent decades has been dramatic. Numbers have almost doubled each decade since 1960. However, the figure reached a peak in 1998/99 (1,583,000 students) and started to decrease slowly due to the remarkable reduction in the size of the youth cohort reaching higher education age (CU, several years).

The current drop in student numbers is extremely important. For the first time in the recent history of Spanish higher education, there is no guarantee that there will be a demand for university places, irrespective of the quality of the service offered by the institutions. This is bound to have a considerable impact on institutions' attitudes towards improving the quality of their teaching and services. The question is whether institutions and staff that have always lived in periods of growth will find it easy to adapt to a new era of stability in which the efficient use of available resources becomes the main objective.

On the other hand, access to higher education is relatively open to all social classes. An analysis of the socio-economic background of higher education students shows a fair representation from middle and upper class groups. Lower socio-economic groups (unskilled, agricultural and industrial workers) also have access to higher education, though they are still underrepresented (Mora, 1997). The number of women exceeds that of men. In 1970, the proportion of women enrolled in higher education was just 26 %, but by 1986 numbers reached 50 % and they have continued to rise to currently stand at 53.3 % of the higher education population (CCU, 2003).

Spanish universities, then, are currently in a position that could be considered as promising. Yet it is the general consensus in academic and governmental sectors that an additional effort must now be made to improve the overall quality of the institutions and their programmes. If in the last few years considerable efforts have been made to stimulate the growth of higher education, quality improvement is clearly the main goal for the near future. Quality assessment and accreditation have become central issues on the higher education agenda and in the policies of central and regional governments.

19.3   Quality Assessment and Accreditation

19.3.1   Initial Experiences in Quality Assessment

The Act that devolved autonomy to universities in 1983 (LRU) made a general statement about the need to incorporate some formal system of quality assessment for universities. But several years passed before this principle started to be implemented. In the early 1990s, several studies analysed the experiences of quality assessment in other countries. At that time, there were three main models in Europe: the Dutch, the British, and the French. The Dutch assessment model was primarily programme-centred and based on self-study and external visits (Vroeijenstijn, 1995). Experts recommended this approach for Spain as well as adding institutional assessment of research and management. Based on these assumptions, the 'Experimental Programme for Assessment of the Quality in the University System', which included these elements, was launched in 1993.

The Experimental Programme evaluated teaching, research, and institutional management in several universities (García et al., 1995; Mora, 1997b). As an experimental project, the primary purpose was to try out various methods and make proposals for change based on the experience gained. The experiment proved to be extensive enough to draw meaningful conclusions. In general, the Experimental Programme attained its main objectives: (a) testing the accuracy of a methodology and (b) extending the culture of assessment in Spanish universities. On the other hand, some weak points were found, such as: (a) lack of institutional data for quality assessment, (b) lack of support from leaders in some universities, and (c) methodological problems as a consequence of the inexperience of the assessors. Generally speaking, the project rapidly created and extended quality assessment in universities as a first step towards improving institutional quality.

Immediately after the Experimental Programme, the European Union launched the *European Pilot Project for Evaluating Quality in Higher Education*. This was also a pilot project to test a common methodology among European universities. The methodology was very similar to the one used in the Experimental Programme. The European Project modified the methodology and adapted it to a broader European context. However, the most important result of the project was probably the recommendation made by the European Commission in 1998 (EC, 1998) to establish a common system of quality assessment in European universities based on self-study and external visits, although each country could reorganise the process to maintain idiosyncratic national characteristics. This European proposal had an important impact in Spain as it convinced some sceptical people, especially politicians from central and regional governments, to support quality assessment in universities.

After this short but intensive experience, several points became clear to those involved in the process. First of all, universities needed to control the quality assessment effort, but some kind of agreement and co-operation with governments had to be reached, especially concerning the consequences of assessment. Second, the basic *methodology employed* (self-study, external visits, and a final report) was adequate. Third, research and management needed to be evaluated using similar processes. Fourth, the importance of *overcoming the reluctance* of some people towards assessment – and having the *support of the university leaders for the project*. Finally, *the results of the process needed to have internal and external consequences*. Although the main consequence of the assessment process had to be the improvement of quality, universities and departments needed to have some kind of incentive to participate and implement the recommendations.

19.3.2   The Programme for Institutional Assessment of Quality in Universities

In 1995, the Council of Universities approved the *Programme for Institutional Assessment of Quality in Universities*, hereafter referred to as the PNECU (CU, 1995). The PNECU formally institutionalised quality assessment in Spanish universities as an extended and continuous process for the entire university system.

Objectives

The PNECU had four stated objectives:

- promoting quality processes in Spanish universities;
- providing universities with methodological tools for this assessment process that would be both homogeneous throughout the country and similar to processes used elsewhere in Europe;
- providing society, and especially students, with relevant and reliable information about the quality of the institutions, their programmes, services and scientific levels; and
- providing accountability to regional government.

Organisational Structure

The PNECU was headed by the Council of Universities, a national organisation composed of representatives from regional and national government and the rectors of all the universities. A Technical Committee comprising officials from the Council of Universities and assessment experts was in charge of the process. The PNECU evaluated teaching (in programmes), research (in the departments related to programmes assessed in teaching), and management (in services also related to the programmes).

The PNECU lasted for six years (from 1995 to 2001). Although the programme was not compulsory, almost all universities participated in its first year. The universities which had taken part in the previous pilot projects participated more actively with an extensive assessment of programmes. Universities that did not have this experience took part at a more basic level.

Methodology

The methodology was the same as that which had been used in previous Spanish projects. The first step was a *self-study* carried out by the Assessment Committee of each university. This report had a double purpose: to provide reliable information on the evaluated unit and to develop awareness of quality issues in the university community. The second step was a *visit* by an External Committee composed of experts in the field (academic and non-academic). It interviewed leaders, staff, and students in each evaluated unit and compared their findings with the self-study report. This External Committee sent a report following each visit to the Council of Universities. Thirdly, the universities issued a *report synthesising* the self-study and the External Committee report. A general report on the programme's activities was published every year by the Council of Universities.

The Technical Committee prepared written guidelines to standardise the process in participating universities. These guidelines defined criteria and procedures and established the main points to be assessed and summarised in the committee reports. But the reports could use a different structure. Some universities with more sophisticated internal quality procedures used the criteria provided by the European Foundation for Quality Management (EFQM) for their self-study report.

Criteria for report structure. All the reports had to use reliable data but also had to focus on the analysis, opinions, and judgements of those involved in the evaluated units. They had to contain recommendations for improvement. The reports included the following sections: description and context of units evaluated; information on aims and objectives; information on resources, structure, and results; judgements by the Assessment Committee on the strong and weak points of the unit; proposals and recommendations for improvement; and relevant quantitative indicators.

Criteria for teaching assessment. The teaching assessment report had to include the following: the structure of the programme, teaching procedures, student and staff characteristics, and resources and outcomes.

Criteria for research assessment. Research was assessed in the following areas: the department's research objectives, human and material resources, research activity, productivity, quality indicators (see García et al., 1995, where these indicators were defined), and research outcomes.

Criteria for the assessment of the management of units and services. The assessment of management had to focus on the following: economic and administrative efficiency, decision-making procedures, student services structure, and facilities in general.

19.3.3   The Final Assessment of the PNECU

When the PNECU came to an end after six years, a final report was drawn up (CCU, 2002). Some of its most noteworthy conclusions are reported below.

Organisational Aspects

- Most universities took part in the assessment process. Only recently-established universities, which were advised to participate at a later date, did not take part.
- The Autonomous Regions of Andalusia and Catalonia reached an agreement with the Ministry of Education, Culture and Sport that allowed them to organise and carry out the university quality assessment programmes in their regions (assessment, decision-making, funding and follow-up).

- The process used in the PNECU allowed various different units, such as programmes, departments and services, to be assessed. In total, 939 programmes, along with their corresponding departments and services, were assessed by the PNECU. In addition, 30 departments and 46 service units were assessed independently. During the programme, approximately 64 % of all programmes which fulfilled the requirements (age of institution or programme) were assessed.

- In addition to the agencies mentioned above, others are now operating or being created, such as the *Axencia para la Calidade do Sistema Universitario de Galicia* (Agency for the Quality of Galicia's University System), the *Agencia de Qualitat Universitaria de les Illes Balears* (Agency for the Quality of the University System in the Balearic Islands) and the agencies for the Quality of the University Systems in Castile and Leon, the Valencian Region or the Madrid Region.

- The Ministry of Education, Culture and Sport provided the PNECU with € 4.5 million to fund the programme. However, the total cost of assessment was greater since there were two other sources of funding. On the one hand, the universities themselves covered most of the expenses and on the other, some autonomous regional governments had supplementary funds at their disposal that were specifically for the PNECU.

Methodological Aspects

- The independent nature of the process and the fact that neither the government nor the institutions under assessment had any influence on the results were important features inherent to the PNECU.

- In general, more emphasis was placed on teaching than on research, and more attention was given to both teaching and research than to services. To a certain extent, this bias was due to the methodology itself, which took the programme as the basic unit of analysis. This explains the structure of this report, in which greater attention is paid to teaching than to the other two aspects. This is partly justified by the fact that teaching processes in Spanish universities are in greater need of assessment.

- Most of the programmes' self-assessment reports concluded that the institutional assessment process was useful insofar as it helped to clarify the strategic objectives of the units assessed, to obtain systematic knowledge of how they worked and to formulate improvement proposals. In this respect, the most highly valued methodological aspect was the fact that the university community was enriched by the experience of carrying out the self-assessment report.

- One of the most obvious strengths of the assessment process was the fact that both the external assessment reports and the final programme reports put forward improvement proposals. This aspect has been strengthened by significant technical advances in formulating improvement actions in the successive rounds of the PNECU. These are becoming more and more accurate when it comes to prioritising, establishing deadlines, implementing means of assessment and assigning responsibility. In addition, the programmes suggested formulating specific plans of action based on their improvement proposals.

- One of the main problems faced by the units assessed was the lack of information and the unreliability of the data required for assessment. Throughout the PNECU, there have been general improvements in this type of information and an increase in its use in the internal administration of the institutions. However, more work needs to be done along these lines and agreements need to be reached between all the administrative departments in order to improve the flow of information required (in institutions as well as in public administration departments) for internal decision-making and above all, to provide more relevant information to the general public.

- Despite the fact that the assessment of services has had the least impact because of its scope, it has been important because of what it implies in terms of knowledge and behaviour in line with the EFQM excellence model which is so closely followed in the business world and in public administration. However, it is important that efforts be maintained in order to adapt the new assessment models to the specific needs of university administration.

- The methodology used in the PNECU was sound, but improvements must be made in terms of writing reports and training all the participants in order to increase the credibility of the process.

Results

- The PNECU has developed the university community's awareness of quality and quality assessment. This greater awareness has led to the creation of administrative support bodies, but a quality culture has not yet developed among university staff in general. This quality culture must be introduced from top to bottom. But a bottom-up approach is necessary if it is to develop effectively. For this to produce visible improvements, the university needs to operate and be organised according to processes in which objectives, customers, products and services are the common denominator. It should be remembered that any change in the culture of an organisation is a long-term process.

- The PNECU has made a considerable impact if we consider the number of institutions and people involved. However, emphasis must be placed on linking assessment results to the proposed improvements and on promoting such links. This is considered to be one of the weaknesses of the process. This aspect must be worked on by the universities themselves and by those responsible for higher education policy. The positive attitude created could easily turn into one of rejection if work is not carried out along these lines.

- The creation, participation and co-ordination of Autonomous Agencies in the whole process were the most prominent features of the PNECU. This has helped to bring assessment closer to the decision-making process, which is largely the responsibility of the Autonomous Regions. As a result, the LOU (Organic Law on Universities) has been decisive in encouraging the existence of these agencies all over Spain by giving them new and important responsibilities. Co-ordinating all these new units will be one of the main challenges of assessment processes in coming years.

- As a result of the PNECU almost all Spanish universities have the infrastructure required for quality assessment (technical units, rector's offices, etc.). This allows them to meet the challenges posed by the creation of a single European Higher Education Area foreseen in the Bologna Declaration and the accreditation of academic programmes foreseen in the LOU. In addition, it will help them to deal with other challenges regarding institutional quality, adaptation and improvement policies.

- Assessment has helped to bring courses into closer contact with their socio-economic environment in two ways. Professionals have been made members of external assessment committees. This has always been viewed positively.

In summary, several important goals have been reached over a relatively short period of time. First, university leaders and staff now accept the assessment process. Second, many of the improvement proposals are being implemented, especially in the fields of teaching and management. Third, new offices are being established very rapidly in the universities to support these processes. Finally, the publicity given to the whole process is promoting and stimulating a *quality culture* in Spanish universities.

These elements are encouraging all institutions to develop more strategies for change and to support improvement proposals. The main question now being raised by all participants is *what is the purpose or the tangible results of these activities?* If they do not find a satisfactory answer to this question soon, their interest and collaboration – which are crucial in this internal-external assessment methodology – will rapidly diminish. Since the required reports contain improvement proposals, they must quickly lead to some discernible consequences and rewards. Once needs are detected, institutions must develop and implement improvement strategies, but it is difficult to go ahead with improvements and additional assessment if in this first stage no tangible results or rewards can be seen.

This has led some universities to move from Quality Assessment to Quality Assurance. Assessment Committees have now become permanent Quality Committees, and assessment processes are being included in the annual agenda of many institutions. This process is in its initial phase and the institutions are already adopting many different approaches. The involvement of institutional leaders in the movement for quality assurance is the main factor that determines the speed and depth of these changes.

19.3.4   The Second Plan for the Quality of Universities

In the light of previous experiences, the Second Plan for the Quality of Universities (*Plan de Calidad de las Universidades*, PCU) was launched in 2001 to pursue the improvement of the assessment process. The general objectives of the PCU are to develop and improve systems for quality assessment of Spanish universities, including transparency and relevant information on the standards reached by each university that can serve as a basis for programme accreditation. Special attention should be paid to designing methodologies for quality assessment and accreditation in order to provide objective information that can be used by different bodies, departments, universities, public administration and citizens in general for decision-making in their areas of responsibility.

While institutional quality assessment is developed and improved in higher education institutions, regional governments must assume a leading role in the management of the PCU in conjunction with the Council of Universities, providing resources and facilities for the management of assessment processes to be carried out adequately and encouraging planning processes as an essential strategy to promote change and improvements in universities.

Objectives

The general objectives of the PCU are:

- To encourage institutional assessment of higher education quality.
- To promote and consolidate a legal framework in which regional governments play a leading role in the management of the PCU in order to encourage regional Assessment Agencies and establish a Network of Agencies that is coordinated by the Council of Universities.
- To develop homogeneous methodologies for quality assessment that are integrated in the current practice of the European Union in order to guarantee a standardisation of assessments.

- To provide objective information on the standards reached by each university that can be used by different bodies as the basis of decision-making in their areas of responsibility.
- To devise an accreditation procedure and a system of indicators that can provide quantitative and qualitative information on the assessment of programmes, departments and universities and inform society as a whole and the institutions themselves.

Organisational Structure

The PCU will be carried out over six years and its modality, conditions and requirements will be revised every year. The Council of Universities is responsible for the management and the co-ordination of the PCU. The Autonomous Regions, together with the Ministry of Education, will be able to set up and consolidate Assessment Agencies to carry out the PCU independently.

The Council of Universities, which is responsible for the management and co-ordination of the PCU, carries out its tasks with the aid of a Technical Committee and a Management Office. The Technical Committee is composed of Council of Universities officials, a representative from each of the regional agencies and several experts in quality assessment.

The Assessment Process

The assessment process, as is current practice in most European countries, follows a mixed methodology of internal (or self-assessment) and external assessment. A report is drawn up for each phase of the assessment, and then a final report summarises the strengths and weaknesses and the improvements proposed for institutional assessment.

The units to be assessed are the study programmes, departments and services of the university. In some cases, very similar programmes or services can be assessed as a whole.

Internal assessment or self-assessment is carried out by the Assessment Committees of the respective universities and gives rise to a report which describes the objective situation of the unit assessed as well as the opinion of the university itself of its strengths, weaknesses and ways to improve the services it offers.

The external assessment phase is carried out by the External Assessment Committee. This Committee draws up a report, called the External Committee Report, which is based on the information provided by the Assessment Committee and also from the information they collect *in situ* from interviews with representatives of the different groups involved in the assessed unit.

The report of the External Assessment Committee, with any observations that the Assessment Committee wishes to add, is submitted to a wide public for assessment programmes, before drawing up the Final Report, which establishes a plan of action for improvement. The Final Report is disseminated more widely in the unit assessed, i.e. the Quality Committee of the University assessed.

A follow-up of the assessment process and results needs to be set up. It should take place between the third and the fourth year, at the end of the first assessment process.

Teaching Assessment

Teaching assessment includes the study programme together with adequate planning which takes the situation of the institution into consideration as well as its social and economic relevance and cohesion with the teaching-learning process. A guide establishes the standard guidelines and formulae for the collection of data and opinions on the following points:

- Context of the programme.
- Aims and objectives.
- Training programmes.
- Human resources.
- Facilities and resources.
- Teaching development.
- Academic performance.
- Improvement proposals and self-assessment.

Research Assessment

The basic units of research assessment are the areas of knowledge or departments. This assessment includes the following:

- Context.
- Objectives formulated.
- Institutional structure.
- Available resources.
- External and internal relations.

The final assessment results should be suggested and the strengths, weaknesses and proposals for improvement found in the unit assessed need to be defined. Standard guidelines for the collection of data include the structure and characteristics of teaching and research staff, obtaining of funding (projects, contracts, etc.), participation in national and international research programmes, conferences, etc. and publications in scientific journals, books, patents, technical reports, etc.

Service Unit Assessment

In addition to the elements that are directly related to teaching and research, the assessment of the university's other services and management is also considered in the PCU. Guidelines for the assessment of other services are based on the EFQM (*European Foundation for Quality Management*). Needs and the current situation are analysed in this assessment process:

- To encourage strategic planning in the development of management and the setting up of well-defined objectives in this domain.
- To establish mechanisms to evaluate, offer incentives and motivate the non-academic staff responsible for governing the development of service management.
- To acknowledge commitment to improving services. This commitment is more noticeable, due to the staff profile in terms of youth, human values, experience, dedication, effort and above all a positive attitude towards change.
- To establish mechanisms to evaluate the co-ordination between the centres and Central Services and the users and staff.
- To set up mechanisms to measure the degree of user satisfaction with the services provided and to gather suggestions for improvement.

System of Indicators

The Council of Universities defined and approved a catalogue of indicators in order to improve the information and to establish mechanisms for emulation among institutions (*benchmarking*). The indicators are:

- Supply
  - Distribution of study programmes
- Demand
  - Percentage of new entrants (first option) out of all new entrants
  - Average grade of access of the 80th percentile
  - Average grade of access
- Human resources
  - Percentage of full-time academic staff (tenured teachers, associates and assistants, excluding scholarship holders)
  - Percentage of academic staff with a doctorate
  - Percentage of tenured academic staff
  - Non-academic/academic staff ratio

- Financial resources
  - Personnel expenditure as a percentage of total expenditure
  - Distribution of expenditure per enrolled student
  - Distribution of expenditure per corrected enrolled student
- Physical resources
  - Vacancies in libraries
  - Vacancies in computer laboratories
- Processes
  - Lecturing time
  - Student/teacher ratio
  - Practical offers in the programme
  - Percentage of students in large groups in the programme (greater or equal to 80 students)
  - Percentage of students in small groups in the programme (less or equal to 20 students)
  - Percentage of tenured staff involved in courses for new students
- Results
  - Dropout rate
  - Graduation rate
  - Return rate
  - Success rate
  - Average duration of studies
  - Average number of research bonuses of academic staff in the programme.

19.3.5   The New Accreditation Scheme

The PCU considered the possibility of initiating accreditation and certification processes as pilot projects. However, the promulgation of the LOU was what formally brought about obligatory accreditation for all official degrees and voluntary quality certification for the services and programmes that wished to be included. The LOU pays special attention to quality assurance in Spanish universities. A whole section of the law is devoted to issues concerning quality. In addition, the LOU has set up ANECA as the body in charge of accrediting official degrees at the national level. ANECA is also responsible for quality assessment in Spain (in association with the agencies of those autonomous regions which have them). ANECA is therefore responsible for the PCU, which does not necessarily mean that its present organisation will remain unchanged. In any case, the most innovative aspect is accreditation, which will be examined in the following sections.

The Concept of Accreditation

The definition of 'accreditation' is firmly established in the world of industry: a process by means of which an accreditation agency 'accredits' that another certifying agency meets certain set quality standards in procedures to award quality certification. In the world of higher education, the term accreditation may be regarded in a similar light if we consider universities as agencies which award academic qualifications. In this respect, university accreditation aims to ensure that the qualifications awarded by universities (in fact by the degree programmes) comply with minimum quality requirements. Thus, accreditation is basically a means of assessing results, which demands the existence of quality criteria and standards. These quality levels are established by setting up quality criteria and standards for each type of programme. In principle, there can only be two possible outcomes (a degree is either accredited or non-accredited), although other possibilities do exist: non-accredited, not yet accredited, accredited and accredited with excellence.

The Objectives of Accreditation

The main objective of accreditation is the assessment of educational programmes (all types of programmes taught by universities) in order to guarantee all citizens that each qualification fulfils certain quality criteria.

In addition to this fundamental objective, there are two other:

- To inform citizens: to provide information on the quality levels and other features of the programmes that are required to make decisions.
- To inform public authorities: to provide information to the public authorities, in the case of public institutions, on whether the resources they receive have been used correctly.

In addition to these three objectives of accreditation, there are other implicit objectives that are also important when it comes to explaining the current interest in accreditation. These are:

- To encourage university institutions to take an interest in quality. Experience shows that assessment processes have not gone far enough to bring about a real interest in quality in all institutions and in all the different bodies of these institutions. Assessment, which entails consequences, just like accreditation, will help make everyone take a greater interest in quality.
- To improve the quality of the degrees themselves. Assuring accreditation, especially with excellence, will be a means of maintaining interest in the quality of the programmes.

- To promote the mobility of students and professors. In some European countries (Spain, for example), students' domestic mobility is very low, but mobility between different European countries is even lower. In order to encourage mobility and to attract students from other countries, an accreditation system that provides information about quality levels and guarantees them, would be very useful.

The ANECA Plan of Action

ANECA's accreditation programme will be responsible for implementing all aspects of the LOU which must be fulfilled by all official degrees. More specifically, it will be in charge of re-accrediting official degrees specified by the LOU. The degrees will be re-accredited when they fulfil the minimum requirements set out by ANECA. This has three important consequences:

- The administrative criteria currently required for accreditation cannot be the same as those required for re-accreditation. Re-accreditation must be much more ambitious and be used as a powerful tool to improve the university system. In addition, re-accreditation must help to bring the Spanish university system in line with the European higher education area. Hence it is necessary to define accreditation criteria and make them public in advance.

- In addition to this system of accrediting minimum quality requirements, another system could be developed which accredits excellence. This could be a simple procedure if it used the same instruments as those for accrediting minimum conditions.

- According to the LOU, re-accreditation does not necessarily need to be repeated, whereas accreditation is basically a decision that has limited validity. It is therefore essential that there should be a legal mechanism making it obligatory for re-accreditation (understood as the accreditation of minimum requirements) to be repeated after a certain length of time.

Implementing the ANECA accreditation process requires the following three consecutive steps:

- A full definition of the concept of accreditation, of its objectives and its results.
- Once accreditation has been clearly defined, the objectives each degree will have to attain need to be specified. Although these will be generic objectives, they must be explicit enough for degrees to recognise them as feasible goals to which they can adapt.
- These objectives must be given the status of regulations, so that universities are legally obliged to reach them.

In order to reach these objectives, a design group has been set up which is in charge of proposing definitions and deciding on the basic criteria that should characterise the accreditation process. In addition, the National Accreditation Committee has been established and includes eminent academics and professionals. In this initial design phase, it aims to validate the process and the accreditation criteria.

Pilot Experiences in Accreditation

It is essential to set up accreditation pilot schemes in order to determine the model to be used, fine-tune the methodologies and discover any logistical problems that may arise. Groups of experts will be in charge of the design and implementation of these pilot projects. To do this, we already have the experience of a pilot project in Computer Engineering, which began under the PCU. Using this project as a reference, a pilot project will be launched in each of the other four fields of study (experimental sciences, social sciences and law, humanities and health sciences). The corresponding work groups will need experimental accreditation instruments so that a limited round can take place to 'experimentally' accredit one or two degrees in each of the fields of study during the 2003/04 academic year. Once this experimental phase is over, a formal accreditation process could be introduced as from 2004/05, although there may be certain restrictions. It seems unlikely that obligatory accreditation will commence before 2005 or 2006.

19.4   The Underlying Forces in the Accreditation Process

The move towards quality assurance in Spanish universities is recent but extremely positive and promising. In just a few years, quality has been formally implemented in the higher education system and in the daily dealings of a growing number of institutions. But quality assessment, for all its success, is threatened by bureaucratisation and frustration.

First, a process of this nature that is centrally organised could be considered by some as an additional formal, and perhaps unnecessary, requirement. The danger is that the process may become too bureaucratic if it is not well explained. The capacity of the ANECA and other regional agencies to develop a dynamic structure to overcome these problems is crucial to circumvent this threat. Universities must incorporate quality assurance as an internal tool for continuous improvement.

Second, the implementation of the recommendations and follow-up of the process is also essential. If those involved in the assessment and the university community in general do not feel that this is a worthwhile process, with matching consequences and rewards, growing feelings of frustration could be a danger in future.

A mechanism to keep positive pressure on the quality assurance movement, albeit not the only one (accreditation could be the other), is to link assessment results directly to funding. This is a very controversial issue that many policymakers and researchers do not recommend because it is regarded as a threat to the fairness of a process and system that should be solely 'improvement focused' (Vroeijenstijn, 1995). But if universities are not compensated or rewarded in some way for attaining high standards of quality and performance, their commitment to quality assurance processes could be cut short. The biggest challenge, however, is to determine how to link the results of these programmes with funding. Several local initiatives could serve as examples. One, which has been adopted in several regions, is the application of funding formulae that incorporate a variable related to quality in the allocation of public funds among universities (Mora and Villarreal, 1996). Another promising approach, which has been adopted in other regions, is *contract-programmes*. This approach involves a contract between the regional government and each institution whereby universities are funded to achieve a set of specific goals. These contracts are designed to reorganise the whole institution from a quality perspective. Whatever the method employed, a system of rewards is needed to firmly embed a quality assurance programme in Spanish universities in the new millennium.

On the other hand, the accreditation process that will soon be underway may prove to be a significant incentive to convince institutions and their employees of the need to improve. The objectives set out in the accreditation process must be an instrument that can be used to put pressure on institutions in this search for efficiency.

19.5 The Influence of Internationalisation on the Process of Accreditation

Certain factors will have an enormous impact on the development and on the definition of the accreditation process and must therefore be taken into account. They are:

- The influence of the Bologna process.
- The internationalisation of accreditation.
- The definition of the skills to be accredited.

The following proposals have been put forward to deal with these three issues:

- To define accreditation exclusively for programmes which have been adapted to the new designs. This must be flexible in order to allow the experimental accreditation process to begin as soon as possible (even if the programmes are not fully adapted).
- To establish and maintain a work group with representatives from other European countries that have already started accreditation processes. This aims to develop compatible methodologies, which may in future lead to systems of mutual accreditation recognition.

- To carry out studies on the professional skills required by graduates. These could then be used as a point of reference to include skills in the accreditation process. These studies would mainly be based on detailed questionnaires on skills carried out by students, graduates and employers.

Approaches to Accreditation

The accreditation process in Spain is strongly influenced by the latest European developments. It is accepted that methodology needs to transcend national boundaries. It is not logical that issues affecting the whole of Europe (mobility, transparency, international recognition, etc.) should be solved by independent, national accreditation systems. At present, the idea of a European accreditation agency is not considered feasible because of the considerable differences that exist between the various education systems. Perhaps the most widely accepted principle would be that of national accreditation systems based on similar criteria that could be acknowledged by different countries.

The criteria being considered in order to take the first steps towards degree accreditation appear in a document by the work group of the *Joint Quality Initiative* on shared descriptors defining the characteristics of a degree ('Dublin Descriptors', JQI, 2002). This document describes the common objectives that must be reached by any type of programme that awards *Bachelor's* and *Master's* degrees. Other specific characteristics that are unique to each country and each area of knowledge can be added, but the characteristics defined are generic and should be common to all countries and all fields of study.

It is important to emphasise that the principles that define the programmes in all European initiatives are not based on course length or course content (which is something that must be decided independently by the universities themselves). Instead, a degree's value is determined by the skills acquired by its graduates (regardless of how or when they are acquired). According to this procedure, as long as it produces results, an educational programme will be assessed positively.

19.6   Other Assessment Schemes

The *individual activity of academics* is evaluated through several mechanisms with differences for teaching or research activities with repercussions or with no repercussions on earning, and with direct or indirect effects on promotion (Mora and Vidal, 1998). The assessment processes for academic staff are the following.

Assessment for teaching productivity bonus (tenured staff). The teaching activities of tenured professors are evaluated by their universities every five years. Because of the lack of reliable standards in the assessment of teaching, all professors (with extremely rare exceptions) are assessed positively. Only in cases of clear misbehaviour is evaluation negative. This mechanism has become an additional method for rewarding seniority since professors receive a permanent increase in their salaries for each positive assessment.

Teaching activity assessment (all academic staff). In most universities, students carry out an annual survey on each teacher and each course. Overall results of the survey are published, but only the assessed teacher and the university itself have access to personal data. This survey has two positive effects: a) universities detect problems caused by teachers' lack of pedagogical abilities or by some type of conflict between students and teachers; b) it affects teachers' attitudes, and encourages the fulfilment of basic teaching duties. But whether the results of these assessments should influence promotion or working conditions of academic staff is an issue that is largely debated and has not yet reached a consensus, although some universities take these results into account in promotion procedures.

Assessment for research productivity bonus (tenured staff). National panels composed of experts for each group of disciplines are in charge of the assessment of individual research activity. For each period of six years, professors can present their most relevant publications to the corresponding panel in the hope of obtaining positive assessment. Unlike the evaluation of teaching activities, this evaluation is relatively strict, and 'research periods' are frequently evaluated negatively. Hence, positive assessment has become an internal symbol of prestige among academics, even over formal categories of professorships. But the most important effect is that many universities have established a certain number of positive assessments as a prerequisite for promotion among tenured professors.

Accreditation of contracted staff. The LOU has established a formal system of 'accreditation' for those who are applying for certain contractual positions in a university. The ANECA and other regional agencies are carrying out this procedure with panels of experts that are reviewing the CVs of the candidates. First results are not yet known.

Assessment of teaching, research and managerial activities for regional productivity bonuses. Some regional governments have established systems of global assessments of activities of academic staff to grant their specific productivity bonuses. These procedures are too recent (or are in process of implementation) to be analysed in depth.

As we can observe, academic staff in Spain are frequently assessed by means of several mechanisms. Accreditation may take some results of the assessment of the academic staff as criteria for accrediting programmes but only research assessments are reliable enough to be taken in account.

References

CCU (2002). Informe Final del PNECU, http://www.mec.es/consejou/calidad.

CCU (2003). http://www.mec.es/consejou/estadis/index.html.

CU (1995). Programa de Evaluación Institucional de la Calidad de las Universidades. Madrid: Consejo de Universidades.

CU (several years). Anuario de Estadística Universitaria, Madrid, Consejo de Universidades.

EC (1998). Recommendation, http://europa.eu.int/eur-lex/es/archive/1998.

García, P. , Mora, J. G., Pérez, J. J., & Rodríguez, S. (1995). Experimenting with institutional evaluation in Spain. Higher Education Management, 7, 1, 111-118.

JQI (2002). BaMa Descriptors, http://www.jointquality.org.

Mora, J. G. (1997). Equity in Spanish higher education. Higher Education, 33, 3, 233-249.

Mora, J. G. (1997b). Institutional Evaluation in Spain: an On-going Process. Higher Education Management, 9, 1, 59-70.

Mora, J. G. (2001). The Academic Profession in Spain: between the civil service and the market. Higher Education, 41, 1-2, 131-155.

Mora, J. G., & Vidal, J. (1998). Introducing Quality Assurance in Spanish University. In Gaither, J. (ed.), Quality Assurance in Higher Education, New Directions on Institutional Research, San Francisco, Jossey-Bass.

Mora, J. G., & Villarreal, E. (1996). Funding for Quality: A New Deal in Spanish Higher Education. Higher Education Policy, 9, 2, 175-188.

Mora, J. G., García-Montalvo, J., & Garcia-Aracil, A. (2000). Higher education and graduate employment in Spain, European Journal of Education, 35, 2, 229-237.

Neave, G., & van Vught, F. (1991). Prometheus Bound. Oxford: Pergamon.

Vroeijenstijn, A. I. (1995). Improvement and Accountability: Navigating between Scylla and Charybdis. London: Jessica Kingsley Publisher.

Woodhouse, D. (1996). Quality Assurance: International Trends, Preoccupations and Features. Assessment and Evaluation in Higher Education, 21, 4, 347-356.

20 From Audit to Accreditation-Like Processes: The Case of Sweden

STAFFAN WAHLÉN

20.1 The National Higher Education System in Sweden

20.1.1 Size of the Higher Education System[1]

The higher education system in Sweden has grown considerably in the last ten years. The number of students has increased by over 60 %. In the academic year 2000/01 there were 330,200 students (268,100 full-time equivalent students) in undergraduate education, 72,100 of whom were new entrants. This was the highest number of beginners yet recorded, and numbers grew again in 2002/03. It can be added that the major rise in enrolment has been among students in somewhat older age groups than previously. Three out of every five students are women. Generally speaking, students in higher education are older in Sweden than in many other countries. Over 50 % are 25 years of age or older.

There were 18,100 active postgraduate students, 3,200 of whom were beginners. This is an increase of more than 30 % compared to ten years ago.

Like in most other countries the participation rate has gone up considerably during the last two decades. The government established a goal in the year 2000 of 50 % of 25-year-olds having participated in higher education. This goal was to be reached 'in a few years'. In these terms, the rate was 20 % in 1981/82 and well over 40 % in 2001/02.

20.1.2 Higher Education Institutions

As a result of the 1977 higher education reform a number of new government-funded higher education institutions were established. At present, the higher education sector consists of the following institutions:

The state-run part of the sector comprises eleven universities plus the Karolinska Institute (medicine and health education) and the Royal Institute of Technology, seven independent colleges of visual and performing arts and 16 university colleges,

---

1 Data are from *Swedish Universities and University Colleges. Annual Report 2002*. National Agency for Higher Education and refer to the year 2001, unless otherwise indicated.

S. Schwarz and D.F. Westerheijden (eds.),
Accreditation and Evaluation in the European Higher Education Area, 445–464.
© 2004 *Kluwer Academic Publishers. Printed in the Netherlands.*

including the Stockholm Institute of Education and the Stockholm University College of Physical Education and Sports. Most of these have the right to award Master's degrees, and a few are allowed to award doctors' degrees in certain fields. In all, there are 36 state-run higher education institutions.

Chalmers University of Technology, the Stockholm School of Economics and the University College of Jönköping are run by private sector governing boards. There are also nine smaller private higher education institutions which are specialised in certain areas (health science, theology, music education) and have the right to award certain undergraduate degrees.

20.1.3 Main Types of Degrees

Sweden has a system of credit points. One week of successful full-time studies is equivalent to one credit point. One academic year usually confers 40 credit points.

The government has established which degrees may be awarded by higher education institutions. Undergraduate degrees are divided into general and professional degrees.

General degrees: A *University diploma* ('högskoleexamen') is awarded after at least 80 credit points. A *Bachelor's degree* ('kandidatexamen') is awarded after studies totalling at least 120 credit points, 60 of which must be in the major subject. The major subject must include a thesis comprising at least ten credit points. A *Master's degree* is awarded after studies totalling at least 160 credit points, at least 80 of which must be in the major subject. The major subject must also include a thesis comprising a total of 20 credit points, or two theses of ten credit points each.

Professional degrees: There are some 60 professional degrees of varying length with specific objectives stated in the Degree Ordinance. Medical degrees (220 credit points), engineering degrees (180 credit points), law degrees (180 credit points) and teaching degrees (from 140 to 220 credit points) are some examples.

Postgraduate degrees: A *Doctor's degree* is obtained after studies totalling 160 credit points after a Bachelor's, or more commonly, a Master's degree. The most important part is the thesis, which must comprise at least 80 credit points, but in most cases confers between 100 and 120 credit points.

20.1.4 Main Types of Programmes

Programmes are usually professionally oriented leading to a professional degree (see above). They vary in length from two years (rare) to six years. Most of these programmes are in engineering, teaching and health care, including medicine and different specialities of nursing. Many institutions also develop their own local programmes.

For general degrees (see above) students may combine different courses to design their own degree, provided they follow the general principles regarding the number of credit points and theses. Two-thirds of the students follow this track.

20.1.5   Transition of Students from Higher Education to Work

Most students leave higher education with (the equivalent of) a Bachelor's degree. However, it is difficult to say what proportion continue to the master's level, since it is possible to go straight for a master's degree without the intermediary step of a bachelor. In fact, only 31 % of those who earned a Master's degree in the year 2001 had a previous degree, according to figures from Statistics Sweden. 16 % of those who completed a bachelor's degree went on to further studies in the year 2000.

Recent statistics show that 94 % of those who completed undergraduate education in 1998/99 were working in March 2002. The corresponding share for postgraduate education was 95 %. This is an increase of six percentage points compared to four years earlier. Those with undergraduate or postgraduate degrees were reasonably successful in finding work in an occupational field that corresponded to their education. Approximately 90 % of degree holders were working in the 'right' occupational field.

22 % of women and 18 % of men had been unemployed at some point after they had completed their education. This share has decreased over the past four years, and long-term unemployment among graduates is low. In late 2002 it represented 2.3 % compared to the overall rate of 4.2 %.

There are no reliable statistics on labour market acceptance of different degree types, but it seems that graduates with professional degrees find it reasonably easy to find employment.

There is no professional accreditation of graduates. However, those who are going to work in the health professions require a licence. Those who graduate from health programmes (medicine, nursing, etc.) usually obtain their licences automatically after having completed their degrees. For physicians, however, an internship of 18 months is required, and several other professions have similar demands.

20.1.6   Governance and Steering of Higher Education

Higher education is state-financed. Students do not pay tuition fees, nor does the government have any plans to introduce such fees. Higher education institution boards are appointed by the government, and the majority of their members, including the chairpersons, are external to the institution and usually represent industry, government agencies, trade unions or other organisations. The government also appoints the rector. Parliament (The *Riksdag*) allocates funding for undergraduate education and, where applicable, for postgraduate education and research. The institutions' allocations also include funding for premises. Allocation for undergraduate education is based on the number of students *and* their academic performance.

Each institution is an autonomous government agency reporting directly to the government. The main legal framework regulating the activities of the institutions is contained in the Higher Education Act and the Higher Education Ordinance. On the basis of these documents each institution develops its own rules in accordance with its special needs.

The National Agency for Higher Education was established in 1995 as the national agency for matters relating to higher education institutions. Its tasks include quality assessment, supervision, research and analysis, evaluation of foreign education and provision of study information. It has no role in the allocation of funding.

20.2   Evaluation, Accreditation, and Approval

In Sweden, accreditation, approval and evaluation processes and procedures are very closely linked. It is thus appropriate to begin by briefly describing evaluation schemes and then accreditation and approval schemes.

The major tasks of the National Agency for Higher Education are evaluation and accreditation (approval). As from 1995 it has carried out two major types of evaluations: institutional audit and programme (subject) evaluation. In 1992 a system of validation (approval) of academic professional programmes and degrees was introduced, which was taken over by the Agency in 1995. Since 2001 the Agency has been responsible for a major programme and subject evaluation scheme, which includes accreditation elements.

20.2.1   Institutional Audit

Types of Units

The national academic audit scheme involves all public higher education institutions in Sweden, i.e. the eleven universities plus the Karolinska Institute and the Royal Institute of Technology, the seven independent colleges of visual and performing arts and the 16 university colleges. It also covers the privately run Chalmers University of Technology, the Stockholm School of Economics and the University College of Jönköping.

It includes teaching at both the undergraduate and postgraduate levels and research as well as areas like leadership, administration and decision-making processes and student participation in these processes. Individual subjects and disciplines are not part of the scheme, except as indications of how the institutional quality systems function at that level.

The Actors

As indicated above, it is the National Agency for Higher Education that owns the evaluation process. It may be discussed to what extent the Agency is an independent unit. In the Swedish political context, the government funds the agencies, defines their tasks, and appoints their directors. The government also determines the general orientation of the Agency's tasks. However, it does not control the results of investigations and reports prepared by agencies. Nor can it control the way agencies work or are organised. It can, thus, reasonably be argued that the evaluations of the National Agency are politically independent and that, in fact, it both controls and is in charge of the evaluation scheme.

The review teams usually comprise five or six members. They are academics who hold, or have recently held senior posts, such as rector or dean. At least one member is a representative of external stakeholders. In the case of technological universities, it may be the CEO of an industrial enterprise, in the case of an ordinary university, it may be the head of a public organisation. A student is always included in each team.

The government is a stakeholder of the process. The audit reports do not have financial consequences, but the government, naturally, can draw its own conclusions and use the results as it sees fit. It is clear, also, that students can use the outcome to choose their university, in the same way as enterprises may decide to support or not support a university on the basis of a report. It is, however, unclear, whether this has actually been the case.

Rules and Regulations and their Implementation

So far, there have been two three-year cycles of audits of Swedish higher education institutions. There is currently a moratorium while a six-year evaluation cycle of programmes and subjects is taking place (see below).

The general legal regulations governing evaluation are included in the Higher Education Ordinance. Decisions regarding procedure, the stages of the processes and information on outcomes are left to the National Agency. There is no appeals or objections procedure.

The process is planned over a three-year period, with 13 to 14 institutions audited each year. The timetable is worked out with the institutions. The audit of a particular institution is then launched by the Agency officer in charge, who contacts the management and organises a meeting to begin the process. The institution prepares a self-assessment during some six months. In the meantime, an audit team is appointed by the Agency, which reads the self-assessment report and prepares a site visit, which takes place about two months later. During the site visit, which lasts between two and five days depending on the size and complexity of the institution, the teams meet with various groups within the institution. These groups include the rector and the board, student representatives, faculty representatives, selected departments and units. The main objective is to ascertain how far the institutional quality system functions at various levels. After the site-visit, a report is prepared over a period of two months. It is approved by the Head of the Agency and then made public. The whole process thus takes between ten months and a year.

The printed report is distributed to the government, to all higher education institutions, student organisations and the media. It is also published on the Agency's web site.

20.2.2 Accreditation Schemes

In order to facilitate understanding of the accreditation processes in Sweden it is necessary to describe further the degree-awarding rights of universities and university colleges. The 1993 Higher Education Act gave universities the right to award all degrees including doctoral degrees, whereas the university colleges were only allowed to award Bachelor's degrees. The right to award professional degrees is limited to specific universities and university colleges.

There are two major kinds of accreditation schemes carried out by the National Agency for Higher Education. One, which was introduced in 1992, is initiated by an institution that wants to upgrade its right to award degrees from a Bachelor to a Master or to award a professional degree. Both kinds involve a yes-or-no decision by the Agency. For questions concerning the right to award doctoral degrees and the upgrading of a university college to university status, the evaluation is made by the Agency and the decision is taken by the government. It should be noted that the purpose of this kind of accreditation activity is to establish whether the institution in question provides education of at least minimum standard for the degree in question.

The other scheme is a six-year cycle of programme and subject evaluation which began in 2001. For each programme evaluated, a decision is made as to whether the institutions in question will be allowed to retain the right to award degrees in the specific field.

Accreditation on the Basis of Application

Since 2001, all university colleges except those of visual and performing arts, two others and the private colleges have been granted the right to award Master's degrees. Thus, most applications today are for the right to award professional degrees, the right to award doctoral degrees in certain areas or being granted university status. In the latter two cases research and postgraduate training naturally constitute a large part of the basis for evaluation. When it comes to accrediting undergraduate programmes the level and extent of research activities are also a criterion, in addition to teaching and infrastructure.

This scheme applies to any subject/discipline or programme, depending on the needs and ambitions of the institution.

The stakeholders are the institution applying for the right to award and the students wishing to obtain the degree in question. The (local) employers are also concerned. It is taken for granted that the institution investigates the needs of the particular programme before launching an application process.

The reviewers are appointed by the Agency, which owns, controls and is in charge of the implementation of the scheme. Thus, the reviewers are appointed by the Agency. They consist of subject experts from other Swedish higher education institutions than the one that is applying. In some cases, a student is also a member of the review team.

It is clear that the government is a customer. In cases of applications for postgraduate degrees and university status, a positive outcome will also lead to costs that have to be met by the state. Again, the students and local employers may be beneficiaries of a new degree.

The Higher Education Ordinance states which degrees are awarded at which institutions. Any institution that wishes to award a degree which it is not eligible to award must apply to the National Agency, and once the degree has been accredited, it will be included in the Ordinance. The procedural rules were first established by the National Agency in 1992 and have been progressively revised since then. They include the following stages:

1. Application by institution.
2. Appointment of the evaluation team.
3. Site visit to confirm (or not) the impression of the application.
4. Report including decision by the Chancellor of the Swedish Universities.

There are no formally established rules for the duration of the process, nor is there any formal way of appeal against the decision. The information is publicly available in a report, to be found on the Agency website, and sometimes in a printed version.

It is one of the tasks of the Agency to carry out evaluations leading to accreditation of programmes and subjects/disciplines. Thus, the costs of experts, including their fees and travel expenses, are met by the Agency. Other costs, e.g. preparing the application, arranging the site-visit, have to be paid for by the institution.

Over the years, the practical application of these principles has changed somewhat. For example, today there is usually not one group for each evaluation/accreditation, but a single one for each broad subject area (e.g. teacher education), which is summoned whenever a specific application is submitted. The time frame from application to decision is generally about three to four months. It varies, however according to the complexity and size of the task.

Application for University Status

Since 1995, university colleges have had the right to apply for full or partial university status.

As in the process described above, the institution applying for university status and its students are the most important stakeholders. The (local and regional) employers and business and industry are also concerned. The government, too, has a legitimate interest in developing advanced research and higher education across the country. At the same time, it is aware that a positive outcome leads to additional costs that have to be met by the state. So the government has to balance the ambition to develop research and higher education and the need to keep within the budgetary frames.

A number of university colleges have adopted a vision stating that they intend to attain university status by a certain year. This means that they base their development and action plans on this vision and strive to achieve the necessary research excellence.

The process as a whole is owned by the government and the institution submits its application to it. The government also makes the final decision. The evaluation process is owned by the Agency, which controls the scheme and is in charge of its implementation. Thus, the reviewers are appointed by the Agency. They consist of Swedish and international experts, from Swedish higher education institutions other than the one applying. In some cases a student is also a member of the review team.

Accreditation as Part of Programme and Subject Evaluation

In the year 2001, a new model of national reviews of higher education was introduced. All undergraduate subjects/disciplines and national programmes of higher education at all higher education institutions in Sweden were to be evaluated over a period of six years in a comparative perspective. The corresponding postgraduate programmes were also to be included in this process. Research was not, however, to be included in the exercise, partly since evaluation of research is the task of another organisation, the Swedish Research Council.

The general idea behind the exercise as well as the general structure were developed by the government and presented in a government Bill (government Bill 1999/2000: 28). The purpose was to provide a detailed picture of the quality (as opposed to quality assurance and quality enhancement activities) of Swedish higher education institutions. The scheme was partly a result of student pressure and student needs. Students had complained that the quality audits provided information on what measures higher education institutions take to ensure the quality of their activities but not on the quality of the various subjects. Other interested parties in this debate were the government itself and other stakeholders such as employers.

There are no specific legal regulations governing the evaluations/accreditations other than the government bill stating that there should be a programme/subject evaluation system with an accreditation element.

The details of the scheme were worked out by the National Agency in co-operation with the institutions, but it is the Agency that owns the procedure and makes the decisions and is in charge of the activities. Thus, the Agency appoints the reviewers after consultations with the institutions. The reviewers are subject experts from Sweden and, to a large extent, from other Nordic countries.

The costs of the review teams are met by the Agency. The institutions and departments have to foot the bill for the self-evaluations (see below) as well as for the time the staff spends on various preparatory meetings and meetings with the review teams. This has caused a certain amount of irritation on the part of some institutions and departments, which maintain (in vain) that this is an extra burden added to their already heavy workload and should be financed by supplementary funding.

The procedure follows a familiar pattern:

- Self-assessment by the department (or other unit in charge of the subject, discipline or programme). The self-assessment is supported by guidelines prepared by the Agency in consultation with the institutions. The guidelines outline quality aspects that are considered to be especially important for higher education provision (see below). The self-assessment phase results in a report submitted to the Agency.

- An external review team is appointed by the Agency. There are consultations with the institutions to ascertain that there are no conflicts of interest. Each team must include prominent teachers/researchers, a student, a postgraduate student and, in relevant cases, a representative of stakeholders (employers, etc.). A chairperson is appointed for each team, and an Agency official functions as project leader and secretary.

- The review team reads the self-evaluation report and conducts an on-site visit in order to check the impressions given by the self-evaluation report in discussions with members of staff, students and faculty administration.
- A report containing a formal decision by the Chancellor of the Swedish Universities on each institution's right to award the relevant degree (accreditation decision). It is not possible to appeal against the decision. The report also provides recommendations for the further development of the subject. It is printed and widely distributed and also put on the Agency's website with an English summary.
- After three months a national conference on the review is held with the participation of the institutions involved in the review and the accreditation procedure. After another two to three years there is a follow-up.
- The formal duration of the whole process is one year.

The actual process is to a considerable extent carried out in consultation with the institutions. As has been pointed out above, this applies to the practical application of the model, such as the timetable for the exercise. Before the review process was initiated, the Agency identified the various programmes, disciplines or subjects offered at the various institutions. The great variety of nomenclature and structure necessitated close co-operation between the Agency and the institutions in this task. Thus, similar programmes are offered at different institutions under different names, and similar names are sometimes used for different programmes. An entity reviewed could be a subject or discipline (History or French or Computer Science). It could be a programme or set of programmes such as engineering or teacher education. Before the evaluation process of a particular area is initiated there is another check that the programmes, etc. involved are actually comparable.

In the six-year programme each programme, subject or discipline is evaluated in the same period at all the institutions that provide it in order to give an overall picture of that area at a given time. The overall timetable for the process, i.e. which programme is to be evaluated/accredited which year, is prepared in co-operation between the Agency and the institutions and is revised, whenever necessary. There will typically be ten to twelve programmes, etc. (defined broadly) reviewed each year.

The process begins each year in October/November with meetings between the Agency officers and the departments from the various institutions responsible for the specific programmes under review. At these meetings, the various elements of the review process are described and discussed, and the departments are given the possibility to influence the time frame (within reason) and the actual implementation, such as the order in which they are to be visited. The general guidelines are adapted to the special needs of each subject. The departments are also given the opportunity to provide names of suitable members of review teams, but it must be emphasised that the Agency makes the final decision in this respect.

As a basis for the self-evaluations and for the review a set of aspects has been developed over the years, which are regarded as fundamental for higher education processes. These aspects, which are covered in each assessment, include:

- Prerequisites for educational programmes
  - Recruitment of students and different student groups: students' prior knowledge, competition for study places, composition of student body with regard to gender, age, social and ethnic background.
  - Teacher competence including teaching skills, research expertise, leadership and administration; provision of opportunities for staff development.
  - Goals, contents and organisation of programme or courses: development and renewal.
  - Library and other information support.
  - Facilities and equipment.
- Educational process
  - Teaching and learning and students' working situation: teaching methods adapted to student needs. Support and supervision of undergraduate and postgraduate theses.
  - Teachers' working situation and responsibilities with regard to teaching, research and administration.
  - Programme structure: links to current research, integration of theoretical and applied knowledge and relevance for future professional life. International aspects.
  - Examination modes.
  - A critical and creative environment for learning.
  - Departments' own quality assurance and enhancement. National and international networking.
- Results of education
  - The departments' system for the monitoring of courses and programmes and the results evidenced by the system. National and international benchmarks.
  - Quality of examination results, especially undergraduate theses.
  - The departments' system for follow-up of quality assurance activities, follow-up of former students and their professional success, questionnaires to employers and the results evidenced by the system.
  - Pass rates.

The size of the review teams varies according to the size of the undertaking. In the case of, for example, Archaeology, it would consist of one chairperson, two other academics, one student, one postgraduate student, one other stakeholder representative and an Agency project leader. Other, larger, areas will have several co-operating teams and a co-steering group.

The first two years of the six-year cycle have shown that one year is often not enough for the completion of a review. It is our experience that from the first meeting between the Agency and the departments, which may be described as the kick-off of the self-evaluations and the whole project, it takes about 16 months to reach the decision and publish the report. In most cases it is the sheer number of site-visits that causes the prolongation. Often, one group will have to visit 20 institutions across the country, a process that in itself takes between two and three months.

Before being published, the report is checked with the departments for factual content. In the cases of institutions threatened with 'de-accreditation' information is given to the rector three days in advance of the formal decision. A decision on 'de-accreditation' gives the institution the chance to submit an action plan within six months for the improvement of those conditions that are deemed unacceptable. In the case of Bachelor's and Master's degrees, the right to award the degree in question is revoked if the action plan is unacceptable or if measures have not been taken within a certain specified period of time. This has not happened in the present system. Only the government has the power to give or revoke the right to award doctors' degrees. That has not yet happened, and the rules for that eventuality are still unclear.

Accreditation by Non-Government Affiliated Accreditor

The subject of accreditation in higher education is discussed widely in certain educational sectors in Sweden. This is particularly true of business studies and engineering. So far, the only non-official organisation that has been successful in gaining access to the Swedish higher education market is EQUIS (European Quality Improvement System), a European organisation that accredits business schools. The purpose of this kind of accreditation is to ascertain whether the schools in question offer an internationally comparable high standard provision, and, if they do, to give them the distinction of accreditation. So far, three Swedish business programmes (schools) have been approved by EQUIS. A Public Administration programme was recently accredited by the European Association for Public Administration Accreditation (EAPAA).

20.2.3   Approval Schemes Other than Accreditation Schemes

It is a matter of definition whether in Swedish higher education there are schemes to approve subjects, programmes or institutions without accreditation. One arrangement may possibly be described as involving such a procedure. It concerns the approval of foreign institutions for the purpose of giving Swedish students the right to receive state study assistance.

The scheme is a collaborative undertaking between the Swedish National Board of Student Aid and the National Agency for Higher Education. A student who wants to study abroad may apply for a state study grant for studies at a foreign institution. If it is a well-known institution which is already in the files of the Board, a positive answer will be given (provided that the student fulfils the other requirements for assistance). If the institution is not recognised by the Board, the National Agency for Higher Education carries out an investigation to find out whether it is recognised by the higher education authorities in its own country and what status it is considered to have. The decision on whether to accept the provision by the institution or not is based on that information.

20.3   Analysis of the Relationship between the Range, Actors and Rules and Regulations of the Processes

20.3.1   Accreditation on the Basis of Application

Driving Forces

When the accreditation model was introduced in 1992, it was intended to provide an opportunity for the smaller university colleges to offer higher undergraduate and, possibly, postgraduate programmes. It was thus an ambition of the *government* to develop higher education in all parts of the country and to improve the participation rate. It can thus be seen as an incentive to improve regional development.

It was also seen by the government and the *National Agency* as a guarantee that programmes at higher undergraduate and postgraduate levels were not initiated unless their quality was more or less equivalent to that offered at traditional institutions. Thus, the review teams were, and still are, mostly made up of representatives of such institutions, normally professors of high standing. This has been a matter of debate in some circles, since they are sometimes seen as preservers of tradition, sceptical of new education and research structures, and it has been questioned whether the teams should not also always include academics teaching at the undergraduate level.

The Political Agenda

There is in Sweden, like in most countries, a continual debate on (higher) education. When the university colleges were first built up in the late 1970s and the 1980s the discussion focused on quality versus opportunity. The government aimed to establish a unitary system, and it was thus necessary to ensure that the system was consistent. In this light, one can wonder why the accreditation model based on application was not introduced until 1992. However, the year 1992 saw the beginning of a major expansion of higher education and greater institutional autonomy. Against that background, it was necessary to have an instrument to control the development of higher education institutions.

It can, in fact, be shown that the university colleges have contributed quite substantially to economic and social development in the regions. At the same time, there are, of course those who have argued that the money needed to develop the new institutions would have been better spent on developing further research and education at established universities. This, indeed, is an additional reason for developing a quality assurance system. As will be discussed below, the implications of the current quality assurance system have been different for universities and university colleges.

Consequences for Higher Education Institutions, Scholars and Students

For the *university colleges* the possibility of applying for the right to award higher degrees was important. The scheme was very clearly seen as a means to develop teaching and research, thus leading to a higher degree of legitimacy nationally and possibly internationally and was thus an important incentive for them. As has been pointed out above, the ambitions of many of the university colleges have gradually increased, and several aimed to be upgraded to university status.

For these institutions it is also a means to attract more and better students. All higher education institutions are national, but students are mainly recruited regionally. With more attractive programmes accredited for higher levels of study it becomes possible to recruit good students both from the region and from the whole country, and, possibly from abroad. It may also contribute to the possibility of creating an academic environment which may attract good scholars and teachers. But not all large universities are happy about the competition created by the new institutions. More resources for them means less money for the universities.

The accreditation scheme gives the *scholars* at the new institutions the chance of conducting more and better research and provides more research-based teaching in those areas that are accredited.

Students who are already studying at the university college have the advantage of being able to pursue studies at higher levels without having to transfer to a university. The drawback is, of course, that the system does not encourage academic mobility.

Other stakeholders include regional authorities and regional business and industry. As has been mentioned above, they have benefited from the development of 'their' university colleges through better opportunities to recruit graduates with higher degrees.

20.3.2   Accreditation as Part of Subject or Programme Evaluation

Driving Forces

There are three essential elements behind the establishment of the evaluation/accreditation system in the year 2001.

The first is the concern for academic quality, especially regarding undergraduate and graduate education (research has its own quality assurance system). This was, in fact, one of the most important reasons for introducing an audit system already in 1995. The argument, in Sweden, like in other countries, is that if the higher education institutions are largely autonomous organisations financed by the government, there must be an assurance that the taxpayers' money going into higher education is well spent and that the goals are met. At the same time, the system must be sufficiently flexible to contribute to development. This ambivalent relationship is important, but difficult to maintain. It is argued, in particular, that an accreditation scheme that is applied to all institutions may lead to standardisation in an environment that requires diversity to develop.

The second is concern for students. The academic audit model assesses the institutions' own quality assurance, which does not provide students with information on quality at the discipline/programme level in a comparative perspective. The decision to focus on the programme/subject level and to include an accreditation element was prompted by an enquiry on student influence and satisfaction. The report found, amongst other things, that students' need for information required a different evaluation policy. The National Agency for Higher Education was charged with developing and implementing such a policy.

The third is international legitimacy and student mobility. In particular, the accreditation processes in the United Kingdom and the United States have sometimes caused problems for Swedish graduates to find employment or even to conduct postgraduate studies in those countries with a Swedish undergraduate degree.

The Political Agenda

There is a domestic debate on accreditation and ranking of higher education institutions and programmes. Several professional organisations (see above under Accreditation on the basis of application) and a few political parties have argued that accreditation is a necessary tool for both graduates and employers and that it has to be carried out by 'independent' organisations. The question is what is meant by 'independent'. There is a case for maintaining that neither professional organisations nor a government-financed institution such as the National Agency for Higher Education are fully independent.

Swedish magazines have conducted a few rankings of institutions, a few business schools have been accredited by an external body (EQUIS), and one school of public administration has undergone a similar process. These activities play a certain role in the debate, but there are no signs that they will develop into a major force (see also under *Sweden, Bologna and GATS*).

There is a national debate on the quality differences between universities and university colleges and the need to establish that degree programmes which do not provide minimum quality are not offered. Not least, the universities have maintained that the quality of university colleges is not high enough and that the money spent on keeping them alive would be much better spent on improving the budgets of the large universities. This is to a certain extent also a political debate.

The introduction of the ambitious evaluation/accreditation system is meant to solve some of the problems raised in this debate. It is true that the evaluations/accreditation reports are not the basis of rankings of either institutions or programmes/disciplines. However, they can be used to gather information at the national level on several aspects that could be considered to be significant quality indicators. The reports also give assurance that degrees are not awarded in programmes that do not provide minimum quality. As is pointed out below, there is, however, no consensus on the question of quality indicators.

Consequences for Higher Education Institutions, Departments and Scholars

So far, out of a total of about 200 degree programmes, the right to award degrees has been questioned in 14 cases. This has led to a debate and criticism of the method used and the criteria applied. But it has also resulted in hectic activity on the part of the universities concerned, and action plans have been submitted. In no case has the right to award a degree actually been revoked. In a few cases, the universities in question are now discussing whether to close them down themselves. Follow-up studies by the Agency also show that measures have been taken in other fields, as a result of the evaluations. In that sense, the scheme can be regarded as successful.

The general structure of the methodology as described in Section 20.2 above was established from the outset. The criteria and implementation were, however, discussed in meetings between representatives of institutions and the National Agency. Similar meeting are still held annually in order to come to an agreement about possible revisions. One debate concerns the standards by which programmes and disciplines are judged. University colleges maintain that they are evaluated according to standards that apply to large universities and that the particular advantages for smaller institutions are not always considered. One example is the better chances to develop cross-disciplinary programmes and interdisciplinary research. The members of the review committees are often professors from well-established universities, who may (consciously or unconsciously) apply these standards. This is a problem that will have to be solved. It may be added that universities, too, sometimes offer education in small environments without always making use of the possibilities of their resources.

For higher education institutions the introduction of the scheme has in many cases resulted in additional work, and led to complaints from many quarters. It could be maintained that institutions ought to have their own systems to ensure the quality of their educational provision. Some institutions have concluded that the establishment of the accreditation system has made such measures unnecessary. But all institutions have had to build up structures to support the departments' handling of the self-evaluations, and, perhaps more importantly, to utilise the results of the accreditation/evaluation reports, whether they be negative or positive, and to include these results in their overall planning. It is worth noting that this has been done in a number of cases. The universities and university colleges have also been able to compare their provision with that of other institutions. This was not possible before.

The implementation of the model has in several respects been more problematic for the universities than for the university colleges. As has been discussed above, the latter have become used to similar processes over a period of ten years, in addition to regular academic audits. They have benefited from the chance to offer higher degrees, and thus improve their status in the system. The universities, on the other hand, have become used to being subjected to the audits once every three years, and to other evaluation activities, unless they have initiated them themselves. And the internal administration of a considerable number of more or less simultaneous accreditation processes including self-evaluations, site visits and follow-up is probably more cumbersome for them. It comes as no surprise that there is currently a discussion in the universities and some university colleges on a simplified model that focuses on results rather than on processes.

For the departments the scheme has also meant additional obligations in a context of diminishing resources per full-time student equivalent. Some have complained and demanded extra funding for self-evaluations and other tasks involved. A number of scholars have noted that the extra work involved has increased their workload. But it has also been pointed out that the self-evaluations (more than the accreditation reports) have contributed to self-reflection and improvement of the educational programmes. The possibility of comparing their own provision and achievement with those of other departments is also seen as an added bonus.

Consequences for Students and Other Stakeholders

The scheme has probably made it easier for students to make an informed choice of where to study. The information about accreditation decisions and quality judgements is publicly available in print and on the Agency' website, which has a special site for this purpose.

Currently, however, the Agency has no knowledge of the extent to which and how students actually use the information. But they have been given an instrument to contribute to the improvement of their own environment and study conditions by participating in self-evaluations.

Projections for the Future

Reviews have an impact as soon as an evaluation is initiated, and when the results are published things may already have changed considerably. The time between the initiation of an accreditation project and the publication of a report is about 15 months. It is therefore essential, that higher education institutions and the National Agency publish current data regularly. It is foreseen that institutions will take this responsibility and that, in future, the Agency (or perhaps several organisations) may evaluate and accredit institutions on the basis of their ability to meet this responsibility.

Students (and other stakeholders) have maintained that the information they are given is still not sufficient, and that the reports are too bland. There is thus, on the one hand, pressure to intensify the process, and on the other to conduct the activities in a way that is less costly for the institutions. Any future change will have to take this conflict into consideration.

20.4 Accreditation and Evaluation Schemes in Relation to Europe and Globalisation

20.4.1 Sweden, Bologna and GATS

The accreditation and evaluation schemes in Sweden are clearly influenced by ideas regarding the development of higher education in Europe. As a member of the European Network for Quality Assurance in Higher Education (ENQA), Sweden has participated in several projects on these themes. The most recent example is the development of a method to ensure the quality of quality assurance agencies (ENQA Occasional Paper no 4, 2002). The Dutch/Flemish Joint Quality Initiative is also part of the new debate on quality assurance.

The European and international character of Swedish higher education is reasonably well developed and the evaluations/accreditations have many international perspectives. The National Agency for Higher Education makes considerable efforts to recruit European members of evaluation teams, although, for language reasons, they tend mostly to come from other Nordic countries.

Further, the emerging Bologna degree system will no doubt also influence Sweden, although the changes which will have to be introduced are not of a magnitude that needs special attention in accreditation schemes, as is the case in other countries. However, the Ministry of Education is now conducting an enquiry into the degree structure, which may lead to an adaptation to the system now being developed across Europe.

The GATS agreements are being discussed, but it is not clear what consequence they will have for Swedish higher education and accreditation.

20.4.2 Sweden and European and International Examples of Accreditation/ Evaluation Models

When first developing its evaluation system in the mid-1990s, Sweden made an inventory of various models across Europe (in particular the Netherlands and the United Kingdom), the United States and Canada. Also, the European pilot project 1994–1996, in which Sweden participated, was of importance.

It is obvious that the models applied in this country are now quite similar to those of many other countries and that they may be described as eclectic. Thus, the use of self-evaluation is a common feature and the peer review team has been used in the evaluation of research across the world for a long time. The public report is also common in many European and other nations. The current Swedish model is probably, however, unusual in that it aims to cover the entire degree system in a comparative perspective. European co-operation within the framework of ENQA has contributed to further co-operation among agencies. This does not necessarily lead to the adoption of exactly the same types of evaluation models, as can be seen from, for example, the different approaches applied in the Nordic countries. But it does contribute to mutual understanding and partial adoption of the methodology of other countries.

20.5 Other Quality Assessment Activities in Higher Education

There are a number of examples of different kinds of assessments carried out locally by the higher education institutions. Besides local quality assessment of subjects or programmes, they may concern, for example, staff policies and student or teacher satisfaction. At the national level there are a few other assessment activities within the sphere of higher education. Two examples can be mentioned here.

The first is a national student survey based on questionnaires distributed to a large number of students at all the higher education institutions called 'Through Student Eyes'. It is a survey of various aspects of quality in higher education, including the extent to which higher education promotes learning and personal development.

Other characteristics of teaching and learning are also examined, such as critical thinking, analytical capacity, examinations, oral and written fluency and degree of commitment to studies. The survey will be repeated every second year in order to follow trends and developments. A similar study of the working conditions of academic staff will be published shortly and one on postgraduate students is just being launched.

The second is thematic evaluations of aspects of teaching and learning and conditions in higher education institutions. They concern internationalisation, gender equality, social and ethnic diversity and the ways in which these are considered. These evaluations are carried out in a similar manner to academic audits. Thus, institutions write self-evaluations on the basis of instructions issued by the Agency. An expert review team is appointed by the Agency after consultations with the institutions. They go through the self-evaluations and visit all institutions over a limited period of time to obtain a comparative view of the state of affairs. The team writes a report which is published and discussed at a conference to which institution representatives are invited. On one occasion, the three institutions which were considered most successful were specially commended.

21   Accreditation and Related Regulatory Matters in the United Kingdom

JOHN BRENNAN & RUTH WILLIAMS

21.1   UK Higher Education

There are currently nearly 2 million students studying in the UK's 167 higher education institutions. This reflects substantial growth and diversification during the 1990s. Of the more than 160 institutions, 132 are in England of which 77 are universities, 14 are general colleges and 41 are specialist colleges, e.g. in music or art and design. There are 14 universities in Scotland and four higher education colleges. Wales has a federal university with eight constituent colleges, one other university and four colleges. Northern Ireland has two universities. The UK universities include the former polytechnics and some higher education colleges 'upgraded' to university status in 1992/93. Of the 2 million students studying in UK higher education in 2000/01, 1.5 million were undergraduates (mainly bachelor's programmes) of whom just over 1 million studied full-time. Of nearly half a million postgraduate students, 172,000 were full-time and 276,000 were part-time. Over 100,000 of the postgraduate students were from overseas. Participation of the age cohort stands at 43 % and the government target is to reach at least 50 % by 2012.

The status of UK universities is of private institutions that are funded substantially by public funds (only the small University of Buckingham is fully private.) As such, they have traditionally enjoyed high degrees of institutional autonomy with funding being the major regulatory tool available to government. Other higher education institutions have traditionally had closer ties with local tiers of government although these were loosened in the late 1980s as part of the more general Thatcherite attack on local government. The post-1992 universities (former polytechnics) have governing bodies that must accord with certain statutory requirements but these, as with the councils of the older pre-1992 universities, are self-reproducing and not subject to any direct state control. Additionally, more than 10 % of higher education is conducted in colleges that are formally part of the 'further education' system. This is the terminology used to refer to post-school education below the level of higher education. But many colleges contain a mixture of 'further' and 'higher'.

The main degree types are the three- or four-year bachelor's degree (the normal first degree), the master's degree and the PhD. There are differences in Scotland (see below). Master's degrees have typically been of two sorts: the one-year 'taught' master's degree and the two-year 'research' master's degree. The doctorate would

S. Schwarz and D.F. Westerheijden (eds.),
Accreditation and Evaluation in the European Higher Education Area, 465–490.
© 2004 *Kluwer Academic Publishers. Printed in the Netherlands.*

normally be three years following a bachelor's degree although initial registration for a master's would be the normal route to a doctorate. These are all full-time durations and all degrees are also available by part-time study over longer periods. In Scotland, reflecting a different education system at school level and the fact that traditionally Scottish students entered higher education a year younger than those elsewhere in the UK. Initial study of four years to an honours bachelor's degree has been the norm although there is also a three-year 'ordinary' bachelor's degree. This contrasts with the 'honours' bachelor's degree after three years in other parts of the UK. The honours classification of the UK bachelor's degree is an important element as it is a crucial indicator of academic achievement and subsequent employment opportunities. Recently, considerable emphasis has been given to a new two-year qualification: the Foundation degree. Two-year higher education qualifications are not entirely new. Higher National Diplomas and Certificates have existed for a long time as has a two-year Diploma in Higher Education. Most of these qualifications have a vocational emphasis and are meant to provide direct routes into employment as well as entry routes into higher level programmes. An attempt to bring a greater degree of order into the qualifications structure has seen the creation of the 'national qualifications frameworks' (see section 21.2.4).

It is important to emphasise that matters of programme type and content are left to the judgements of individual institutions although attempts to introduce some degree of conformity have recently been made with the introduction of 'subject benchmarks'. That said, programmes may be organised along academic subject lines or professional/vocational lines. A very common development during the 1990s was the introduction of modular degree programmes (along with semesterisation) that afforded individual students considerable choice over what to study and the possibility of constructing unique programmes reflecting personal interests and aptitudes. There may be a shift away from this approach following criticisms of its consequences for both the academic and the social aspects of the student experience.

Around 60 % of students go straight into the labour market after the bachelor's degree and approximately 7 % are unemployed or seeking further study or training. Many of the rest take postgraduate courses of one sort or another. Particularly common are diplomas linked to entry to professions such as teaching or social work where possession of a diploma is a pre-requisite for entry. Other postgraduate courses (e.g. in areas such as law, accountancy and engineering) are linked to the entry requirements of particular professional and statutory bodies (PSBs). Some would regard these courses as postgraduate 'in time' rather than postgraduate 'in level'. Other postgraduate courses may have less clear labour market links but may still possess considerable vocational relevance, for example courses in information technology or in aspects of business management. There is very little long-term unemployment of graduates although the transition from higher education into suitable graduate-level employment can take a few years for some. The higher education-labour market linkage in the labour market is a looser one in the UK than in many European countries. Many labour market opportunities for graduates are not regulated by specific qualification requirements and employers regard degrees as evidence of the broad levels of ability and competence of the holders rather than a specific occupational competence. That said, there has been considerable emphasis in recent years on making graduates 'more employable' through a variety of curriculum and other initiatives.

As stated above, UK higher education institutions have traditionally enjoyed much greater autonomy from the state than has been common in other parts of Europe. It follows therefore that considerable powers rest with their governing bodies. These differ between the old (pre-1992) and new (post-1992) universities. In the case of the old universities, the constitution of the governing body or council is defined in the university's Charter and Statutes. These differ between institutions. The University Commissioners (a government body) reviewed these around 1990 and produced a model statute. The aim was to remove excessive variation between university governing bodies on matters such as size, powers, membership, etc. But its recommendations were only advisory. One important symbolic (and rarely practical) aspect of old university statutes is the role of the 'visitor' (often the Queen). The visitor is the ultimate authority on matters of complaint and appeal by members (staff and students) of the university.

In new universities, the authority of the visitor is vested in the governing body itself, i.e. they must resolve matters of appeal and complaint within the university. (There may of course be ultimate recourse to a court of law.) The powers and composition of the governing bodies of new universities were defined in the 1992 Education Act, building on the 1988 Act which gave the former 'public' local authority run polytechnics the status of independent (private) corporations. A major difference between them and the pre-1992 universities lies in the absence of senates, or bodies of equivalent authority, in the latter. The equivalent advisory boards of new universities ultimately only have advisory status.

However, most people working in higher education would claim that it has been steadily eroded in recent years. The introduction of new national quality assurance arrangements is widely considered to be an important aspect of that erosion. Greater accountability in state funding arrangements would be another. Although high levels of institutional autonomy have been a traditional feature of higher education in the UK, this should not be confused with the autonomy of the individual academic. While this is also generally regarded as high, it is also the case that institutional power is greater than in many HE systems, and the individual professor will be constrained by the collegial, and increasingly managerial, authority of his/her institution.

21.2   Accreditation and Other Schemes

21.2.1   Accreditation

'Accreditation' is not a widely used term in UK higher education, being mainly associated with the work of (some of) the professional bodies and (some of) the university arrangements for approving courses in non-university institutions without their own powers to award degrees. Professional bodies evaluate programmes in their particular fields and this leads to an approval by the professional body. This approval relates to the labour market status of the qualification awarded, in particular whether a 'licence to practise' is involved, in whole or in part. It does not relate to the programme itself. Non-university institutions without the power to award their own degrees must seek 'validation' from a university or other degree-awarding institution. Universities are both responsible for the evaluation and the subsequent formal approval of their own degrees. These responsibilities and evaluations by individual universities also extend to the degrees of any higher education colleges or other organisations which prepare students for the degrees of the 'accrediting' or 'validating' (the more commonly used term) university. Thus, university X will review the programmes in college Y prior to their formal approval by the university.

Accreditation of Programmes by Professional and Statutory Bodies (PSBs)

Professional and statutory bodies are organisations that approve or recognise specific programmes which lead to a professional qualification or licence to practise. Many such bodies receive their authority from the Crown on the advice of the Privy Council, which may also be involved in other matters such as the approval of regulations. Accreditation of programmes of study that lead to a professional title (for example, law, medicine and the various branches of engineering) is carried out by PSBs. Accreditation is intended to ensure that a programme of study provides some, or all, of the competencies needed for professional practice. This leads to an approval decision and recognition that in some cases carries statutory weight. However, it is important to understand that this does not affect the course's right to exist. The university's right to offer courses as it thinks fit is not limited. Qualifications awarded to students on completion of courses not recognised by the appropriate professional body might well be of limited value in the labour market but the situation varies between occupational areas. Such a qualification (i.e. not recognised by the professional body) might well be sought after, especially if it was awarded by a prestigious university.

PSBs have a number of roles which will vary according to the individual PSB. Among the roles are the following:

- specifying the nature of the education and training required for entry to the profession
- assessing required knowledge, competence and values
- ensuring the suitability of providers of professional education and training
- specifying continuous professional development.

PSBs will vary in terms of their involvement in higher education and the accreditation of programmes of study. Most PSBs accredit programmes of study while others, to a much lesser extent, will accredit centres or schools of higher education institutions.

PSBs are concerned with curriculum content of both initial and professional education and training. Many, however, will also take into account the wider institutional environment, such as resources and internal quality assurance processes. Minimum standards are specified at the initial level whereas more detailed specifications are made at the professional level. Over the last decade or so there has been a growing tendency for PSBs to delegate the provision of 'suitable' initial level education to higher education institutions. However, most will undertake initial accreditation visits (while a minority will limit their involvement to desk exercises). Re-accreditation reviews take place from anything between two to ten years depending on the PSB, although the common time frame is five yearly. Most reviews take the form of a visit and these make use of peer review procedures.

Professional bodies) are different from statutory bodies. Statutory bodies (e.g., General Medical Council and English National Board for Nursing, Midwifery and Health Visiting) are established by the government, mostly through statute, to exercise control over a particular profession. Unlike professional bodies (e.g., the Royal Institute of British Architects), they do not offer membership to professional practitioners, although some maintain a register of practitioners. Professional bodies are of two sorts: 'those for which membership is compulsory for practice within the profession (such as solicitors) and those where membership is advantageous but where it is possible to practice without being a member of the professional body (such as electrical engineers)'. Professional bodies have authority to withdraw accreditation whereas statutory bodies must recommend to the Privy Council that a qualification from a higher education institution should no longer be registered.

In the recent past, some PSBs conducted their reviews in conjunction with subject review undertaken by the Quality Assurance Agency for Higher Education (QAA). The recent changes in QAA procedures from subject review to institutional audit (see section 21.2.4) imply that some PSBs that relied on QAA subject review will now need to involve themselves in their own review visits. What form this will take remains to be seen – the following statement was made in a HEFCE document regarding the new arrangements:

It will be for each PSB to determine, in consultation with higher education institutions and the QAA, whether it undertakes such reviews separately from the arrangements covered by this paper, or as reviews undertaken jointly with the QAA. Opportunities for collaborative arrangements between individual PSBs and the QAA will continue to be explored and encouraged. Where such reviews are conducted in accordance with the QAA method, they could form part of – rather than being undertaken in addition to – other separate reviews.

The approach taken to accreditation varies from PSB to PSB. Two examples are provided below, one for law and the other for engineering.

(1) The Law Profession. The law profession comprises separate two bodies, one for solicitors and the other for barristers. Different bodies represent the different countries of the UK, reflecting the differences in the legal systems. In England and Wales, the *solicitors'* professional body is the Law Society; in Scotland and Northern Ireland, the professional bodies are separate but take the same name. The *barristers'* professional body is the General Council of the Bar and there are separate bodies for England and Wales, and Northern Ireland; in Scotland, it is known as the Faculty of Advocates. The professions are responsible for laying down the qualification regulations governing those seeking to qualify as a solicitor or barrister. The following sections describe the system operating in England and Wales.

To qualify as a solicitor or barrister, there are two stages: i) the academic stage and ii) the vocational stage[1]. One of the main routes for completing the academic stage is through the law degree where the 'seven foundations of legal knowledge' must be studied and passed. (The other routes are via a non-law degree supplemented by the Common Professional Examination or a Postgraduate Diploma in Law, and the non-graduate route.) The law degree must be of a standard, which has been approved by The Law Society.

The Law Society and Bar Council act jointly in respect of the initial or academic stage of training. In a joint statement of 1999 (effective from 2001), the two bodies will recognise a programme of study as satisfying the requirements of the academic stage if a number of conditions are met by a higher education institution. These condition include the following:

•   Are adequate learning resources provided?
•   Does the institution have degree awarding powers conferred by the Privy Council?

---

1   The vocational stage comprises the Bar Vocational Course for barristers and the Legal Practice Course for solicitors. Both are one year full-time or two part-time. The purposes of the courses are to prepare trainees for practical experience in the areas of law and for the more specialised training in the year long 'pupillage' for barristers and the training contract with a firm of solicitors.

- Do the standards of achievement expected of students conform to or exceed the QAA benchmark statement for law?
- Are the external examiners satisfied by the programme of study?

In addition, information must be supplied by the institution to the professional bodies about the programme to permit a visit to discuss the programme with the institutional representatives, the programme team and the students. Recognition can be withdrawn from a programme that fails to comply with the conditions set out in the joint statement of meets the minimum standards prescribed by QAA.

(2) The Engineering Council. The Engineering Council (EC) is a UK-wide organisation and promotes and regulates the engineering profession in the UK and is responsible for the Register of Chartered Engineers. The EC is established through a Charter and has Bye-Laws which set out its governance and obligations. Regulation of the profession is achieved through the professional 'Engineering Institutions', of which there are 35 (e.g., civil, mechanical, structural, etc). Engineering Institutions undertake assessments of individuals and of education and training programmes in higher education institutions.

The Institutions, subject to the licences they hold from the EC, may place individuals on the Register. Entry to the Register means satisfying the appropriate membership requirements; these are determined through the EC's Standards and Routes to Registration whose application by the Engineering Institutions is regularly audited by the EC. Registration requires a satisfactory educational base (preferably through an accredited course), initial professional development and a professional review. This paper is concerned with the educational base.

To become a Chartered Engineer (CEng) or member of another professional Engineering Institution, engineering students are required to follow a framework of educational preparation – the educational base – as defined by the EC. The requirements for CEng are:

- The four-year full-time undergraduate programme (MEng) fully accredited for CEng.
- The three-year full-time undergraduate programme (BEng) accredited for CEng *plus* an accredited or approved 'Matching Section' (one-year full-time or equivalent) to achieve equivalence with MEng graduates.

The Engineering Council normally licenses the Institutions to accredit or approve programmes of study leading to BEng or MEng qualifications. *Accreditation* involves 'periodic quality audit' through a peer review process comprising a panel made up of members of academe and industry. The process involves scrutiny of documentation and a visit to the higher education institution. The panel will focus on entry to the programme, the process of teaching and learning, resources, the assessment strategy and the outcomes achieved. *Approval* processes relate to educational provision which is short of full accreditation such as Matching Sections. Accreditation and approval are undertaken in recognition that the processes rely principally upon the internal quality assurance systems of higher education institutions.

A programme of study should only require one accreditation visit either by one or more professional engineering institution. Amongst other things, the Engineering Institutions are responsible for

- Selecting and training members of accreditation panels
- The constitution of panels
- The form of submission from the higher education institution seeking accreditation of its programme(s)
- The criteria against which an accreditation judgement will be made.

Accreditation judgements are valid for five years when 'further consideration' is required. This can take the form of a formal re-accreditation process, an arrangement for continuing periodic audit and review, or evidence obtained by other bodies – it is up to the higher education institution to decide.

University Accreditation of Higher Education Outside the University

Partnership arrangements between higher education institutions and between higher education institutions and public or private non-academic organisations, both in the UK and overseas, have been developing since the 1980s. They are seen as providing a means of extending opportunities for large numbers of students. Arrangements will vary, but the main partners will be the awarding institution (i.e., with degree awarding powers) and the providing institution or organisation (i.e., providing the higher education programme, but without degree awarding powers). In all cases, accreditation (or validation, terminology varies between universities) is the result of an evaluation process conducted by peer review.

The awarding institution is responsible for the quality and standards of all the awards that are granted in that institution's name. Partnership arrangements are subject to institutional audit by the Quality Assurance Agency for Higher Education (QAA), the quality assurance body for the UK (see below). The QAA will examine i) the way in which the institution manages the quality of programmes offered in its name by a partner organisation, and ii) the ways it ensures that the academic standards of its awards gained through study with partner organisations are the same as those gained through study with the institution itself. If the partnership is overseas or is on a large scale, the Agency has in the past undertaken separate reviews to the institutional audit. The QAA's code of practice for the assurance of academic quality and standards in higher education includes a section on 'collaborative provision'

– the term used by QAA for such partnerships. The code outlines a set of precepts (key issues) with accompanying guidance. The code is meant to cover various forms of collaborative provision, although the word 'collaborative' is not defined more widely than those arrangements 'involving the provision of programmes of study and the granting of awards and qualifications'. The code comprises 38 precepts arranged around the following headings:

- Responsibility for, and equivalence of, academic standards
- Policies, procedures and information
- Selecting a partner organisation
- Written agreements
- Agreements with agents (a third party employed by the awarding institution to facilitate a collaborative arrangement)
- Assuring academic standards and the quality of programmes and awards
- Assessment requirements
- External examining
- Certificates and transcripts
- Information for students
- Publicity and marketing.

Arrangements for accreditation vary within the above framework between institutions. Some colleges and organisations receive accreditation from several universities, relating to different programmes. Below are two examples of university accreditation arrangements. The first, the Open University, is the largest but not a typical accreditor. The second, the University of Sussex, is more typical of university accrediting.

(1) Accreditation by the Open University. An organisation that wishes to offer a programme of study leading to a validated[2] award of the Open University (OU), must first be approved at institutional level as being suitable to do so – this process is called 'accreditation'. To become accredited an organisation must meet a set of principles which cover the following:

- A suitable environment
- Independence of institutional ownership from the exercise of academic authority
- Clear academic structures
- An effective quality assurance system

---

2 'Validation' is the process by which the programmes of study of accredited organisations are approved to lead to an OU award.

- A challenging learning environment
- Relationships with the wider academic community.

Organisations will be required to show how they meet these principles through documentary evidence – the 'submission'. Often the validation of a programme of study will be combined with the institutional accreditation. The process involves initial dialogue between the OU and the organisation which may or may not lead to a formal submission for accreditation. Once the formal submission has been received, a visit will be made by a panel of expert advisors with knowledge of quality assurance, senior management and teaching in higher education (these are drawn from across the higher education sector rather than from its own academics). The purpose of the visit is to explore and clarify the information provided in the documentary evidence. A report is produced which, if successful, will recommend accreditation and an Accreditation Agreement will then be negotiated. This agreement will outline responsibility for the validation and review of programmes, the approval of external examiners, maintenance of quality assurance records, and the provision of information to the OU.

All accredited institutions and their programmes are re-accredited or re-validated within six years. However, peer review panels may limit approval to a shorter term - whatever they deem appropriate. Additionally, an interim review to follow up a limited agenda of issues, often carried out by a smaller panel comprising the chair and an officer from the University, is sometimes required.

(2) Accreditation by the University of Sussex. The University of Sussex has a set of criteria and procedures for partner institutions that wish to seek accredited status. Through accredited status, the University recognises the partner institution's own internal processes for the approval of new programmes of study leading to an award of the University and the review and modification of existing programmes leading to an award. In other words, unlike the OU, the University of Sussex, once accredited status is conferred, will not conduct validation or re-validation events, but will delegate authority for the approval of the curriculum to the partner institution. However, the University will remain responsible for the academic standards of all awards granted in its name.

To become accredited, a partner institution must meet a number of criteria:

- Have a commitment to quality assurance and operate an effective system
- Operate as a self-critical academic community
- Have experience of delivering programmes leading to a University of Sussex award
- Understand and comply with the University's policies and practices
- Have a well developed administrative structure and professional staffing

- Have effective systems for identifying and disseminating good practice
- Have processes and procedures that are subject and responsive to external academic points of reference
- Have the University as its principal validating authority.

To become accredited, partner institutions are required to submit an analytical account outlining the institution's case based on the above criteria. If successful, the institution will undergo an audit conducted by the University to establish that the functions for which the institution is seeking accredited status are being discharged effectively. If successful at the end of this stage, a visit to the institution will be undertaken by an accreditation panel comprising internal and external members. Once all stages have been completed and accredited status conferred, an agreement is entered into which sets out a number of obligations that the partner institution must fulfil, including the provision of reports of programme approval and review events, nominations and appointments of external examiners, the provision of annual monitoring reports, and an annual statement that the obligations have been discharged properly.

Renewal of accredited status will be at intervals no greater than five years and will comprise a self-evaluation report submitted by the partner institution followed by an accreditation panel visit.

21.2.2 Approval of Institutions, Degree-Types, Programmes

The institutional 'right to exist within the system' has two elements in the UK context. The first is the right to a university (or university college) title. The second is the right to award degrees. The latter can be separated into the right to award degrees for taught courses and the right to award research degrees. The important point to note is that both rights, once awarded, cannot be removed without a special Act of Parliament. (This is the case in England. There are no such powers referred to in the case of Scotland.) It follows therefore that many universities received these rights quite long ago and according to the procedures in place at the time. Thus, the old universities (i.e. pre-1992) operate under a Royal Charter while the new universities (i.e. post-1992) and certain other higher education institutions operate under an Instrument of Government and Articles of Government. The authority for the award of and amendment to royal charters, instruments and articles resides with the Privy Council – one of the oldest parts of Government. It is also responsible for approving the use of the title 'university' and the granting of degree awarding powers. The powers of certain professional bodies also derive from the Privy Council (see above). Currently, such advice regarding the award of university titles or degree awarding powers would be made on the basis of very thorough evaluation and review procedures by the national Quality Assurance Agency for Higher Education and, in the case of university titles, an evaluation of the financial stability of the institution by the relevant higher education funding council. (Separate councils exist for England, Scotland and Wales.)

Applications are considered against criteria agreed between the QAA and government, and are applicable throughout the UK. The criteria cover such issues as governance and management, quality assurance, administrative systems, and other specific criteria relating to the type of application (i.e., taught or research degree awarding powers or university title). Applications for degree awarding powers or a university title can only be made if an institution is able to demonstrate that its provision or institutional audit has not been subject to an unsatisfactory outcome as a result of a review by the quality assurance body in the last five years (see below for details of these processes). The 2003 Government 'White Paper' on *The future of higher education* indicated that the criteria for degree awarding powers will be examined and modernised to reflect the increasing diversity of higher education, although 'there will be no relaxation of the high standards that have to be reached before taught degree awarding powers are granted'.

It should be noted that recent applications for the award of a university title have mostly ended in failure. For example, the Bolton Institute, a large well-established institution in the north-west of the country already possessing degree-awarding powers, had its application for a university title turned down in 2001 following a special institutional audit by the QAA. The conclusions of the report, and therefore the reasons why the Institute was turned down, are not public. The most recent successful application for the award of a university title was the University of Gloucestershire in 2001. Again, the report is not a public document.

At the level of degrees and programmes, approval is the responsibility of the individual university. Procedures vary but are subject to periodic audit by the QAA. Procedures include arrangements for regular monitoring and periodic review, often involve external inputs. But they are formally a matter for the individual university.

21.2.3 Approval Outside the Accreditation Scheme

There are hardly any examples of this in the UK case. The Archbishop of Canterbury is one of a small number of bodies and individuals who have a traditional authority to award certain specific degrees. Concerns about 'bogus degrees' surfaced at the end of the 1980s and the government department (DfES) issued 'recognised and listed body orders' to attempt to regulate new providers. A specific case was the creation of an American institution – now Richmond College – which attempted to establish itself as Richmond University. This was prevented – it would have been acceptable if there had been a parent Richmond University in the USA. The solution was for the institution to be renamed Richmond College and to seek accreditation from the UK Open University, whose degree awarding powers were used for Richmond students. This example illustrates the UK arrangement well. Anyone can establish a college or institute. But the title of university is protected, as is the authority to award degrees.

21.2.4   Evaluation Schemes: The Quality Assurance Agency for Higher Education

Evaluation of universities and other institutions with degree awarding powers is the responsibility of the Quality Assurance Agency for Higher Education (QAA). It was created in 1997. The QAA's mission is 'to safeguard the public interest in sound standards of higher education qualifications and to encourage continuous improvement in the management of the quality of higher education' (Strategic Plan 2003-05, March 2003). Consistent with the UK emphasis upon institutional autonomy, the focus of QAA evaluation is the way in which an institution safeguards and ensures quality and standards. It is not attempting to make a direct judgement about quality or standards. The Agency will express varying degrees of 'confidence' in the institution and although such judgements have no formal status for the recognition of the institution or its programmes, they may affect the institution's reputation and the funding decisions of the relevant higher education funding councils.

The QAA is a UK-wide organisation, but operates in a devolved context. The Agency has devolved responsibilities in Scotland and Wales, operating through QAA Scotland and the Advisory Committee for Wales, respectively. The QAA works on behalf of the different national higher education funding councils and has contractual agreements with each – the Higher Education Funding Council for England, the Scottish Higher Education Funding Council, the Higher Education Funding Council for Wales and the Department of Education Northern Ireland.

The QAA is formally 'owned' by all UK higher education institutions, which pay a subscription and the heads of the institutions are the company's shareholders. However, much of its funding and 'powers' are effectively delegated to it by the higher education funding councils. The Governing Body of the QAA has a 'controlling' external (non HE) membership in the majority. Thus, the QAA is intended to be independent although its owners could theoretically decide to close it down. The QAA has around 50 staff. Its reviewers ('auditors') are drawn from higher education institutions and receive training from the Agency. QAA reports are published and therefore have potential to influence all 'customers' and stakeholders. However, generally they have received little attention outside the higher education institution concerned, except for a few celebrated critical cases. New arrangements introduced in England and Northern Ireland in 2003 place greater emphasis on the publication of information on quality and standards. Although this will be the responsibility of individual higher education institutions, the QAA will have a role in 'auditing' the information provided. (The following sections refer to the arrangements in England

and Northern Ireland. New developments in arrangements in Scotland and Wales are different and are described at the end of this section).

The main procedures operated by the QAA are institutional audit, qualifications frameworks, subject benchmark statements, programme specifications and codes of practice.

Institutional Audit

The new approach, introduced in 2003, focuses on institutional audit – a review of the way in which an institution safeguards and ensures quality and standards. Where areas of concern are identified, the audit will be followed up by reviews at subject level.

In addition, institutions are now expected to collect and make publicly available information about the quality and standards of their programmes. This includes summaries of external examiners' reports, results of student feedback surveys, internal programme reviews and so on.

Audit aims to examine three areas:

- The effectiveness of institutions' internal quality assurance processes and with reference to the QAA's *Code of Practice* (see below)
- The accuracy, completeness and reliability of the information published about the quality and standards of its programmes, and with reference to *programme specifications* (see below)
- Examples of the institutions' internal quality assurance processes in operation at programme level or across the institution as a whole (covering some 10 % of the institution's provision), and with reference to the *qualifications frameworks*, the *Code of Practice* and *subject benchmark statements* (see below).

The audit visit normally lasts about five working days and covers the overall management of an institution's quality and standards and more specific areas of enquiry. In particular, the audit will focus of the following aspects relating to quality and standards:

- Publicly available information
- Internal systems for the management of information
- Internal reviews and their outcomes
- Students' experiences as learners
- The academic standards expected and achieved by students
- The use made of the qualifications framework, the Codes of Practice, subject benchmark statements and programme specifications (see below)
- The quality assurance of teaching staff.

Judgements will be made by audit teams on the confidence in the 'soundness of the institutions management of the quality of its programmes and the academic standards of its awards' and the reliance placed on the 'accuracy, integrity, completeness and frankness of the information that an institution publishes' about its programmes and awards. Auditors will be required to report any areas of concern, make recommendations for further consideration by the institution, and identify areas where a full subject review is necessary or where an action plan needs to be implemented by the institution.

After completion of the audit and the publication of the report, the Agency will follow up areas of weakness through institutional progress reports. As with previous approaches to reviewing quality and standards at subject level, in extreme unsatisfactory cases, the Agency will revisit an institution; if again the outcome is unsatisfactory the Higher Education Funding Council for England would withdraw its funding (although there has yet to be a case where this has occurred).

In helping to define clear and specific standards for higher education institutions, the QAA has established a number of points of reference for reviews and public information. These are the qualifications frameworks, subject benchmark statements, programme specifications and the Code of Practice.

Qualifications Frameworks

The frameworks for England, Wales and Northern Ireland – and a parallel one for Scotland – have been designed to provide an easier understanding of higher education qualifications by ensuring a consistent use of qualification titles. The frameworks include qualifications such as Bachelor's degree with Honours, Master's and Doctorate degrees and describe the achievements and attributes represented by these main titles. The frameworks are intended to help students and employers understand the meaning and level of qualifications. They also aim to provide public assurance that qualifications bearing similar titles represent similar levels of achievement.

Subject Benchmark Statements

Subject benchmark statements set out expectations about standards of Bachelor's degrees with honours in broad subject areas. They are intended to be an explicit statement of the conceptual framework that gives a discipline its coherence and identity. They define what can be expected of a graduate in terms of the knowledge, skills and other attributes needed to develop understanding in the subject. They are benchmarks of the level of intellectual demand and challenge represented by an honours degree in the subject area concerned. Benchmark statements are intended to help higher education institutions when they design and approve programmes and to help external examiners and academic reviewers to verify and compare standards.

They also provide information for students and employers. However, benchmarks are not intended to be prescriptive. Institutions are merely required to take them into account in designing their programmes.

Programme Specifications

Programme specifications are standard sets of information that each institution provides about its programmes. Each specification describes what knowledge, understanding, skills and other attributes a student will have developed on successfully completing a specific programme. It provides information about teaching and learning methods, assessment, and career opportunities on completion. Specifications will also explain how a particular programme relates to the qualifications framework. In providing this information, it is intended that prospective students should be able to make comparisons and informed choices about the programmes they wish to study. Programme specifications also provide useful information for recruiters of graduates.

Code of Practice

The *Code of Practice* sets out good practice relating to the management of academic quality and standards. The *Code of Practice* comprises 'precepts or principles' that institutions should demonstrate, together with guidance on how they might meet these precepts. The Code to date covers:

- postgraduate research programmes
- collaborative provision
- students with disabilities
- external examining
- academic appeals and student complaints on academic matters
- assessment of students
- programme approval, monitoring and review
- career education, information and guidance
- placement learning
- recruitment and admissions.

21.2.5   Developments in Scotland and Wales

In Scotland, a new process of enhancement-led institutional review (ELIR) has been in development to start from 2003/04. ELIR is a new national strategy focusing explicitly on the enhancement of the learning experience of students. It comprises five inter-related elements:

i)   a framework for internal review at subject level

ii) a set of public information provided by institutions

iii) involvement of students in quality management (as members in review teams for the ELIR process, as representatives in institutions and through national surveys of the student experience)

iv) quality enhancement engagements involving a structured programme of developmental activities with the sector

v)   the institutional review process – an enhancement-led process through peer review.

A number of reference points will be used during the ELIR process, which include the qualifications framework for Scotland, the code of practice and subject benchmarks (see above). The ELIR process itself comprises four stages: i) an annual meeting between the Agency and the institution, ii) production of a *reflective analysis* by the institution, iii) the ELIR visit and a public report (which will express a level of confidence) and iv) sector-wide feedback and workshops held annually on themes emerging from ELIR.

In Wales, the Higher Education Funding Council for Wales has adopted a new quality assurance and standards framework to come into operation from 2003/04. The focus of the approach is on institutional audit and the removal of subject-level reviews. In addition, HEFCW has emphasised the need for comparability of judgements with England. The approach is similar to the one adopted for England and Northern Ireland, but with some differences (e.g. institutions will not be required to publish summaries of external examiner reports and internal programme reviews).

21.2.6   Other Evaluation Schemes

Internal review. Most evaluation is actually done within institutions on the authority of the institutions. Most have arrangements for the regular review of departments or programmes, usually involving inputs from external peers. These reviews are generally seen as part of quality enhancement activities although if major concerns arise out of a particular review, actions would probably be taken by the institution and these could include the closure of a department or programme. Until 2001, reviews at subject level were carried out by the QAA. These led to published gradings with reputational implications for the institutions and, *in extremis*, could lead to the withdrawal of funding by the funding council. This external review process has now been replaced by reliance on institutional review procedures and the publication of information based on them. From time to time, most institutions also review central services such as library and student support services.

External examining. Part of internal review procedures, external examining constitutes the most traditional aspect of quality assurance in UK higher education. Institutions appoint examiners from other higher education institutions to oversee the examining and the award of degrees on specific programmes. External examiners typically read a sample of the students' assessed work and provide written comments on the standards of achievement and the consistency of internal marking. They will normally attend the examination board within the awarding institution that determines the award of degrees on the particular programme. As part of the new quality assurance arrangements, external examiner reports (or extracts/summaries of them) will be published by the higher education institution.

Access to Higher Education courses are provided by further education colleges and other providers, including some universities. These courses are aimed at mature students, normally lacking formal entry qualifications, from under-represented groups to help them progress to higher education. The QAA manages the scheme that recognises these courses. Consortia are established which are responsible for developing, validating and reviewing Access to Higher Education courses. These are called Authorised Validating Agencies (AVAs). The QAA 'licenses' the AVAs to recognise courses and to issue awards to successful students.

Research Assessment Exercise (RAE). Public funding for research in higher education institutions is provided through the 'dual support' system that comprises two streams of funding:

- Funding for the research infrastructure (e.g., staff salaries, premises, computing and library costs) from the UK funding bodies
- Funding for the costs of individual research projects from the research councils.

The RAE is a means of rating the quality of research in higher education institutions and distributing the funding for the research infrastructure selectively across higher education institutions. The RAE, as well as being a tool for selectively distributing research funds, is used to promote high quality – the research submitted by higher education institutions is assessed against a benchmark of international excellence for each subject concerned. Since 1986 the process has been developed and refined. The process itself operates through peer review and subject 'experts' make up the panels for each of the 69 'units of assessment' (subject disciplines). Experts are nominated by research associations, learned societies, PSBs and other organisations, and selected by the funding councils.

Higher education institutions are able to make submissions in as many subjects as they choose. The submissions comprise information about research active staff and details of research output for these staff (up to four items – books, papers, journals can be submitted for each researcher). Each panel defines its own criteria for assessing submissions and these are published in advance. Panels do not visit institutions. Each submission is assessed and awarded a quality rating on a seven point scale ranging from 5* (quality that equates to attainable levels of international excellence in more than half of the research activity submitted and attainable levels of national excellence in the remainder) to 1 (quality that equates to attainable levels of national excellence in none, or virtually none, of the research activity submitted). Upon completion of the panels' work, the outcomes are published to provide public information on the quality of research in UK higher education institutions.

Financial audit. Institutions also undergo systems of financial audit by the higher education funding councils. Although no approval decisions hang on the results, the continued flow of government money ultimately does.

21.3   Analysis

21.3.1   Overview

Until a Government Act in 1988, reference was often made to the 'public sector' of higher education in the UK. This referred to local authority run colleges and polytechnics and contrasted with the 'private sector' of the universities. Today it is formally possible to see virtually all UK higher education institutions as private, albeit substantially dependent on 'public' funding. (The OECD refers to UK universities as 'state funded private institutions'.)

The UK tradition has been to preserve an arms-length relationship between higher education and government in the interests of university autonomy and academic freedom. (And the separation of government from state – in the form of the Sovereign – is a further mechanism of protection of universities from political interference.) While this formal autonomy may perhaps account for the sometimes high levels of belligerence from individual vice-chancellors, it might be argued that the autonomy is more apparent than real. Overall, higher education institutions are dependent on various government monies for about 80 % of their funding. Only a few receive more than 50 % of their funding from other sources. In many ways, it has been through its various funding mechanisms and incentives that UK government has attempted to steer and control higher education.

But it is also the case that there is probably consensus that central control should be limited. Much is made of control and steerage through the market. With well over 100 separate institutions and a tradition of students leaving home to study, institutional competition exists at quite high levels. Thus, evaluation judgements that impact upon the reputation of the institutions can have great effect on the institution's competitive position.

In summary, emphasis in the UK is placed upon the maintenance of sound, competent, well-managed institutions. The strength of university managements and administrations should be noted in the UK case with a growing emphasis upon responsiveness to markets and the role of public information to inform these markets. Evaluation is seen by Government as having an increasingly important role to play in providing information for higher education's markets.

21.3.2   Recent History

Quality assurance arrangements for higher education have been extremely unstable since the early 1990s. They have been criticised by higher education leaders, been under pressure from politicians and been generally unpopular with most academics. They have changed several times over this period. The main phases are described briefly below.

The 'Ancien Regime'

At the start of the 1990s, the only external system of quality assurance in place in the universities was that of external examining. This was a voluntary self-regulatory arrangement to be found across the whole of higher education with the one exception of the University of Oxford. External examiners were responsible to the higher education institution whose courses they were examining. Politicians had been making it clear that they did not regard this system as sufficiently rigorous, especially as far more extensive national systems existed for the other sector of higher education, by now the larger, i.e. the polytechnics and colleges. The general perception was that this was all a part of the Thatcherite attack on the public sector in general and on the professions in particular. Thus, it was regarded as a very specific problem to Britain.

The polytechnics and colleges, as well as having external examiners, were subject to the validation and accreditation requirements of the Council for National Academic Awards (CNAA), a chartered body set up in 1964 to ensure the standards of academic awards in higher education outside the universities. The CNAA, with its degree-awarding powers, had considerable authority over the polytechnics and colleges which it exercised through linked peer review processes of institutional and programme review. This was becoming increasingly unpopular with the large and mature institutions that now comprised the 'public sector' of higher education. On the other hand, the Thatcher Government did not regard this essentially academic body as sufficiently tough on the institutions for which it was responsible. A celebrated charge of 'Marxist bias' in the teaching of sociology in one of the polytechnics saw the Government turn to its preferred instrument of quality scrutiny – Her Majesty's Inspectors. The Inspectorate operated in all public sector educational institutions, from schools to polytechnics. But at the end of the 1980s, the Government transformed their predominantly advisory role into a genuinely inspectorial one, involving the observation of teaching and with potential consequences for institutional funding.

Recognising their exposed position in comparison to the surfeit of regulation in the polytechnics and colleges, the universities' representative body, the Committee of Vice-Chancellors and Principals (CVCP), set up its own quality assurance system administered by a new body, the Academic Audit Unit. This was a voluntary system under which universities 'invited' the AAU to audit their internal arrangements for ensuring quality and standards. This it did through a peer review process of visits to universities. The autonomy of each individual university was to be jealously safe-guarded. There was to be no question of the AAU making judgements of what the quality and standards of universities actually were. If the aim of the CVCP was to prevent the Government introducing its own evaluation system for universities, it must be judged a failure. It did however introduce the concept of academic audit into higher education with long-term consequences for the approach to evaluation in the UK.

Dual Evaluations in a Unitary Higher Education System

In 1992, the Government abolished the old higher education 'binary line', awarding university titles to all of the polytechnics, some of the larger higher education col-leges and the so-called 'central institutions' in Scotland. However, in setting up a unitary system of higher education, the government established a dual system of evaluation. The AAU was transformed into the Higher Education Quality Council (HEQC), a body owned by the institutions through the CVCP and the equivalent body for the higher education colleges – the Standing Conference of Principals (SCOP). It continued the process of audit (now called 'quality audit') and took on some of the quality enhancement functions of the CNAA. The latter was closed down although some functions for research and development and an accreditation service for non-university institutions were transferred to the Open University. In parallel to the institutionally owned HEQC, the Government established quality assessment committees in each of the national higher education funding councils. These took over the methods and many of the staff of the Inspectorate to introduce a system of teaching quality assessment at subject level across all higher education institutions. The funding councils had, and still have, a statutory responsibility for the assessment of higher education quality.

Thus, for the rest of the decade, higher education institutions were subject to the external audit of their quality assurance procedures by the HEQC – with visits ap-proximately every five years – and the assessment of their teaching on a subject-by-subject basis by the funding council assessors. The latter process continued to be largely based on the observation of teaching practice and resulted in public gradings of the quality of teaching in each institution. Both audit and assessment made use of peer review, auditors/assessors being drawn from higher education institutions and trained in the appropriate methods by the respective agencies. The external examining system continued as did professional accreditation and research assessment. The much-vaunted autonomy of UK universities was looking a bit thin!

A New Agency

The dual arrangements for audit and assessment were extremely unpopular in higher education. They took up a lot of time and resource during a period when higher education was expanding fast and the unit of resource was plunging. Assessment in particular, with its observation of teaching and its numerical gradings, was the cause of considerable tensions within institutions even though high grades were celebrated and used extensively in institutional publicity materials.

A joint review of the arrangements was made by the funding councils and the CVCP and this led to the creation in 1997 of the Quality Assurance Agency for Higher Education. Initially, the new agency continued to operate the dual procedures of institutional-level audit and subject-level assessment (now called subject review and with much less emphasis on the observation of teaching). It was claimed that their operation by a single body would be more efficient and would make fewer demands on the institutions. Despite several tinkerings with the assessment methodologies, the arrangements remained unpopular. Moreover, public and political attention was shifting away from process to outcome and calls were made for evaluation processes that would be more effective in the enhancement of quality. The fact that subject review had uncovered hardly any cases of really poor quality was also used by its opponents to argue that it was an onerous and unnecessary burden.

In a wider context, the Labour Government was continuing its Conservative predecessor's policies of introducing greater competition and consumer choice into the public sector. Consequently, it was not keen to see the removal of subject review with its gradings and consequent league tables of institutions, essential in the view of New Labour enthusiasts to inform markets, ensure competition and hence efficiency and quality improvement. If then evaluation had to produce information to inform the public, it was clear that subject review would need to be replaced by something that would also deliver consumer information. A number of influential vice-chancellors argued that institutions could do this for themselves by publishing selective extracts from the information that they held about themselves. A committee was established to consider this proposition and to make recommendations for the kinds of information to be published. The Committee's report was accepted by the funding councils and the Government and its recommendations are in the process of implementation. Subject review is being run down, replaced for an interim period by review-style 'disciplinary engagements' but lacking the controversial gradings aspect. However, institutions are expected to operate their own internal systems of review and these should include some external peer input. Information from these reviews, from external examiners and from student feedback questionnaires are among the sources of institutional data that higher education institutions are expected to publish on the web-sites.

21.3.3 Whose Victory?

This brief history is necessary to record in order to understand why evaluation has been subject to so much controversy in UK higher education in recent years. To a considerable extent it can be seen as a long running battle between several governments and university leaderships. The generals have been the higher education funding councils on the one hand and the universities' representative bodies (the CVCP re-branded itself as Universities UK a few years ago) and the front-line troops have been the thousands of academic staff who have spent much time evaluating each other. In what sense then is it possible to talk about victory or defeat in this battle? On the one hand the hated teaching quality assessments have gone. On the other, external evaluation is still present and a new system, as yet untried, will expose possibly even more of the inner workings of higher education institutions to public scrutiny.

If a victory is to be claimed, it probably has to go to the government side. Given the starting point of the vice-chancellors of opposition to almost any form of external evaluation, the present arrangements represent a fairly comprehensive system of external scrutiny. The fact that much of the evaluative work will be done by the institutions themselves should not disguise the reality that it is being externally driven, and to an agenda dictated by government. Moreover, the notion that there should be some form of externally monitored quality assurance is now almost universally accepted by academics.

This agenda has been one of exerting control over a fast-growing and expensive area of the public sector. The traditions of relative (and symbolic) autonomy of universities in the UK go a long way to explaining why governments wanted to exert control and why universities wanted to resist it. Control mechanisms common elsewhere in Europe – e.g. over university curricula, over staffing – were entirely absent in the UK. Evaluation (or quality assurance as the more generally used term in the UK) became a principal tool for the state to acquire more control and it was seen as such by the universities.

Evaluation – especially by state controlled bodies – was objected to in principle, because it resulted in gradings and rankings, and because it was seen as consuming vast amounts of time and resource. Those operating the various evaluation procedures would stress the quality improvement potential of evaluation and while much was undoubtedly changed for the better within institutions as a result of evaluation, it was largely out of sight from the generals fighting the battle. Insofar as a quality improvement function was acknowledged, it was felt to be something which institutions could achieve for themselves much more effectively than through the efforts of an external body.

21.3.4 Consequences

Away from the noise of battle, the twin procedures of institutional audit and subject assessment have produced many changes in higher education institutions. Especially for the older pre-1992 universities, they were responsible for the establishment of internal quality assurance procedures which formalised and standardised practices which, where they had existed at all, had been informal and local rather than systematic and institution-wide. These practices would include the better documentation of courses and the requirements made of students, new monitoring and review arrangements, more systematic data collection and analysis (including student performance and feedback data), action plans to chart the effectiveness of changes made. New 'quality' committees were established as were specialist administrative units to support their work. Managers at all levels across the institutions found themselves with new responsibilities for quality and evaluation.

At the level of individual teachers, some counter pressure to the dictates of research assessment has been achieved. External evaluation has pushed teaching up the agenda of academic departments. Teaching and learning have been discussed by staff where previously they had been the private business of individuals. Staff appraisal and development systems have looked at teaching in a more systematic way. Related national developments such as the creation of an Institute for Learning and Teaching and the subject-focused Learning and Teaching Support Networks have given further impetus to looking at the teaching function in higher education.

How far all of this has really improved the learning experiences of students is less clear. There is probably rather less really poor teaching than had existed previously. Student views are probably taken more into account although a lack of action on student feedback is a common complaint. Courses are better documented and objectives and expectations more clear. Whether these improvements compensate for the decline in resources for teaching is another matter, but given that the latter would have happened anyway, these changes were probably even more necessary.

Looking outside the institutions towards other stakeholders and society in general, the effects of the evaluation systems have probably been to reinforce the already strong sense of stratification of higher education institutions in the UK. The gradings of subject assessment and research assessment have been used to create league tables of institutions. While these have mainly reinforced existing reputational hierarchies, they have given added credence to them. In a sense the post-1992 'unitary' system has become more stratified than the old 'binary' system (of universities and polytechnics). It remains to be seen whether plans to publish even more comparative data on institutions will further reinforce these hierarchies or challenge them, or at least give recognition to diversity of type and function.

An important claim for external evaluation systems was that they were essential for continued government support for higher education and that funding settlements would be in part dependent on the higher education sector having effective mechanisms of accountability for the vast sums of public money it consumed. It is difficult to really test this claim although it may be noted that the recent Government strategy announcement on higher education was financially quite generous.

It should be noted that in the context of the larger comparative project, activities that can properly be called accreditation have been left largely untouched by the controversies and changes to national evaluation arrangements. Professional bodies have continued to accredit programmes using mechanisms broadly recognisable to those which have existed for decades. Various attempts to better integrate their procedures with those of the QAA and its predecessors do not appear to have achieved a lot. (Professional bodies constitute another largely independent actor in the evaluation scene and have had no overwhelming interest in seeing their autonomy and authority diminished by closer collaboration with other actors.) University accreditation of other institutions and programmes has been affected by QAA guidelines and its reviews of 'collaborative provision'. These have not been particularly controversial although in the case of international partnerships they may have limited the entrepreneurial zeal of certain universities.

However, in the UK, the QAA can be seen as the body, and institutional audit (or its equivalent in the different countries) as the process that brings together the different accreditation and evaluation schemes. Institutional audit focuses on the ways in which an institution safeguards and ensures the quality and standards of its awards. For example and as described above, audit does this through examining institutional procedures for internal review, how institutions act upon the reports of professional and statutory bodies, what action they can take in the light of external examiners' comments, and how well an institution manages its partnership arrangements within the UK and abroad.

21.4   International

There has been little apparent influence of European or wider international developments on accreditation and evaluation procedures in the UK. Rather, the influence has been seen in the other direction with UK models exported to other countries (largely to former colonies). Insofar as key actors have looked outside the UK for inspiration, it has been towards the US or Australia rather than across the English Channel to the rest of Europe. The recent Government strategy paper makes virtually no reference to Bologna and European issues although references abound to notions of 'world class' and 'international excellence'.

That said, individuals from UK quality agencies are active in the various international forums to do with accreditation and evaluation. But while there may be an awareness of the international issues and contexts, it is rarely visible in domestic debates.

The one area where there has been international activity has been with regard to the overseas collaborations of UK higher education institutions. These come within the remit of the QAA and are audited in quite rigorous ways. The basic principle has been that quality and standards should be equal to the institution's UK provision. This is an issue of ongoing concern and debate, especially with regard to the extent to which UK institutions have the mechanisms to discharge their responsibilities when working with other institutions in other jurisdictions. As more and more countries establish their own accreditation or evaluation systems, the potential for a clash of regulatory procedures becomes more likely. It may be that this will make the British more interested in a possible harmonisation of evaluation practices but there are few signs of this to date.

International issues are also of interest to professional bodies and there are signs of international accreditation/evaluation developments in several fields. A European system for the review of business and management programmes has been in existence for some time (EQUIS – European Quality Improvement System). As at November 2002, twelve UK business schools have been awarded the European Quality label.

21.5   Other Quality Assessment Activities

Staff appraisal systems have been in existence in UK universities for some years now. They differ to some extent between institutions but tend to emphasise a staff development function. They do however also contribute to promotion decisions. (They generally take the form of an annual interview with a senior colleague which reviews the achievements and difficulties of the last year and sets objectives and targets for the next.)

They do not relate directly to other evaluation or quality assessment activities other than in the sense that any recent evaluation experiences would probably be discussed during the annual interview. The introduction of systematic staff appraisal arrangements was at the prompting of Government in return for a more favourable funding settlement.

About the Contributors

Alberto Amaral, Professor, Director of CIPES, Centre for Research in Higher Education Politics. Scientific research area: emergence of private higher education; diversity and diversification in the Portuguese higher education system; managerialism and governance in higher education. Comparative studies of the higher education systems of Portuguese speaking, European and South American higher education.

Harilaos Billiris, Professor. M.A. in Physics and Astronomy, doctorate in Engineering. Professor Billiris has taught Geodesy for over 25 years at the National Technical University of Athens (NTUA). He is director of the Higher Geodesy Laboratory and Secretary-General of the Hellenic National Committee for Geodesy and Geophysics. He is involved in the Evaluation processes in his School and NTUA. Substitute of the National representative at ENQA.

John Brennan, Professor of Higher Education Research and Director of the Centre for Higher Education Research and Information at the UK Open University. Author (with Tarla Shah) of 'Managing Quality in Higher Education', Open University Press, 2000.

Silvia Capucci, Professor, Deputy Director of CIMEA (Centro Informazione Mobilità Equivalenze Accademiche) della Fondazione Rui, Rome, Italy.

Thierry Chevaillier, Senior Lecturer in economics at the University of Bourgogne (Dijon, France) and a member of IREDU, Institute for Research on the Economics of Education. His research interests are higher education finance and resource allocation in higher education. He has been involved in several international comparative studies on various aspects of higher education in Europe and is an expert to Eurydice.

Ewa Chmielecka, Dr. hab., Foundation for the promotion and accreditation of economic education, Warsaw, Poland.

Marcin Dąbrowski, Foundation for the promotion and accreditation of economic education, Warsaw, Poland.

Carlo Finocchietti, Dr., Director of CIMEA (Centro Informazione Mobilità Equivalenze Accademiche) della Fondazione Rui, Rome, Italy.

Margarita Jeliazkova, M.Phil., Research Associate at the Center for Higher Education Policy Studies, University of Twente, the Netherlands. Current research interests include quality management in higher education, comparative public policy, evaluation methodology, higher education policy in Central and Eastern Europe.

Maureen Killeavy, Dr., University College Dublin. Her research interests centre on teacher education and related areas. Serves as External Examiner for various institutions and programmes. Member of several national commissions, among others member of the National Policy Advisory and Development Committee.

Cornelia Klepp, Mag., graduated in Pedagogy at the University of Klagenfurt in 2000. Doctoral studies with focal point on international and comparative educational research. Working in the field of educational research and political education at the Faculty for Interdisciplinary Studies (IFF).

Dorte Kristoffersen, Deputy Director and Director of Development at the Danish Evaluation Institute. Evaluation and quality assurance of education.

Birutė Victoria Mockienė, Ph.D. candidate in Higher Education Economics at the Center for the Study of Higher Education, Pennsylvania State University, USA. She is involved in the development of the Graduate Certificate in Institutional Research, and the study on collaborative accreditation. Held positions of the Deputy Director of the Lithuanian Center for Quality Assessment in Higher Education and the Head of the Lithuanian ENIC/NARIC from 1995 through 2003.

José-Ginés Mora, Professor, Director of the Centre for Higher Education Management (CHEM), Technical University of Valencia.

Hans Pechar, Associate Professor at the Faculty for Interdisciplinary Studies (IFF), University of Klagenfurt, and head of the Department for Higher Education Research. His research topics are comparative higher education and economics of higher education.

Andrejs Rauhvargers, Professor, Secretary-General of the Latvian Rectors' Council and President of the International Committee of the Lisbon Recognition Convention.

Maria João Rosa, CIPES, Centre for Research in Higher Education Politics, Matosinhos, Portugal.

Christina Rozsnyai, M.A., M.S. She has been working as a Programme Officer for the Hungarian Accreditation Committee since its inception in 1992.

Angelika Schade, Dr., Managing Director of the German Accreditation Council. Her former positions include lecturer (European integration and development of education in Europe) and researcher (topics: Educational systems in Europe and beyond, Quality assurance in education).

Stefanie Schwarz, Dr., Senior researcher at the Centre for Research on Higher Education and Work, University of Kassel, Germany. She carries out international empirical higher education research projects on the topics of Bachelor and Master, Accreditation, Evaluation, Student Financing, and Organisational Studies of Higher

Education. Stefanie Schwarz serves as a member of expert groups on the implementation of structural reforms in higher education in Germany and Europe and has published several books in the respective fields.

Helena Šebková, Ing. PhD., Director of the Centre for Higher Education Studies, Praha.

Bjørn Stensaker, Political scientist. He works at the Norwegian Institute for Studies in Research and Higher Education (NIFU) in Oslo as head of research in the area of higher education institutions. His research interests include how quality is adapted in higher education, organisational change and studies of institutional management and management systems.

Jussi Välimaa, Ph.D., Professor. One of the main academic goals of Professor Välimaa is to develop higher education research theoretically with the help of empirical studies.

Dirk Van Damme, Professor of Education at Ghent University. Director of the Flemish Inter-University Council.

Staffan Wahlén, Senior Advisor at the National Agency for Higher Education, Sweden. He has a background in English linguistics, but has been working in the field of quality audit, quality assessment and higher education pedagogy since the early 1990s at the National Agency and the Ministry of Education and Science. He has published articles, mostly on quality audit, in various international journals.

Don F. Westerheijden, Dr., Senior Research Associate at the Center for Higher Education Policy Studies, University of Twente, the Netherlands. He co-ordinates research, training and consultancy projects related to quality management. He is an executive editor of the journal *Quality in Higher Education*. In addition, he has edited and contributed to books on quality assessment in higher education as well as produced a number of articles on the topic.

Ruth Williams, Senior Policy Analyst in the Centre for Higher Education Research and Information of the UK's Open University. Her main research focus in the Centre is on systems and methods of quality assessment, assurance and evaluation. She undertakes policy-related research for higher education policy bodies both within the UK and internationally. Recent work has focused on the collection of student feedback and its use in the quality assurance of teaching and learning.

Higher Education Dynamics

1. J. Enders and O. Fulton (eds.): *Higher Education in a Globalising World.* 2002
   ISBN Hb 1-4020-0863-5; Pb 1-4020-0864-3

2. A. Amaral, G.A. Jones and B. Karseth (eds.): *Governing Higher Education: National Perspectives on Institutional Governance.* 2002   ISBN 1-4020-1078-8

3. A. Amaral, V.L. Meek and I.M. Larsen (eds.): *The Higher Education Managerial Revolution?* 2003   ISBN Hb 1-4020-1575-5; Pb 1-4020-1586-0

4. C.W. Barrow, S. Didou-Aupetit and J. Mallea: *Globalisation, Trade Liberalisation, and Higher Education in North America.* 2003   ISBN 1-4020-1791-X

5. S. Schwarz and D.F. Westerheijden (eds.): *Accreditation and Evaluation in the European Higher Education Area.* 2004   ISBN 1-4020-2796-6

KLUWER ACADEMIC PUBLISHERS – DORDRECHT / BOSTON / LONDON